T0289991

HIV/AIDS: Molecular and Cell Biology of Opportunistic Infections

HIV/AIDS: Molecular and Cell Biology of Opportunistic Infections

Editor: Eliza Blair

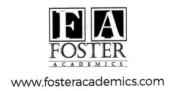

www.fosteracademics.com

www.fosteracademics.com

Cataloging-in-publication Data

HIV/AIDS : molecular and cell biology of opportunistic infections / edited by Eliza Blair.
   p. cm.
Includes bibliographical references and index.
ISBN 978-1-64646-602-3
1. HIV infections--Molecular aspects. 2. AIDS (Disease)--Molecular aspects.
3. HIV infections--Cytopathology. 4. AIDS (Disease)--Cytopathology.
5. Opportunistic infections--Cytopathology. I. Blair, Eliza.
RC606.6 .H58 2023
616.979 2--dc23

Foster Academics,
118-35 Queens Blvd., Suite 400,
Forest Hills, NY 11375, USA

ISBN 978-1-64646-602-3 (Hardback)

Contents

Preface

The human immunodeficiency virus (HIV) causes a life threating condition known as acquired immune deficiency syndrome (AIDS). The first stage of HIV infection is acute infection, following latency and then AIDS, which is the last and critical stage. Patients of AIDS generally have fully dysfunctional immune systems and they acquire a number of severe illnesses known as opportunistic infections (OIs). These illnesses occur in HIV patients with greater severity. Various OIs include tuberculosis (TB), pneumonia, toxoplasmosis, salmonella infection and candidiasis. These infections are caused by various germs, which can be transmitted through contaminated water and food, body fluids and air. AIDS normally takes years to grow following an infection with the human immunodeficiency virus (HIV). Infected AIDS patients are more likely to acquire cancers, such as Kaposi's sarcoma, cervical cancer, and cancers caused by damaged immune-system known as lymphomas. AIDS patients can benefit from certain medications like antiretroviral medicines. This book contains some path-breaking studies on the molecular and cell biology of opportunistic infections in HIV/AIDS. It will provide comprehensive knowledge to the readers. This book will serve as a reference to a broad spectrum of readers.

This book is a comprehensive compilation of works of different researchers from varied parts of the world. It includes valuable experiences of the researchers with the sole objective of providing the readers (learners) with a proper knowledge of the concerned field. This book will be beneficial in evoking inspiration and enhancing the knowledge of the interested readers.

In the end, I would like to extend my heartiest thanks to the authors who worked with great determination on their chapters. I also appreciate the publisher's support in the course of the book. I would also like to deeply acknowledge my family who stood by me as a source of inspiration during the project.

Editor

1

Pneumocystis jirovecii Pneumonia in AIDS Patients

Jose M. Varela[1], Francisco J. Medrano[1],
Eduardo Dei-Cas[2,3] and Enrique J. Calderón[1]
[1]*Instituto de Biomedicina de Sevilla and CIBER de Epidemiología y Salud Pública,
Internal Medicine Service, Virgen del Rocío University Hospital. Seville,*
[2]*Parasitology-Mycology Service (EA4547), Centre of Biology Pathology, Lille-2 University
Hospital Centre, Faculty of Medicine, Univ. Lille Nord de France,*
[3]*Biology & Diversity of Emerging Eukaryotic Pathogens, Institut Pasteur de Lille, Lille,*
[1]*Spain,*
[2,3]*France*

1. Introduction

Pneumocystis pneumonia (PcP) in humans is caused by the opportunistic eukaryotic pathogen *Pneumocystis jirovecii* (previously known as *Pneumocystis carinii* f. sp. *hominis*), which has recently been reclassified as a fungus because its cell wall composition and gene sequences (Edman, 1988, Stringer, 1989). This atypical uncultured fungus remains a major cause of illness and death in patients who have HIV infection. PcP has been the most common AIDS-defining opportunistic infection in the United States and Europe during more than two decades. Before 1989, 60-80% of AIDS patients presented with PcP, and the infection was estimated to be the cause of the death of 20-25% of these patients (Dei-Cas, 2000). Nowadays, despite the introduction of *Pneumocystis* chemoprophylaxis and advances in the treatment of HIV infection, mainly the development of highly active anti-retroviral therapy (HAART), PcP remains as a major opportunistic infection in patients with AIDS. While, the incidence of PcP among individuals with HIV infection has decreased in developed countries, the prevalence of AIDS-related PcP in developing countries remains high and poorly controlled. AIDS-related PcP continues to be an overwhelming illness among individuals who are unaware of their HIV infection, those without access to antiretroviral therapy, among patients who are intolerant or nonadherent to therapy, those who do not comply with prophylactic medications and in cases of failure of prophylaxis, probably relate to the emergence of drug-resistant strains (Calderon, 2010b).

2. Epidemiology

Pneumocystis jirovecii is probably one of the more frequent infectious agents faced by humans in everyday life. Today, it is recognized as an extracellular, obligate, host-specific, yeast-like parasitic fungus virtually restricted to lung tissue that can be directly transmitted among susceptible hosts by the airborne route. It is established that human PcP in not a zoonotic disease, and this notion has important implications for the epidemiology of *P. jirovecii* (Calderon, 2009). Although early studies reported the isolation of *Pneumocystis* DNA from the air surrounding apple orchards and the surface of pond water, no *Pneumocystis* forms were identified in environmental samples by microscopic analysis, and it is uncertain whether there is an ecological niche for *Pneumocystis* outside mammalian hosts (Wakefield, 1996). Animal sources of *P. jirovecii* can be excluded, because the *Pneumocystis* organisms that infect mammalian species are characterized by strong, close host-species specificity (Aliouat-Denis, 2008). Thus far, the human being is the only known reservoir host for *P. jirovecii*, and humans probably acquire the infection only from other humans (Calderon, 2009).

Serologic studies have shown that specific serum anti-*Pneumocystis* antibody can be detected in most children early in life, indicating frequent exposure to this organism (Respaldiza, 2004). On the basis of this finding, disease in immunocompromised persons has long been thought to result from reactivation of latent infection acquired in childhood. However, animal and human studies have shown that elimination of *Pneumocystis* often occurs after infection, implying that the persistence of latent organisms is limited (Morris, 2002). Recent demonstration of *P. jirovecii* transplacental transmission may explain the accumulating evidence that the primary infection is widely acquired very early in the life and support the commonly held view that human infants are a major natural reservoir for *P. jirovecii*, since they can remain colonized as their immune response matures (Montes-Cano, 2009).

Colonization with *P. jirovecii* in adults has recently gained attention as an important issue for understanding the complete cycle of human *Pneumocystis* infection (Calderón, 2010a). In general, colonization is defined as isolation of an infectious agent that does not result in sufficient damage to cause clinical disease, but that may alter host homeostasis. In the specific case of *Pneumocystis*, colonization is currently defined as the detection of the organism or its DNA in respiratory samples from subjects without signs or symptoms of pneumonia (Morris, 2008).

Among adults, *Pneumocystis* colonization has been well documented in both HIV-infected and non–HIV-infected individuals, and certain populations appear to have a higher risk of colonization. Studies have shown that individuals who have an underlying HIV-infection or another cause of immunosuppression and those who are not immunosuppressed but have chronic lung disease may often be colonized by *P. jirovecii* (Calderón, 2009). These groups at risk for carriage probably represent a major species-specific reservoir of infection, although transient *Pneumocystis* colonization has been also identified in healthy individuals that could behave as a sort of dynamic reservoir for future *Pneumocystis* infection in other susceptible subjects (Medrano, 2005).

Several outbreaks of PcP have been reported in hospitals. Molecular analyses of *Pneumocystis* in some of these studies suggested nosocomial acquisition of the infection (de Boer, 2007, Olsson, 2001, Rabodonirina, 2004). In addition, *Pneumocystis* colonization has been found more frequently in health care workers in close occupational contact with patients with PcP than in those who had no occupational exposure (Vargas, 2000, Miller 2001). On the other hand, a recent study has provided molecular evidence that airborne transmission of *P. jirovecii* from colonized immunocompetent carrier hosts to susceptible persons may occur (Rivero, 2008). Therefore, interindividual airborne transmission seems to occur in humans in both hospitals, as a nosocomial infection, and in the community.

3. Pathogenesis

Basic knowledge on *Pneumocystis* has been hampered by the lack of a reliable in vitro culture system. However, through the use of molecular techniques and experimental models of PcP in immunosuppressed animals, many progresses have been made over the last decades in our understanding of the complex pathophysiology and pathogenesis of this fungal infection.

At the histopathological level has been shown that the proliferation of *Pneumocystis* is accompanied by anatomical and physiological changes. In animal models, alterations in alveolar-capillary permeability are followed by degenerative changes in type I pneumocytes, restorative hypertrophy of type II pneumocytes and diffuse alveolar damage leading to pulmonary fibrosis (Walzer, 1993). Studies in humans have also shown changes in the permeability of the alveolar-capillary membrane, pulmonary diffusing capacity and vital capacity in total lung (Coleman et al., 1984). These changes depend on the ability of *Pneumocystis*, demonstrated in animal models to induce in the very early stages of the infection alveolar macrophage activation, increased pro-inflammatory cytokines and changes in pulmonary surfactant even when small amounts of microorganisms are present (Prevost et al., 1998).

In the infected host, *Pneumocystis* organisms dwell almost exclusively within lung alveoli. Within some hours after experimental intra-tracheal infection, Pneumocystis trophic forms attach to the alveolar epithelial cells. The host immune response against the infection involves complex interactions between CD4+ and CD8+ T-cells, alveolar macrophages, neutrophils and soluble mediators that facilitate clearance of the infection. Disease only occurs when cellular and/or humoral immunity is defective.

3.1 Interactions of *Pneumocystis* with alveolar host cells

Trophic forms adhere tightly to alveolar type I cells through interdigitation of their membranes with those of the host. The binding of *Pneumocystis* to the epithelium is facilitated by interactions with proteins of the alveolar fluid, such as fibronectin and vitronectin that bind to the surface of *Pneumocystis* and mediate the attachment to integrin receptors present on the alveolar epithelium. In infected tissues, type I alveolar cells with adherent *Pneumocystis* appear vacuolated and eroded (Benfield et al., 1997). However, studies of cultured lung epithelial cells have shown that the adherence of *Pneumocystis* alone does not disrupt the structure or barrier function of alveolar epithelial cells, although proliferative repair of the epithelium is reduced. It is therefore unlikely that the adherence of *Pneumocystis* to alveolar epithelium is by itself responsible for the diffuse alveolar damage in severe pneumonia (Benfield et al., 1997; Thomas & Limper, 2007). Rather, the inflammatory responses in the host are primarily responsible for the compromise of the alveolar-capillary surface (Thomas & Limper, 2007).

Electron microscopic studies have shown that *Pneumocystis* organisms are embedded in protein-rich alveolar exudates, which contain abundant fibronectin, vitronectin, and hydrophilic surfactant proteins A and D. In contrast, hydrophobic surfactant protein B and C are reduced during PcP. Both surfactant protein A and surfactant protein D interact with the Major Surface Glycoprotein (MSG) components of the surface at *Pneumocystis*. Surfactant protein A modulates the interactions of *Pneumocystis* with the alveolar macrophages. In contrast, surfactant protein D mediates the aggregation of the *Pneumocystis* organisms, but because the aggregated organisms are extremely poorly taken up by macrophages, they may escape elimination. Pulmonary surfactant phospholipids, which contribute to the low surface tension in the alveoli, are reduced during PcP, and abnormalities in the composition and function of the surfactant are the result of the host's inflammatory response to *Pneumocystis*, rather than direct effects of the organisms on the surfactant components (Wright et al., 2001; Thomas & Limper, 2007).

3.2 Innate immunity (alveolar macrophages and neutrophils)

Although parasite attachment to lung epithelial cells is essential for *Pneumocystis* infection and propagation, invasion of host cells does not occur (Krajicek et al., 2009). Alveolar macrophages are the first line of host defence to control the infection, since they are the principal phagocytes mediating the uptake and direct degradation of both trophic forms and cysts forms in the lung (Kelly & Shellito, 2010). Macrophages display several potential receptors for glucans, including CD11b/CD18 integrin (CR3), dectin-1, and toll-like receptor 2. The activation of macrophages by *Pneumocystis* is augmented by host proteins such as vitronectin and fibronectin that bind the glucan components on the organism (Vassallo et al., 2001). When there are not opsonins in the epithelial-lining fluid, the uptake of *Pneumocystis* is mediated mainly through the macrophage mannose receptors, pattern-recognition molecules that interact with the surface mannoprotein, MSG (also called glycoprotein A). After they have been taken up by macrophages, *Pneumocystis* organisms are incorporated into phagolysosomes and degraded. Macrophages produce a large variety of proinflammatory cytokines, chemokines, and eicosanoid metabolites in response to phagocytosis of *Pneumocystis*. Although these mediators participate in eradicating *Pneumocystis*, they also promote pulmonary injury (Limper et al., 1997).

Neutrophils alone are unable to control the infection. Unlike other opportunistic fungal infections, *Pneumocystis* disease is rare in patients with neutropenia. Neutrophils are associated with inflammation and, therefore, have been implicated in severity of disease. In fact, decreased pulmonary function and local lung inflammation and damage have been correlated with elevated neutrophil counts in HIV-infected patients with PcP (Kelly & Shellito, 2010). The neutrophils recruited into the lungs release reactive oxidant species, proteases, and cationic proteins, which directly injure capillary endothelial cells and alveolar epithelial cells (Thomas & Limper, 2004).

3.3 Adaptive immunity (T cells and B cells)

Both cellular and humoral immune systems are important in defence against *Pneumocystis* infection.

The activity of CD4+ T cells is pivotal in the host's defences against *Pneumocystis*, since most HIV-infected patients with PcP have CD4+ T-cell counts below 200 cells/mm^3. CD4+ lymphocytes as memory cells coordinate and orchestrate the host inflammatory responses by means of the recruitment and activation of other immune effector cells, including monocytes and macrophages, which are responsible for elimination of the organism. Macrophage-derived TNF-α and interleukin-1 are believed to be necessary for initiating pulmonary responses to *Pneumocystis* infection that are mediated by CD4+ cells. The cells proliferate in response to *Pneumocystis* antigens and generate cytokine mediators, including lymphotactin and interferon gamma (IFN-γ). Lymphotactin, a chemokine, acts as a potent chemoattractant for further lymphocyte recruitment in PcP.

Although T lymphocytes are essential for the clearance of *Pneumocystis*, experimental data suggest that T-cell responses may also result in substantial pulmonary impairment during pneumonia. For instance, in severe combined immunodeficiency (SCID) mice infected with *Pneumocystis*, normal oxygenation and lung function occur despite active infection until the late stages of the disease. When the immune systems in these animals are reconstituted with the use of intact spleen cells, an intense T-cell–mediated inflammatory response ensues, resulting in substantially impaired gas exchange (Wright et al., 1999b). In the absence of brisk lung inflammation, *Pneumocystis* has little direct effect on pulmonary function. In a similar manner, in patients who have undergone bone marrow transplantation the clinical onset of PcP and of most marked alterations in lung function occur during engraftment (Thomas & Limper, 2004).

The CD8+ T cells seem to play also an important role in control of *Pneumocystis* infection since in experimental animal models depletion of both CD4+ and CD8+ cells results in a more severe PcP than only depletion of CD4+ cells. However, their role may be less important than CD4+ T cells since CD8+ T-cell-depleted animals can still clear the infection (Lu & Lee, 2008). *Pneumocystis* infection results in the marked accumulation of CD8+ T lymphocytes in the lung. Although not as extensively investigated as CD4+ T cells, insights into the role of CD8+ T cells in host defence against *Pneumocystis* have been achieved, but that is not nearly enough. Recent data provide the concept that CD8+ T cells, most likely those of the Tc1 phenotype, are critical for clearance of some fungal organisms including *Pneumocystis*, particularly in the context of CD4+ T-cell deficiency or dysfunction. CD8+ T cells have also been shown to play a detrimental role in *Pneumocystis* infection. CD8+ T cells are considered to be part of the damaging inflammatory response in CD4+ T-cell-depleted mice. The presence of CD8+ T cells affected surfactant function and it also has been shown to exacerbate TNF-α production (Steele et al., 2005).

Lastly, a significant role of humoral immune response in the host defence against *Pneumocystis* is supported by the observations that SCID animals require B cells to clear the infection (Burns et al., 1990), and that patients with agammaglobulinemia develop PcP despite of an intact cellular immune system (Alibrahim et al., 1998; Lu & Lee, 2008). B lymphocytes appears to play an important role in the generation of CD4+ memory cells in response to *Pneumocystis* (Lu & Lee, 2008).

3.4 Cytokine and chemokine networks

Various pro-inflammatory cytokines including IFN-γ, tumour necrosis factor alpha (TNF-α), interleukin (IL)-8, IL-1 and IL-6 and chemokines such as RANTES (Regulated upon Activation normal T-cell Expressed, and Secreted), macrophage inflammatory protein (MIP)-1α, MIP-1β and MIP-2 release by macrophages, neutrophils, epithelial cells and lymphocytes are involved in the host immune response and lung damage during *Pneumocystis* disease (Calderon et al., 2007).

INF-γ has a critical role for control lung inflammation during PcP, although is not directly toxic to *Pneumocystis* organisms. This cytokine is produced primarily by CD4+ T cells. There is an indirect correlation between IFN-levels and severity of PcP (Kelly & Shellito, 2010). IFN-γ strongly activates the macrophage production of TNF-α, superoxides, and reactive nitrogen species, each of which is implicated in the host defence against *Pneumocystis* (Wright et al., 1999a).

TNF-α is a potent pro-inflammatory cytokine secreted primarily by macrophage that promotes the recruitment of neutrophils, lymphocytes, and monocytes. Although their recruitment is important for clearance of the organisms, these cells injure the lung by releasing oxidants, cationic proteins, and proteases. TNF-α also induces the production of other cytokines and chemokines, including IL-8 and IFN-γ, which stimulate the recruitment and activation of inflammatory cells during *Pneumocystis* infection (Wright et al., 2004). The cell wall of *Pneumocystis* contains abundant beta-glucans, and studies have confirmed that the production of TNF-α by alveolar macrophages is mediated by recognition of the beta-glucan components of *Pneumocystis*. IL-8 is correlated with both neutrophil infiltration of the lung and impaired gas exchange during severe PcP (Thomas & Limper, 2004).

The most important function of chemokines is to recruit effector cells to the site of injury. Many studies have found an increase in chemokine expression during PcP. In a SCID experimental model of PcP it has been found that expression levels of RANTES, MIP-1α, MIP-1β and MIP-2 were all upregulated after lymphocyte reconstitution of the SCID animal. In addition, the time course of chemokine expression correlates *Pneumocystis* clearance, but also with the lung inflammation (Wright et al., 1999a). Thus, the role of chemokines is essential for the resolution of infection, but overexpression may also result in a hyperinflammatory state and lung damage (Kelly & Shellito, 2010).

4. Clinical presentation and chest radiology

In patients infected with HIV, PcP is a common AIDS-defining illness and occurs most frequently in subjects with a CD4+ count less than 200 cells per mm^3. The symptoms of PcP are nonspecific and PcP in patients with HIV infection tends to run a more subacute indolent course and tends to present much later, often after several weeks of symptoms, compared with PcP associated with other immunocompromising conditions. A more acute illness with symptoms including a cough productive with purulent sputum should suggest an alternate infectious diagnosis, such as bacterial pneumonia or tuberculosis

Patients with PcP often develop dyspnea (95%), which increases over time; cough productive of clear sputum or non-productive cough; low grade or no fever; malaise, and sometimes chest tightness or pain. However, the clinical picture in individual patients is variable and many infectious and non-infectious processes can present identically. Also, the general hallmarks of this disease such as fever, shortness of breath, and diffuse infiltrates do not invariably occur, especially early in the course while the disease is mild (Thomas & Limper, 2004). Acute dyspnea with pleuritic chest pain may indicate the development of a pneumothorax, which has been presented in 2% to 4% of patients (Sepkowitz et al., 1991). In all cases, a high index of suspicion and a thorough history are key factors in early detection of PcP. Physical examination may reveal tachypnea, tachycardia, and cyanosis. Lung auscultation usually reveals few abnormalities with dry cackles or rhonchi present in less than 50% of patients. Individuals with PcP can be hypoxemic with respiratory alkalosis but can also have normal alveolar-arterial gradients if identified early in the natural history of their disease. Elevated serum levels of lactate dehydrogenase (LDH) have been related with PcP and probably reflects lung parenchymal damage but is not specific and elevations can be seen in many pulmonary and non-pulmonary conditions. In general, laboratory abnormalities are less severe in HIV-infected patients than in non-HIV immunosuppressed patients (Hughes, 2004).

Classically, chest radiographic features of PcP are bilateral, symmetric, fine reticular interstitial infiltrates involving the perihilar areas (figure 1a), becoming more homogenous and diffuse as the severity of the infection increases (Thomas & Limper, 2004). Less frequently, PcP may present with unilateral or asymmetrical opacities. Thin-walled cysts or pneumatocele are seen in 10-20% of cases. Pleural effusions and intrathoracic adenopathy are rare. Patients who receive aerosolized pentamidine have an increased frequency of upper-lobe infiltrates, pneumothorax, or cystic lesions. Early in the course of PcP, the chest radiograph may be normal in up to 25% of cases (Schliep & Yarrish, 1999).

A high-resolution computed tomography scan is more sensitive than chest radiograph and is helpful when the chest radiography findings are equivocal. The typical appearance is patchy areas of ground-glass attenuation with a background of interlobular septal thickening or cystic lesions predominating in perihilar areas (figure 1b), even then chest radiographic findings are normal (Nyamande et al., 2007). While such findings are suggestive, they are not diagnostic. However, a negative high-resolution computed tomography scan may allow exclusion of PcP in patients with HIV.

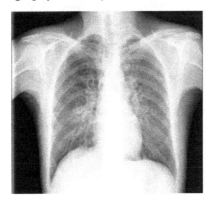 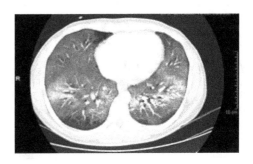

Fig. 1. Radiographic findings of *Pneumocystis* pneumonia in a patient with AIDS. (1a, left) Chest x-ray of a *Pneumocystis* pneumonia showing diffuse infiltrations in both lung fields. (1b, right) Chest high-resolution CT scan of a patient with AIDS revealing diffuse ground glass opacities and thickened alveolar septum in both lungs.

Extrapulmonary manifestations of *P. jirovecii* infection (extrapulmonary pneumocystosis) are distinctly unusual but they has been reported primarily among HIV-infected patients, particularly those who receive aerosolized pentamidine for prophylaxis of PcP and in those with advanced HIV infection who are not taking any prophylaxis. Mainly, during the terminal stage of HIV-related disease *Pneumocystis* organisms may disseminate from the lungs to other organs where they induce secondary visceral lesions. However, sometimes pulmonary infection may not be apparent when extrapulmonary lesions are detected. Lymph nodes, spleen, kidneys, liver, thyroid and bone marrow are the most commonly infected organs, but microorganisms have been also found in the brain, pancreas, skin, heart, muscle and other organs (Ng et al, 1997). For HIV-infected patients, extrapulmonary pneumocystosis limited to the choroid layer or ear (external auditory canal or middle ear) has a better prognosis, with good response to specific treatment, than disseminated pneumocystosis in multiple noncontiguous sites. Lesions are frequently nodular and may contain necrotic material or calcification. Extrapulmonary pneumocystosis in solid organs appears on computed tomography scan as focal, hypodense lesions with well-defined borders and central or peripheral calcification (Schliep & Yarrish, 1999).
Immunorestitution disease (IRD) is defined as an acute symptomatic or paradoxical deterioration of a (most probably) preexisting infection that is temporally related to the recovery of the immune system and it is due to immunopathological damage associated with the reversal of immunosuppressive processes. PcP manifesting as a form of IRD has been described in both HIV and non-HIV immunosuppressed patients (Cheng et al., 2004; Jagannathan et al., 2009; Mori et al., 2009). Among HIV-infected patients, PcP manifesting acutely during the initiation of HAART is a well-recognized phenomenon (Wislez et al., 2001). AIDS-related PcP patients seem to be at risk of clinical deterioration due to IRD if antiretroviral therapy is started within one to two weeks after the initiation of treatment for PcP (Wislez et al., 2001). The onset of clinical deterioration is associated with an increase in the CD4+ lymphocyte count and a reduction in the HIV viral load (Wislez et al., 2001).

5. Prognosis

Despite treatment, mortality of PcP still remains high. Several studies highlight that mortality rates are declining in patients with PcP. However, in other studies, PcP has remained the leading cause of death among those nor receiving o failing to comply with HAART or PcP prophylaxis. Predictors of mortality include older age, recent injection drug use, increased total bilirrubin, low serum albumin, and alveolar-arterial oxygen gradient >50 mm Hg (Fei et al, 2009).

6. Management PcP

There is no universally agreed approach on to the initial management of patients with suspected PcP. Many institutions treat patients with suspected PcP empirically, while others pursue a definitive microbiological diagnosis (Huang, 2004). Since PcP can be rapidly progressive and the mortality rate remains high, early therapy is essential (Calderon et al, 2004; Roblot, 2005). Identification of patients having PcP into mild, moderate or severe disease allows to guide the choice of the drug for the treatment of PcP, as well as, to decide if adjuvant corticosteroids are indicated (table 1) (Miller et al., 1996). In AIDS-related PcP, the typical duration of therapy is at least 21 days because of the risk for relapse with shorter treatment duration. Patients generally improved after 4 to 8 days of therapy. Although the overall prognosis of patients whose degree of hypoxemia requires intensive care unit (ICU) admission or mechanical ventilation remains poor, survival in up to 50% of patients requiring ventilatory support has been reported. Patients with reasonable functional status and severe PcP should be offered ICU admission or mechanical ventilation (CDC, 2009).

	Mild	Moderate	Severe
Symptoms and signs	Dyspnoea on exertion, with or without cough and sweats	Dyspnoea on minimal exertion and occasionally at rest. Cough and fever	Dyspnoea and tachypnoea at rest. Persistent fever and cough
Arterial oxygen tension (PaO2) at rest	> 11.0 kPa (82.7 mmHg)	8.0 to 11.0 kPa (60-82.7 mmHg)	< 8.0 kPa (60 mmHg)
Arterial oxygen saturation (SaO2) at rest	> 96%	91 to 96%	< 91%
Chest radiograph	Normal, or minor perihiliar shadowing	Diffuse interstitial shadowing	Extension interstitial shadowing with or without diffuse alveolar shadowing

Modified of Miller RF, et al., 1996.

Table 1. Grading of severity of *Pneumocystis* pneumonia.

7. Diagnosis of PCP

7.1 Microscopic detection of *Pneumocystis*

The single most important diagnostic tool for *Pneumocystis* infection is a high clinical suspicion. However, specific diagnosis of PcP requires documentation of the microorganism in respiratory specimens. Since *Pneumocystis* cannot be cultured, the diagnosis of PcP relies on microscopic detection of *Pneumocystis* organisms on stained respiratory specimens. Conventional stains such as toluidine blue O (TBO), Grocott's methenamine silver nitrate

(GMS), or methanol Giemsa methods (figure 2) can be used to identify the organism (cysts or trophic forms) but immunofluorescent staining is the most common technique currently used. TBO or GMS stains facilitate rapid parasite detection, even at low magnification, in all kinds of clinical specimens. However, these dyes also stain the cell wall of yeasts or other fungi. For this reason, a good strategy to identify *Pneumocystis* organisms accurately in clinical specimens is to systematically associate the examination of both TBO- or GMS-stained smears and methanol-Giemsa–stained smears from the same specimen (table 2). Actually, methanol-Giemsa (or other equivalent panoptical Giemsa-like stains) makes it possible, on the one hand, to distinguish *Pneumocystis* organisms from other microorganism and, on the other hand, to identify the different *Pneumocystis* life-cycle stages. In fact, Giemsa and other stains with similar cytological affinities, such as Diff Quick or RAL-555, cause the parasite nuclei to stain pinkish purple and the cytoplasm to stain blue (Dei-Cas et al, 1998). They do not stain cystic or sporocytic walls, which appear like a clear peripheral halo around cystic forms. These polychrome stains make it possible accurately to distinguish *Pneumocystis* trophic or cystic forms from other fungi and also from host cells or cell debris. On the whole, the biggest advantage of methanol-Giemsa or Giemsa-like stain methods consists in staining trophic forms and sporocytes, which remain unidentified in TBO- or GMS-stained smears (Dei-Cas et al, 1998).

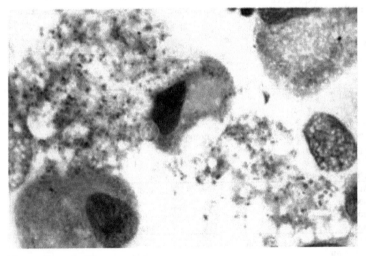

Fig. 2. Stain with methanol–Giemsa stain

Efficiency and cost-effectiveness of the different microscopic stains evoked here vary according to experience of groups, technical protocols, type and quality of the samples, local incidence of PcP, and the number of organisms present (Chouaid et al., 1995) (table 2). It is generally accepted, however, that association of methods that stain cystic cell wall (e.g. TBO or GMS) with panoptical techniques (methanol-Giemsa or analogous staining methods) is usually required (Dei-Cas et al., 2006). Moreover, it is usually recognized that specific antibody staining is mainly helpful to detect *Pneumocystis* organisms in non-BAL smears (e.g. induced sputum, expectorated sputum, gastric wash) and to clarify conflicting light microscopic observations (Aderaye et al., 2008; Cruciani et al., 2002; Kovacs et al., 1998; Limawongpranee et al., 2007).

Typically, the respiratory specimens are obtained by sputum induction or fiberoptic bronchoscopy with bronchoalveolar lavage (BAL). Sputum induction by inhalation of a hypertonic saline solution is the quickest and least-invasive method for definitively diagnosing PcP with a sensitivity between 50-90% and specificity of 99-100%. Sputum induced may also be less sensitive in patients receiving aerosolized pentamidine for prophylaxis. All of the direct organism visualization methods can lead to false-negative results, consequently, a negative sputum induction cannot rule out a diagnosis of PcP. If sputum induction is nondiagnostic or cannot be performed, then bronchoscopy with BAL is the next step. A BAL that is negative for *Pneumocystis* rules out the diagnosis of PcP.

In order to detect *Pneumocystis* organisms in histological sections from lung or other organs, pathologists target usually the cystic forms, since trophic ones are uneasily identifiable in paraffin-embedded tissues. They use therefore GMS and, less frequently, TBO staining procedures adapted to tissue sections. Trophic forms can however be identified in epon-embedded semi-thin sections stained with toluidine blue or other stains (Dei-Cas et al., 1998; Durand-Joly et al., 2000). Furthermore, *Pneumocystis*-specific fluorescein-, phosphatase or peroxidase-labeled monoclonal antibodies available from many suppliers may help to identify *Pneumocystis* organisms in BAL, induced sputum or tissue samples (table 2).

Technique	Suitable kind of sample	Needed experience	Sensitivity	Specificity	Advantages	Drawbacks	Recommended combination with:
Microscopy:							
PC/IC	BALF wet smear	very good	variable	good	rapidity	needs confirmation by other methods	panoptical stain
GMS/TBO							
	BALF air-dried cytospin smear or biopsy (histological section)	average	high	average	cost; rapidity	false positive (poor experienced staffs); identifies only the cystic stages	panoptical stain
Panoptical stains*	BALF air-dried cytospin smear	very good	average	very high	cost; rapidity; identify all *Pneumocystis* stages	limited sensitivity (poor experienced staffs)	GMS/TBO
FL Mab	BALF, IS or sputum air-dried cytospin smear	good	high	good	good sensitivity/ specificity	cost; time-consuming	-
IP/AP Mab	biopsy (histological section), air-dried cytospin smear	good	good	good	good specificity	cost; time-consuming	-
PCR	BALF, IS, OW, NPA, biopsy	average	very high	very high	Helpful in HIV-negative patients; rapidity (real-time PCR assays); non-invasive	cost; positive in colonized patients	-

Technique	Suitable kind of sample	Needed experience	Sensitivity	Specificity	Advantages	Drawbacks	Recommended combination with:
					sampling; genotyping		
BG	serum	average	good	low	rapidity; post-therapeutic control	positive in other deep fungal infections	other tests
KL-6	serum	average	good	low	-	positive in other pulmonary infections	
Serum *Pneumocystis* antibody assay	serum	average	depending on antigen and assay	depending on antigen and assay	helpful in epidemiology studies	positive in people without PcP	other tests

*Giemsa or Giemsa-like stains. BALF: Bronchoalveolar lavage fluid; BG: serum beta-1,3-glucan; FL Mab: fluorescein-labeled Pneumocystis monoclonal antibody; GMS: Grocott-methenamine silver stain; IP/AP Mab: immuneperoxidase/alkaline-phosphatase labeled monoclonal antibody; IS: induced sputum; PC/IC: phase contrast/interference contrast; TBO: toluidine blue stain. KL-6: Mucin like glycoprotein.

Table 2. Laboratory diagnostic methods for *Pneumocystis* pneumonia.

7.2 Molecular detection of *Pneumocystis*

Many *Pneumocystis* PCR assays have been developed during the last two decades. PCR tool revealed highly efficacious to amplify *Pneumocystis* DNA from diverse kinds of clinical specimens (BALF, IS, expectorated sputum, oropharyngeal or nasopharyngeal wash samples, biopsy specimens) (figure 3) (de la Horra et al., 2006; Durand-Joly et al., 2005; Olsson et al., 1993; Wakefield et al., 1990). In the clinical laboratory, the use of molecular methods is mainly warranted to increase the sensitivity of P. jirovecii detection in clinical specimens in order to establish earlier PcP diagnosis, detecting low parasite rates, mainly in non-HIV infected patients with PcP, and detecting *Pneumocystis* DNA in noninvasive samples (Durand-Joly et al., 2005; Respaldiza et al., 2006) (table 2). Moreover, PCR assays followed by direct sequencing or other strategies were used for typing *Pneumocystis* isolates in order to identify parasite strains and to explore correlation between specific genotypes and virulence, transmissibility or drug susceptibility. PCR, especially nested PCR assays applied to noninvasive samples, have also been used to detect *Pneumocystis* colonization either in susceptible individuals or in apparently healthy people, including health care workers in hospitals (Durand-Joly et al., 2003; Medrano et al., 2005; Nevez et al., 2008).

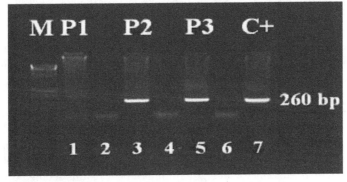

Fig. 3. Nested PCR (mtLSU rRNA region) results.

M: molecular mass marker. Lane 1 (P1) negative specimen. Lanes 3 and 5 (P2, P3) positive specimens of oral wash in cystic fibrosis patients. Lane 7 (C+) positive control. Lanes 2, 4 and 6 negative controls (water).

For PcP diagnosis in humans, conventional or real-time PCR assays based on the amplification of the large subunit of mitochondrial ribosomal DNA (mtLSUrDNA) (Wakefield et al., 1990) are the most commonly used, but many other sequences have been targeted (Major Surface Glycoprotein, Internal Transcribed Spacers, Thymidylate Synthase, Dihydrofolate Reductase, heat-shock protein 70, etc.) (Durand-Joly et al., 2005; Hugett et al., 2008). Comparative evaluating studies are uneasy to perform because of different clinical contexts, sampling methods, laboratory reagents or technical strategies used to DNA extraction, amplification or analysis of results (Durand-Joly et al., 2005).

In general, conventional or real-time *Pneumocystis* PCR assays have represented a significant advance in PcP laboratory diagnosis. Actually, highly sensitive and specific PCR tools, especially real-time PCR assays, improved the clinical diagnosis of PcP allowing an accurate, early diagnosis of *Pneumocystis* infection (Durand-Joly et al., 2005), which should lead to a decreased duration from onset of symptoms to treatment. This period has a recognized impact on prognosis since PcP-associated respiratory failure requiring mechanic ventilation entails significant mortality (Huang, 2004). In addition, PCR assay may reveal PcP in patients with negative microscopic test. For instance, among 62 HIV-negative patients with clinical PcP diagnosed in the Lille University Hospital between 1998 and 2001, 30 patients (48%) had positive PCR results with negative microscopic tests (Durand-Joly, 2002).

Notably, molecular techniques play a significant role when they are applied to noninvasive specimens as IS, oropharyngeal wash (OW, obtained by gargling 10 ml of 0.9% NaCl for >60 seconds) (Respaldiza et al., 2006) or nasopharyngeal aspirates (NPA) (Richards et al. 1994). When DNA sequences used as primers or probe have been adequately defined, the analytical specificity of *Pneumocystis*-PCR assays applied to noninvasive or to BALF samples should usually be of 100% (Durand-Joly et al., 2005). With regard to sensitivity, *Pneumocystis*-mtLSUrDNA PCR showed high analytical sensitivity for the detection of *Pneumocystis* organisms on BALF samples from AIDS patients, with a detection threshold of 0.5–1 organism/μl^{-1} (Tamburrini et al., 1998). The sensitivity of PCR assays applied to OW (or other noninvasive samples) is certainly lower (<80%) than that of PCR on BALF samples (>95%) (Tsolaki et al., 2008). However, OW can be easily repeated in order to monitor the evolution of infection and, potentially, the therapeutic response (Tsolaki et al., 2008).

A significant problem of *Pneumocystis* PCR assays is raised by *Pneumocystis* colonization (Calderon, 2009). Actually, a positive PCR result associated with a negative microscopic test may result from either *Pneumocystis* colonization or PcP. In common practice, this difficulty is often solved on the basis of a careful clinical, radiological and laboratory assessment of the patient pathological condition, as it is usually done to other infectious diseases, especially when their agents are opportunistic pathogens. However, the alternative of quantifying parasite rates was also explored (Larsen et al., 2002). Thus, a quantitative real-time PCR assay that targeted *Pneumocystis* Major Surface Glycoprotein (MSG) multigene family was applied to OW samples, and revealed significant differences between PcP patients and *Pneumocystis* colonized subjects in the number of MSG copies. The authors suggested a cutoff value of 50 MSG gene fragment copies/tube for distinguishing between the two conditions (Larsen et al., 2002). However, quantitative PCR results seemed difficult to use on the field. The main problem was inability to control the volume of the sample. Another difficulty is related with the kind of patients. Actually, it seems difficult to apply a same cutoff to AIDS patients, patients with other underlying diseases or individuals receiving chemoprophylaxis against *Pneumocystis*.

There is no formal agreement about an unequivocal definition of *Pneumocystis* colonization. The notion may however be characterized on the basis of clinical and experimental observations. In clinical practice, the diagnosis of *Pneumocystis* colonization or subclinical carriage is usually retained when *Pneumocystis* DNA is detected by PCR methods in respiratory samples from immunodepressed or immunocompetent subjects without symptoms or signs of *Pneumocystis* infection, and who do not progress to PcP (Morris et al., 2008) In these subjects, *Pneumocystis* organisms are only exceptionally detected by microscopy (Vidal et al., 2006). Interestingly, recent experimental data strengthened the biological significance of *Pneumocystis* colonization (Chabe et al., 2004). They demonstrated that *Pneumocystis* organisms can replicate in the lungs of immunocompetent carriers, stimulate an antibody response and be efficiently transmitted by airborne route to either naive immunocompetent hosts, who will develop a primary infection, or to immunosuppressed hosts, who may then develop PcP (Chabe et al., 2004). In addition, many evidences suggest that beyond PcP, *Pneumocystis* colonization may induce local or systemic inflammation, a condition that could aggravate chronic pulmonary diseases. For instance, *P. jirovecii* pulmonary carriage in patients with chronic obstructive pulmonary disease (COPD) could favor the progression of this disease (Calderon et al., 2007; Morris et al., 2008).

Efforts have been made to associate specific *P. jirovecii* genotypes with virulence, drug susceptibility or other medically important biological properties of parasite strains. Some studies reported some correlation between polymorphism and clinical features (Miller & Wakefield, 1999; Totet et al., 2003). Polymorphism of internal transcribed spacer (ITS1/ITS2) sequences was quite frequently used and more than 30 ITS1 genotypes and 40 ITS2 genotypes with more than 90 haplotypes (combinations of ITS1 and ITS2 types) have been reported (Beard, 2004).

Most polymorphism studies targeted mutations of the *P. jirovecii* dihydropteroate synthase (DHPS) gene, which could potentially be linked with sulfa resistance. Regarding this issue, and since effective *P. jirovecii* culture systems are unavailable, several groups have assessed putative trimethoprim-sulfamethoxazole (TMP-SMX) drug resistance by detecting *Pneumocystis* DHPS mutations. Indeed nonsynonymous DHPS point mutations at nucleotide positions 165 and 171 entail an amino acid change at positions 55 (Thr to Ala) and/or 57 (Pro to Ser) (Friaza et al., 2009). Such mutations confer resistance to sulfa drugs in other organisms, including *Escherichia coli*, *Streptococcus pneumoniae* and *Plasmodium falciparum*. The *P. jirovecii* DHPS mutant form has also been shown to be more resistant to sulfamethoxazole in a *Saccharomyces cerevisiae* model (Iliades et al., 2004), but it is still uncertain if *Pneumocystis* DHPS mutations lead to drug resistance in patients (Huang et al., 2000, 2004; Nahimana et al., 2004). Such mutations were shown to be associated with the use of TMP-SMX or dapsone (two DHPS inhibitors), the duration of sulfa or dapsone prophylaxis and with geographic areas in which sulfamethoxazole or dapsone were commonly used for PcP prophylaxis (Huang et al., 2004; Kazanjian et al., 2000). However, results of studies searching specifically to establish an association between the presence of *P. jirovecii* DHPS mutations and clinical outcomes, such as treatment failure or death, are contradictory (Alvarez-Martinez et al., 2008, Helweg-Larsen et al., 1999; Huang et al., 2004,

Stein et al., 2004; van Hal et al., 2009). Outstandingly, most PcP patients carrying *P. jirovecii* isolates with DHPS mutations responded well to TMP-SMX treatment and survived probably because these mutations may confer a low-level of resistance to sulfa-drugs that is overcome by high drug concentration achieved in lung tissues by sulfamethoxazole (Calderon et al., 2004; Huang et al., 2004).

7.3 Other laboratory diagnostic methods
7.3.1 Beta-D-glucan assay
β-1,3-glucan (BG) is the main structural component of the cell wall of all fungi, including *Pneumocystis* cysts (Thomas & Limper, 2007). Interestingly, high serum BG levels have been reported in patients with PcP (Desmet et al., 2009; Nakamura et al., 2009; Teramoto et al., 2000). Consistently, such levels decreased with effective anti-*Pneumocystis* treatment (Teramoto et al., 2000). Serum BG appeared therefore as a good marker of *Pneumocystis* infection. The potential utility of this assay was analyzed in a retrospective case-control study of patients with suspected PcP comparing BG with microscopic examination on BAL. The BG assay had a sensitivity of 92% and a specificity of 86% for detecting PcP for a ut-off level of 31.1 pg/ml (Tasaka et al., 2007). In a recent study, it has been observed that BG levels in HIV patients with PcP are higher than in non-HIV patients. This could be attributed to the fact that HIV patients have greater numbers of microorganisms that non-HIV patients (Nakamura et al., 2009).

However, BG levels could not be correlated with PcP prognosis, and false positive results could exceed more than 30% (Nakamura et al., 2009). False positive results were reported in patients undergoing bacterial septicemia, hemodialysis with cellulose dialysis membranes, treatment with immunoglobulin, glucan-containing antitumor drugs, amoxicillin-clavulanate, piperacillin-tazobactam or contact with gauze or surgical sponges containing BG (Ponton, 2009). Furthermore, since invasive fungal infections induce also an increase of serum BG, the test should often be associated with laboratory assays aiming at detecting such infections (Desmet et al., 2009). These preliminary studies suggest that in the right clinical setting serum BG may provide a useful noninvasive diagnostic adjunct for patients with *Pneumocystis* infection. However, additional information is necessary to address the general specificity of BG in diagnosing PcP versus other fungal infections in diverse immune-suppressed patient populations and to differentiate among patients with PcP and patients with *Pneumocystis* colonization.

7.3.2 KL-6
KL-6 is a mucin-like glycoprotein expressed on type II pneumocytes and bronchiolar epithelial cells. This marker has reached elevated levels in several studies in patients with PcP. However, the reported false-positive rate and level of detection were not as good as for the BG assay (Nakamura et al, 2009; Tasaka et al, 2007). Recent investigations indicate that KL-6 is more a generalized marker for alveolar epithelial injury (Sato et al, 2004) and high levels have also be found in non-fungal infections such as *legionellosis*, severe tuberculosis and respiratory syncythial virus bronchiolitis, and even in noninfectious interstitial lung disease (Inou et al., 1995; Kawasaki et al., 2009; Sukoh et al., 2001). Therefore, KL-6 elevation in PcP is thought to be related to lung damage and regeneration of epithelium lining and cannot be used as a specified marker of *Pneumocystis* infection.

7.3.3 *S*-adenosylmethionine (SAM)

Some observations suggested that S-adenosylmethionine (SAM), which is a universal methyl donor synthesized from methionine and ATP by SAM synthetase, could stimulate *Pneumocystis* in vitro growth (Clarkson et al., 2004). Since SAM was depleted from both the culture medium and the plasma of rats with PcP, it was hypothesized that *Pneumocystis* cells could scavenge SAM from host fluids due to the lack of SAM synthetase (Clarkson et al., 2004) Consistently, plasma SAM levels were found to be low in patients with PcP and to increase gradually with treatment (Skelly et al., 2003, 2008). These findings strengthened the idea of using plasma SAM levels as a non-invasive PcP diagnostic method. However, recent data showed that SAM-related issue could be more complex than previously thought. Firstly, differences in SAM levels between laboratories could be influenced by the method of measurement. Thus, Wang and colleagues using Chromatography Tandem Mass Spectrometry found generally higher plasma SAM levels than those reported before (Wang et al., 2008). The same group was unable to distinguish patients with acute PcP from the ones without PcP on the basis of plasma SAM levels, though these levels increased significantly with effective anti-*Pneumocystis* treatment. Indeed, the concern needs to be further explored because fasting status, dietary intake of methionine and other medications can affect plasma SAM concentration (Wang et al, 2008). Secondly, and contrarily to the results of previous works (Clarkson et al., 2004), *P. carinii*, *P. murina* and *P. jirovecii* have genes that encoded SAM synthetase (Sam1) (Kutty et al., 2008) . Moreover, the corresponding *Sam1* mRNA is transcribed, and the protein, which is enzymatically active, was immuno-localized in *P. murina* cells. Such data suggest strongly that *Pneumocystis* species do not depend on an exogenous source of SAM to survive (Kutty et al., 2008).

7.3.4 Serological tests

Serum antibody detection constitutes an adjunctive strategy currently used to diagnose systemic fungal infections, even in immunosupressed patients. This strategy was however only rarely used to PcP diagnosis because healthy subjects have frequently significant levels of serum anti-*Pneumocystis* antibody. Moreover, the antibody response against *Pneumocystis* infection is currently highly variable and the results reported by diverse groups are contradictory (Walzer, 2004). In contrast, *Pneumocystis* antibody assays, especially those using recombinant *Pneumocystis* antigens, constitutes an interesting tool in epidemiology (Daly et al., 2009).

8. Treatment

The recommended treatment of PcP has remained unchanged for many years, being Co-trimoxazole, an association of trimethoprim and sulfamethoxazole, the drug of choice as first line of treatment. Regarding which agent of second line must be choice preferably, data are limited (table 3). Drug related toxicities are increasing in HIV-infected patients and organ transplant recipients. Because of the potential for additive or synergistic toxicities associated with anti-*Pneumocystis* and antiretroviral therapies, certain health-care providers delay initiation of HAART until after the completion of anti-*Pneumocystis* therapy, or until at least 2 weeks after initiating anti-*Pneumocystis* therapy, despite some suggestion of potential benefit of early HAART in the treatment of patients with AIDS-related opportunistic infections (CDC, 2009; Zolopa et al., 2009). In order to a correct management of PcP is important to distinguish between progressive PcP, drug toxicity and concomitant infection if clinical deterioration is detected.

Trimethoprim-sulfamethoxazole (TMP-SMX)

TMP and SMX target sequential steps in the folate synthesis pathway. TMP inhibits dihydrofolate reductase and SMX inhibits dihydropteroate synthetase. TMP-SMX is the treatment of choice for PcP in all patients who tolerate this drug, and it achieves the most rapid clinical response of the anti-*Pneumocystis* agents (CDC, 2009; Helweg-Larsen et al., 2009). The recommended dose of TMP-SMX for adults (or children aged > 2 months) is 15 to 20 mg/kg/day of TMP and 75 to 100 mg/kg/day of SMX intravenously every 6 or 8 hours. With renal dysfunction, dosing must be reduced. The bioavailability of TMP-SMX from oral therapy is comparable to parenteral administration (CDC, 2009; Mofenson et al., 2009).

Patients who have PcP despite the use of TMP-SMX prophylaxis, are usually successfully treated with TMP-SMX. In this way, the presence of mutations in the DHPS gene of *P. jirovecii* has been associated with resistance to sulfa drugs, although the clinical outcome is uncertain (Crothers et al. 2005; Huang et al., 2004; Stein et al., 2004). Drug related toxicities from TMP-SMX are greater than that from therapy with other anti-*Pneumocystis* agents. The side effects of TMP-SMX are: rash (30-55%), (including Stevens-Johnson syndrome), fever (30-40%), leukopenia (30-40%), hepatitis (20%), thrombocytopenia (15%), azotemia (1-5%), and hyperkaliemia (Eeftinck et al., 1990; Gordin et al., 1984; Hughes et al., 1995). Nephrotoxicity occurs frequently in the renal transplantation recipient receiving full-dose of TMP-SMX. Liver transplant recipients are particularly susceptible to TMP-SMX toxicity. Leucovorin to prevent myelosuppression is not recommended because its uncertain efficacy and a higher rate of failure (CDC, 2009).

Pentamidine

Pentamidine is an aromatic diamidine that has broad spectrum anti-protozoal activity. This drug inhibits metabolism of P amino benzoic acid, interferes with anaerobic glycolysis, inhibits oxidative phosphorylation and impairs nucleic acid and protein synthesis. It was the first drug reported to treat PcP successfully and subsequent reports have confirmed the efficacy of intravenous pentamidine. Although intravenous pentamidine has been recommended as the main alternative to TMP-SMX for moderate to severe PcP (Gordin et al., 1984), a recent study has found a greater risk of death when pentamidine was used as first and second-line therapy for HIV-associated PcP with compared with TMP-SMX and clindamycin-primaquine (Helweg-Larsen et al., 2009). These findings could be due to toxicities related to pentamidine and the absence of an antibacterial effect, in contrast to TMP-SMX or clindamycin-primaquine, which might act against concomitant bacterial co-infection (Helweg-Larsen et al., 2009).

Pentamidine for children and adults is administered once a day at 4 mg/kg (maximum 300 mg daily) intravenously, infused slowly 1 to 2 hr in 5% glucose; due to its toxicity the dose can be reduced to 3 mg/kg. Aerosolized pentamidine should not be used because of limited efficacy and more frequent relapse, and intramuscular administration is not used due to the related complications (Conte et al., 1990). Side effects of pentamidine include azotemia, pancreatitis, hypo- or hyperglycemia, pancytopenia, electrolyte abnormalities, cardiac dysrhythmia and renal dysfunction (Conte et al., 1990). Pentamidine should be avoided in pancreas transplant recipients due to the potential for islet cell necrosis.

Clindamycin-primaquine

Clindamycin is a lincosamide antibiotic used to treat infections with anaerobic bacteria but can also be used to treat some protozoan diseases. Primaquine is an 8-aminoquinoline anti-protozoan agent. This combination is effective in adult patients with mild to moderate PcP, but data for children are not available (Toma et al., 1998). Clindamycin is given at 600 to 900 mg intravenously or 300-450 mg orally every 6 to 8 hours and primaquine is given orally at 15 to 30 mg/day. Clindamycin component can be administered intravenously in severe cases; primaquine is only available orally. Recently, clindamycin-primaquine appeared superior to pentamidine as second-line therapy for PcP in patients failing or developing toxicity with TMP-SMX (Helweg-Larsen et al., 2009). Side effects of clindamycin include rash, anemia, neutropenia and the development of *Clostridium difficile* colitis. The main toxicity of primaquine is methemoglobinemia, thus, patients should be tested for glucose-6-phosphate dehydrogenase deficiency before administration of primaquine (Larsen, 2004).

Dapsone

Dapsone is a sulfone drug that inhibits DHPS and it is used as alternative therapeutic regimen for mild-to-moderate PcP. Dapsone must be taken with TMP (Medina et al., 1990). Although this association might have similar efficacy and fewer side effects than TMP-SMX, is less recommended due to the number of pills. The dosage of dapsone for adolescents and adults is 100 mg orally once daily (among children aged < 13 years, 2 mg/kg/day). The dosage of TMP for children and adults taken orally is 15 mg/kg/day divided into three doses (CDC, 2009; Mofenson et al., 2009). The most common adverse effects associated to dapsone are methemoglobinemia and hemolysis, especially in those with glucose-6-phosphate dehydrogenase deficiency. Thus, patients should be tested for glucose-6-phosphate dehydrogenase deficiency (Larsen et al. 2004).

Atovaquone

Atovaquone is a unique naphthoquinone that target the cytochome B complex and, thus, inhibits mitochondrial electron transport. This drug was developed clinically in the 1990s and it is available only as oral agent. It is used as second-line agent for treatment of mild to moderate PcP if TMP-SMX cannot be used. The standard dosing regimen for adults is atovaquone 750 mg orally twice a day with food for increasing gastrointestinal absorption (30-40 mg/kg/day for children < 3 months and > 24 months of age; between 3-24 months of age, 45 mg/kg/day are required) (Medina et al., 1990; Mofenson et al., 2009). Mutations of the cytochrome *b* gene have occurred in atovaquone-resistant isolates of *Pneumocystis*, but the clinical significance of gene mutations has not been determined (Kazanjian et al., 2001). The advantages of atovaquone include oral administration and fewer side effects. Disadvantages are its high cost and its bioavailability, although it has been improved with the micronized suspension formulation (Baggish & Hill, 2002). The most frequently reported adverse effects are rash, nausea, diarrhea, elevation of liver enzyme levels and headache. Atovaquone does not cause bone marrow suppression (Larsen et al., 2004).

Trimetrexate

Trimetrexate is an analogue of methotrexate that is an inhibitor of dihydrofolate reductase, and *in vitro* it is 1500 times more potent than trimethoprim (Kovacs et al., 1988). This drug is effective for treating PcP but is available only in an intravenous formulation. Because this drug also inhibits human folate metabolism, leucovorin must be administered concomitantly to prevent cytopenias (Larsen et al., 2004). A clinical trial showed that trimetrexate is less effective but better tolerate than TMP-SMX against AIDS-related PcP (Sattler et al., 1994). Trimetrexate with folinic acid have been approved for use in patients with moderately severe PcP, however, it is not longer available commercially. The dosage recommended for treatment of PcP is trimetrexate, 45 mg/m² intravenously once daily, plus

leucovorin 20 mg/m^2 orally or intravenously four times daily (Sattler et al., 1994)..
Leucovorin therapy must extend for 72 hours past the last dose of trimetrexate. For adults,
trimetrexate may alternatively be dosed on a mg/kg basis, depending on the patient's body
weight: <50 kg, 1.5 mg/kg; 50-80 kg, 1.2 mg/kg, and >80 kg, 1.0 mg/kg. Also, leucovorin
may be dosed on a mg/kg basis (<50 kg, 0.6 mg/kg, and >50 kg 0.5 mg/kg) administered
every 6 hours. Despite the suggestion that leucovorin impairs the efficacy of TMP-SMX,
there is no indication that the coadministration of leucovorin impairs the efficacy of
trimetrexate for PcP (Larsen et al., 2004). In some cases trimetrexate plus leucovorin could be
used as salvage treatment for PcP (Short et al., 2009).

Adjunctive therapies

The use of corticosteroids may reduce pulmonary inflammation response caused by the lysis
of *Pneumocystis* in the lung after initiating treatment of PcP. Corticosteroids have been
related with a significant benefit in terms of preventing deterioration in oxygenation in the
first seven days of therapy, mortality, and reduction of intubations in AIDS patients (Briel et
al., 2005). Corticosteroids are indicated in HIV-infected patients with a moderate-to-severe
PcP who have hypoxemia (the partial pressure of arterial oxygen under 70 mm Hg with the
patient breathing room air or an alveolar-arteriolar gradient greater than 35). In these cases,
corticosteroids should be administered as early as possible within 72 hours after starting
anti-*Pneumocystis* therapy (Thomas & Limper, 2004; CDC, 2009). Recommended dose are
showed in table 3.

Therapeutic use	Moderate to severe *Pneumocystis* pneumonia		
	Drug	Dose	Route
First line	Trimethoprim-Sulfamethoxazole	15-20 mg/Kg daily divided into 3 or 4 doses 75-100 mg/Kg daily divided into 3 or 4 doses	Intravenous
Second line	Primaquine plus Clindamycin	30 mg daily 600-900 mg three times daily	Oral Intravenous
Second line	Pentamidine	4 mg/Kg daily (3 mg/Kg if toxicities)	Intravenous
Salvage therapy	Trimetrexate plus Leucovorin	45 mg/m^2 daily 20 mg/m^2 four times daily	Intravenous Intravenous or oral
Adjunctive therapy	Prednisone Methylprednisolone	Days 1–5: 80 mg daily divided into 2 doses Days 6–10: 40 mg daily Days 11–21: 20 mg daily 75% of prednisone dose	Oral Intravenous
	Mild to moderate *Pneumocystis* pneumonia		
First line	Trimethoprim-Sulfamethoxazole	15-20 mg/Kg daily divided into 3 doses 75-100 mg/Kg daily divided into 3 doses	Oral
Second line	Dapsone plus Trimethoprim	100 mg daily 15-20 mg/Kg daily divided into 3 doses	Oral Oral or intravenous
Second line	Primaquine plus Clindamycin	15-30 mg daily 300-450 mg 3 or 4 times daily	Oral Oral
Second line	Atovaquone	750 mg two times daily	Oral with food

Table 3. Drugs therapy for treatment of *Pneumocystis* pneumonia in adults according to
severity

Novel agents

Novel agents undergoing clinical investigation include echinocandins and pneumocandins, which target synthesis of beta 1,3 glucan, a cell wall compound of *Pneumocystis* and other fungi.

Caspofungin is an echinocandin that acts on the cell wall by inhibiting β-1,3-glucan synthesis and it has been approved for several fungal infections as *Candida* and *Aspergillus* species. Caspofungin has shown activity against *Pneumocystis* in experimental animal models and it has strong activity on cyst forms and weak activity on trophic forms (Powles et al., 1998). Due to TMP-SMX affects only the trophic forms, it has been suggested that the association of TMP-SMX and caspofungin by fully inhibiting the organism life cycle, may provide a synergistic activity against *Pneumocystis*. According to this, it has been reported cases of PcP where the association of caspofungin and TMP-SMX achieved a complete cure of PcP (Utili et al., 2007). However, this promising therapeutic approach needs to be assessed by controlled clinical trials.

9. Prevention

Many studies have demonstrated that PcP can largely be prevented by administration of chemoprophylaxis to susceptible individuals (Di Cocco et al., 2009; Green et al., 2007; Podzamcser et al., 1995; Rodriguez & Fishman, 2004) and according with the American Thoracic Society recommendations patients infected with HIV (Huang et al., 2006) need to receive prophylaxis to prevent disease depending on specific risks to the patient's system. Recommendations for chemoprophylaxis should be based on weighing the efficacy against the risk of adverse events, the risk of developments of antimicrobial resistance, and the cost of the intervention (Roblot et al., 2005). Medications recommended for chemoprophylaxis against PcP are listed in table 4.

9.1 Primary prophylaxis

The majority of recommendations are based in studies performed in HIV-infected patients. Guidelines recommend starting primary prophylaxis against PcP in HIV-infected adolescents and adults, including pregnant and patients under HAART, when the CD4 cell count is less than 200 cells/mm³ or the patient has a history of oropharyngeal candidiasis. Patients with a CD4 cell percentage of <14% or a history of an AIDS-defining illness should be considered for chemoprophylaxis (CDC, 2009). Prophylaxis recommendations for HIV-infected children are age-based. Chemoprophylaxis should be provided for children 6 years or older based on adults guidelines, for children aged 1 to 5 years if CD4 counts are less than 500 cells/mm³ or CD4 percentage is less than 15%, and for all HIV-infected infants younger than 12 months (Zolopa et al., 2009).

TMP-SMX is the recommended prophylactic agent in both primary and secondary prophylaxis for PCP, because of its high efficacy, relative safety, low cost, and broad antimicrobial spectrum (CDC, 2009; Di Cocco et al., 2009; Roblot et al., 2005; Rodriguez & Fishman, 2004). TMP–SMX also is effective in preventing *Toxoplasma gondi, Isospora belli, Cyclospora cayetanensis* and some bacterial infections such us, *Streptococcus pneumoniae, Salmonella, Haemophilus, Staphylococcus,* common gram-negative gastrointestinal and urinary pathogens (Rodriguez & Fishman, 2004). Either one single-strength tablet daily or one double-strength tablet daily are the preferred regimens, but the first regimen might be better tolerated than the second (CDC, 2009). An alternative choice can be one double-strength tablet three times per week (CDC, 2009; Roblot et al., 2005). TMP-SMX at a dose of one double-strength tablet daily confers cross-protection against toxoplasmosis and selected common respiratory bacterial infections. Lower doses of TMP-SMX also likely confer such protection (CDC, 2009; Di Cocco et al., 2009).

For patients who have an adverse reaction that is not life threatening, prophylaxis with TMP-SMX should be reinstituted. These patients might better tolerate reintroduction of the drug with a gradual increase in dose or reintroduction of TMP-SMX at a reduced dose or frequency (CDC, 2009). If TMP-SMX is not tolerated, a second choice would be dapsone given 100 mg daily, dapsone 50 mg daily plus pyrimethamine 50 mg weekly plus leucovorin 25 mg weekly or dapsone 200 plus pyrimethamine 75 mg plus leucovorin 25 mg weekly, aerosolized pentamidine 300 mg monthly administered by an ultrasonic or jet-nebulizer, and atovaquone 1500 mg daily (CDC,2009). Dapsone is effective and inexpensive but

Drug	Dose for adults	Dose for children	Route	Comments
Trimethoprim-Sulfamethoxazole	160/800 mg (DS tablet) per day or 3 times per week 80/400 mg (SS tablet) per day	150/750 mg/m^2 body surface area (max: 320/1600 mg) as single or 2 divided doses 3 times per week	Oral	First choice Weekly regimen is recommended if daily therapy in not tolerated
Dapsone	100 mg per day	2 mg/Kg body weight (max: 100 g) per day 4 mg/Kg body weight (max: 200 g) per week	Oral	Alternative choice Ensure patient does not have Glucose-6 phosphate dehydrogenase deficiency
Pentamidine	300 mg per month	300 mg per month (aged ≥ 5 years)	Aerosol	Alternative choice
Atovaquone	1500 mg per day	30-45 mg/Kg body weight according to age per day	Oral	Alternative choice Take with high-fat meals for maximal absorption
Dapsona + Pyrimethamine + Leucovorin	50 mg per day 50 mg per week 25 mg per week		Oral Oral Oral	Alternative choice Ensure patient does not have Glucose-6 phosphate dehydrogenase deficiency Effective in preventing toxoplasmosis
Dapsona + Pyrimethamine + Leucovorin	200 mg per week 75 mg per week 25 mg per week		Oral Oral Oral	Alternative choice Ensure patient does not have Glucose-6 phosphate dehydrogenase deficiency Effective in preventing toxoplasmosis

Table 4. Prophylaxis regimens for *Pneumocystis* pneumonia.

associated with more serious adverse effects than atovaquone (El-Sadr et al., 1998). Atovaquone is effective, safe and it is effective against *Toxoplasma gondii* but it is more expensive (Rodriguez & Fishman, 2004). The widespread concept that TMP-SMX is contraindicated for prophylaxis in patients treated with methotrexate might be obsolete because the safety of one single-strength tablet daily or one double-strength tablet thrice-weekly has been proved in clinical studies (Langford et al., 2003). However, these patients need to receive folate supplementation besides blood counts and liver-function tests should be closely monitored (Roblot, 2005).

Primary prophylaxis should be discontinued for HIV-infected adult and adolescent patients who have responded to HAART with an increase in CD4 counts major than 200 cells/mm^3 during more than 3 months (Lopez Bernaldo et al., 2001). Prophylaxis should be reintroduced if the CD4 cell count decreases to less than 200 cells/mm^3.

9.2 Secondary prophylaxis
HIV-infected adults and adolescents patients who have developed previous episodes of PcP should receive secondary prophylaxis (Thomas & Limper, 2004). Chemoprophylaxis should be discontinued for adult and adolescent patients when CD4 cell count increases to more than 200 cells/mm^3 for a period of 3 months as a result of HAART (Lopez Bernaldo et al., 2001). Prophylaxis should be reintroduced if the CD4 count decreases again to less than 200 cells/mm^3. If PcP recurs at a CD4 count higher than 200 cells/mm^3, continuing PcP prophylaxis for life would be prudent (CDC, 2009).

10. Conclusions

Pneumocystis jirovecii is an atypical fungus that causes PcP mainly in HIV-infected individuals. Today, PcP is still a major cause of morbidity and mortality among AIDS patients, and constitutes a worldwide problem to public health. While the incidence of PcP among HIV infected individuals has decreased in developed countries, the prevalence of AIDS-related PcP in developing countries remains high and poorly controlled. The epidemiology of this infection is only beginning to be understood. The accumulating evidence suggests that *P. jirovecii* is a highly infectious organism with low virulence that takes advantage of hosts as temporary reservoirs of infection. In this sense, colonization with *P. jirovecii* (that is infection without disease) has recently gained attention as a important issue for understanding the complete cycle of human *Pneumocystis* infection. The clinical presentation in HIV-infected patients may differ from that in other immunosuppressed patients and its diagnosis continues to be challenging. Clinicians must be familiar with its presentation and management because mild cases are sometimes difficult to diagnose. The emergence of highly sensitive and specific molecular methods for PcP diagnosis have represented a significant advance in order to establish earlier PcP diagnosis, detect low parasite rates, and detect *Pneumocystis* DNA in non-invasive samples. Co-trimoxazole is the most effective medication for its prevention and treatment but other alternative medications are also available. Future clinical research should include studying the transmission and epidemiology of PcP in populations worldwide, improving the diagnosis of PcP, improving regimens for prophylaxis and treatment in various patient populations, and determining the significance of the DHPS mutations in various populations and in different geographic locations. Furthermore, the threat of emerging resistance to available anti-*Pneumocystis* drugs highlights the need to continue investigating the biology of this organism in the hope of developing novel treatment strategies.

11. References

Aderaye G, Woldeamanuel Y, Asrat D, *et al.* (2008). Evaluation of Toluidine Blue O staining for the diagnosis of *Pneumocystis jiroveci* in expectorated sputum sample and bronchoalveolar lavage from HIV-infected patients in a tertiary care referral center in Ethiopia. *Infection*, Vol. 36, pp. 237-243, ISSN 0300-8126

Alvarez-Martínez MJ, Moreno A, Miró JM *et al.* (2008). *Pneumocystis jirovecii* pneumonia in Spanish HIV-infected patients in the combined antiretroviral therapy era: prevalence of dihydropteroate synthase mutations and prognostic factors of mortality. *Diagn Microbiol Infect Dis*, Vol. 62, pp. 34-43, ISSN 0732-8893

Alibrahim, A., Lepore, M., Lierl, M. et al. (1998). *Pneumocystis carinii* pneumonia in an infant with X-linked agammaglobulinemia. *J Allergy Clin Immunol*, Vol.101, pp. 552–553, ISSN 0091-6749

Aliouat-Denis CM, Chabé M, Demanche C, Aliouat el M, Viscogliosi E, Guillot J, et al. (2008). *Pneumocystis* species, co-evolution and pathogenic power. *Infect Genet Evol*, Vol. 8, pp. 708-26, ISSN 1567-1348

Baggish AL, Hill DR. (2002). Antiparasitic agent atovaquone. *Antimicrob Agents Chemother*, Vol. 46, pp. 1163-1173. ISSN 0066-4804

Beard CB. (2004). Molecular typing and epidemiological insights. In: *Pneumocystis carinii Pneumonia (3rd edition)*. Walzer PD, Cushion MT (eds.), Marcel Dekker, Inc., New York, 479-504. ISBN 0-8247-5451-4

Benfield, TL., Prento, P., Junge, J. et al. (1997). Alveolar damage in AIDS-related *Pneumocystis carinii* pneumonia. *Chest*, Vol.111, No.5, (May 1997), pp. 1193-1199, ISSN 0012-3692

Briel M, Boscacci R, Furrer H, Bucher HC. (2005). Adjunctive corticosteroids for *Pneumocystis jiroveci* pneumonia in patients with HIV infection: a meta-analysis of randomised controlled trials. *BMC Infect Dis*, Vol. 5, pp. 101. ISSN 1471-2334

Burns, SM., Read, JA., Yap, PL. et al. (1990). Reduced concentrations of IgG antibodies to *Pneumocystis carinii* in HIV infected patients during active Pneumocystis carinii infection and the possibility of passive immunisation. *J Infect*, Vol.20, pp. 33–39. ISSN 0163-4453

Calderon E, de la Horra C, Montes-Cano MA, Respaldiza N, Martín-Juan J, Varela JM. (2004). Resistencia genotípica a sulfamidas en pacientes con neumonía por *Pneumocystis jiroveci*. *Med. Clin. (Barc)*, Vol. 122, pp. 617-619, ISSN 0025-7753

Calderon EJ, Rivero L, Respaldiza N *et al.* (2007). Systemic inflammation in patients with chronic obstructive pulmonary disease who are colonized with *Pneumocystis jirovecii*. *Clin Infect Dis*, Vol. 45, pp. 17-19, ISSN 1058-4838

Calderon EJ. (2009). Epidemiology of *Pneumocystis* infection in human. *J Mycol Med*, Vol. 19, pp. 270-275, ISSN 1156-5233

Calderon EJ. (2010a). *Pneumocystis* infection: seeing beyond the tip of the iceberg. *Clin Infect Dis*, Vol. 50, pp. 354-356, ISSN 1058-4838

Calderon EJ, Gutiérrez-Rivero S, Durand-Joly I, Dei-Cas E. (2010b). *Pneumocystis* infection in humans: diagnosis and treatment. *Expert Rev Anti Infect Ther*, Vol. 8, pp. 683-701, ISSN 1478-7210

Centers for Disease Control and Prevention. (2009). Guidelines for Prevention and Treatment of Opportunistic Infections in HIV-Infected Adults and Adolescents. *MMWR*, Vol. 58, pp. 1-216, ISSN 0149-2195

Chabé M, Dei-Cas E, Creusy C *et al.* (2004). Immunocompetent hosts as a reservoir of *Pneumocystis* organisms: histological and RT-PCR data demonstrate active replication. *Eur J Clin Microbiol Infect Dis*, Vol. 23, pp. 89-97, ISSN 0934-9723

Cheng VC, Hung IF, Wu AK, Tang BS, Chu CM, & Yuen KY. (2004). Lymphocyte surge as a marker for immunorestitution disease due to *Pneumocystis jiroveci* pneumonia in HIV-negative immunosuppressed hosts. *Eur J Clin Microbiol Infect Dis,* Vol. 23, pp. 512-514, ISSN 1058-4838

Chouaid C, Housset B, Lebeau B. (1995). Cost-analysis of four diagnostic strategies for *Pneumocystis carinii* pneumonia in HIV-infected subjects. *Eur Respir J*, Vol. 8, pp. 1554-1558, ISSN 0903-1936

Clarkson AB, Merali S. (2004). Polyamines, Iron, and *Pneumocystis carinii*. In: *Pneumocystis carinii Pneumonia (3rd edition)*, Walzer PD, Cushion MT (eds.), Marcel Dekker, Inc., New York, 577-605. ISBN: 0-8247-5451-4

Coleman, DL., Doder, PM., Goleen, JA. et al. (1984). Correlation between serial pulmonary function test and fiberoptic bronchoscopy in patients with *Pneumocystis carinii* pneumonia and the acquired immune deficiency syndrome. *Am Rev Respir Dis*, Vol.129, pp. 491-493, ISSN 0003-0805

Conte JE, Jr., Chernoff D, Feigal DW, Jr., et al. (1990). Intravenous or inhaled pentamidine for treating *Pneumocystis carinii* pneumonia in AIDS: a randomized trial. *Ann Intern Med*, Vol. 113, pp. 203-209, ISSN 0003-4819

Crothers K, Beard CB, Turner J, et al. (2005). Severity and outcome of HIV-associated *Pneumocystis* pneumonia containing *Pneumocystis jirovecii* dihydropteroate synthase gene mutations. *AIDS*, Vol. 19, pp. 801-805, ISSN 0269-9370

Daly K, Koch J, Respaldiza N *et al.* (2009). Geographical variation in serological responses to recombinant *Pneumocystis jirovecii* major surface glycoprotein antigens. *Clin Microbiol Infect*, Vol. 15, pp. 937-942, ISSN 1469-0691

de Boer MG, Bruijnesteijn van Coppenraet LE, Gaasbeek A, et al. (2007). An outbreak of *Pneumocystis jiroveci* pneumonia with 1 predominant genotype among renal transplant recipients: interhuman transmission or a common environmental source? *Clin Infect Dis*, Vol. 44, pp. 1143-9, ISSN 1058-4838

Dei-Cas E, Fleurisse L, Aliouat EM *et al.* (1998). Morphological and ultrastructural methods for *Pneumocystis*. *FEMS Immunol. Med Microbiol*, Vol. 22, pp. 185-189, ISSN 0928-8244

Dei-Cas E. (2000). *Pneumocystis* infections: the iceberg?. *Med Mycol*, Vol. 38, pp. 23-32, ISSN 1369-3786

Dei-Cas E, Chabé M, Moukhlis R *et al.* (2006). *Pneumocystis oryctolagi* sp. nov., an uncultured fungus causing pneumonia in rabbits at weaning: review of current knowledge, and description of a new taxon on genotypic, phylogenetic and phenotypic bases. *FEMS Microbiol. Rev*, Vol. 30, pp. 853-871, ISSN 0168-6445

de la Horra C, Varela JM, Friaza V, et al. (2006). Comparison of single and touchdown PCR protocols for detecting *Pneumocystis jirovecii* DNA in paraffin-embedded lung tissue samples. *J. Eukaryot. Microbiol*, Vol. 53, (Suppl 1), pp. 98-99, ISSN 1066-5234

Desmet S, Van Wijngaerden E, Maertens J *et al.* (2009). Serum (1-3)-beta-D-glucan as a tool for diagnosis of *Pneumocystis jirovecii* pneumonia in patients with human immunodeficiency virus infection or hematological malignancy. *J Clin Microbiol*, Vol. 47, pp. 3871-3874, ISSN 0095-1137

Di Cocco P, Orlando G, Bonanni L, et al. (2009). A systematic review of two different trimetoprim-sulfamethoxazole regimens used to prevent *Pneumocystis jirovecii* and no prophylaxis at all in transplant recipients: appraising the evidence. *Transplant Proc*, Vol. 41, pp. 1201-1203, ISSN 0041-1345

Durand-Joly I, Wakefield AE, Palmer RJ *et al.* (2000). Ultrastructural and molecular characterization of *Pneumocystis carinii* isolated from a rhesus monkey (*Macaca mulatta*). *Med Mycol*, Vol. 38, pp. 61-72, ISSN 1369-3786

Durand-Joly I. (2002). Épidémiologie moléculaire de la pneumocystose humaine. Caractérisation génétique et phénotypique de *Pneumocystis jirovecii* et espèces proches. *Thesis Dissertation*. Lille, France.

Durand-Joly, I., Soula, F., Chabe, M *et al.* (2003). Longterm colonization with *Pneumocystis jirovecii* in hospital staffs: a challenge to prevent nosocomial pneumocystosis. *J Eukaryot Microbiol*, Vol. 50 (Suppl.), pp. 614–615,ISSN 1066-5234

Durand-Joly I, Chabé M, Soula F, Delhaes L, Camus D, Dei-Cas E. (2005). Molecular diagnosis of *Pneumocystis* pneumonia (PcP). *FEMS Immunol. Med Microbiol*, Vol. 45, pp. 405-410, ISSN 0928-8244

Edman JC, Kovacs JA, Masur H, Santi DV, Elwood HJ, Sogin ML. (1988). Ribosomal RNA sequence shows *Pneumocystis carinii* to be a member of the fungi. *Nature*, Vol. 334, pp. 519-22, ISSN 0028-0836

Eeftinck Schattenkerk JK, Lange JM, van Steenwijk RP, Danner SA. (1990). Can the course of high dose cotrimoxazole for *Pneumocystis carinii* pneumonia in AIDS be shorter? A possible solution to the problem of cotrimoxazole toxicity. *J Intern Med*, Vol. 227, pp. 359-362, ISSN 1365-2796

Fei MW, Kim EJ, Sant CA, et al. (2009). Predicting mortality from HIV-associated *Pneumocystis* pneumonia at illness presentation: an observational cohort study. *Thorax*, Vol. 64, pp. 1070-1076, ISSN 0028-4793

Friaza V, Montes-Cano MA, Respaldiza N, Morilla R, Calderón EJ, de la Horra C. (2009). Prevalence of dihydropteroate synthase mutations in Spanish patients with HIV-associated *Pneumocystis* pneumonia. *Diagn Microbiol Infect Dis*, Vol. 64, pp. 104-105, ISSN 0732-8893

Gordin FM, Simon GL, Wofsy CB, Mills J. (1984). Adverse reactions to trimethoprim-sulfamethoxazole in patients with the acquired immunodeficiency syndrome. *Ann Intern Med*, Vol. 100, pp.495-499, ISSN 0003-4819

Green H, Paul M, Vidal L, Leibovici L. (2007). Prophylaxis of *Pneumocystis* pneumonia in immunocompromised non-HIV-infected patients: systematic review and meta-analysis of randomized controlled trials. *Mayo Clin Proc*, Vol. 82, pp. 1052-1059, ISSN 0025-6196

Helweg-Larsen J, Benfield TL, Eugen-Olsen J, Lundgren JD, Lundgren B. (1999). Effects of mutations in *Pneumocystis carinii* dihydropteroate synthase gene on outcome of AIDS-associated *P. carinii* pneumonia. *Lancet*, Vol. 354, pp. 1347–1351, ISSN 0140-6736

Helweg-Larsen J, Benfield T, Atzori C, Miller RF. (2009). Clinical efficacy of first- and second-line treatments for HIV-associated *Pneumocystis jirovecii* pneumonia: a tri-centre cohort study. *J Antimicrob Chemother*, Vol. 64, pp. 1282-1290, ISSN 0305-7453

Huang L, Beard CB, Creasman J *et al.* (2000). Sulfa or sulfone prophylaxis and geographic region predict mutations in the *Pneumocystis carinii* dihydropteroate synthase gene. *J Infect Dis*, Vol. 182, pp. 1192–1198, ISSN 0022-1899

Huang L. (2004). Clinical presentation and diagnosis of *Pneumocystis* pneumonia in HIV-infected patients. In: *Pneumocystis carinii Pneumonia, 3rd edition,* Walzer PD, Cushion MT (eds.), Marcel Dekker, Inc., New York, 349-406. ISBN 0-8247-5451-4

Huang L, Crothers K, Atzori C *et al.* (2004). Dihydropteroate synthase gene mutations in *Pneumocystis* and sulfa resistance. *Emerg Infect Dis*, Vol. 10, pp. 1721–1728, ISSN 1080-6059

Huang L, Morris A, Limper AH, Beck JM; ATS *Pneumocystis* Workshop Participants. (2006). An Official ATS Workshop Summary: Recent advances and future directions in *Pneumocystis* pneumonia (PCP). *Proc Am Thorac Soc*, Vol. 3, pp. 655-664, ISSN 1546-3222

Huggett JF, Taylor MS, Kocjan G *et al.* (2008). Development and evaluation of a real-time PCR assay for detection of *Pneumocystis jirovecii* DNA in bronchoalveolar lavage fluid of HIV-infected patients. *Thorax*, Vol. 63, pp. 154-159, ISSN 0028-4793

Hughes WT, LaFon SW, Scott JD, Masur H. (1995). Adverse events associated with trimethoprim-sulfamethoxazole and atovaquone during the treatment of AIDS-related *Pneumocystis carinii* pneumonia. *J Infect Dis*, Vol. 171, pp. 1295-1301, ISSN 0022-1899

Hughes WT. (2004). *Pneumocystis* Pneumonitis in Non-HIV-Infected Patients: Update. In: *Pneumocystis carinii Pneumonia (3rd edition)*. Walzer PD, Cushion MT (eds.), Marcel Dekker, Inc., New York, 407-434, ISBN 0-8247-5451-4

Iliades P, Meshnick SR, Macreadie IG. (2004). Dihydropteroate synthase mutations in *Pneumocystis jiroveci* can affect sulfamethoxazole resistance in a *Saccharomyces cerevisiae* model. *Antimicrob Agents Chemother*, Vol. 48, pp. 2617-2623, ISSN 0066-4804

Inoue Y, Nishimura K, Shiode M, et al. (1995). Evaluation of serum KL-6 levels in patients with pulmonary tuberculosis. *Tuber Lung Dis*, Vol. 76, pp. 230-233, ISSN 0962-8479

Jagannathan P, Davis E, Jacobson M, & Huang L. (2009). Life-threatening immune reconstitution inflammatory syndrome after *Pneumocystis* pneumonia: a cautionary case series. *AIDS*, Vol. 23, pp. 1794-1796, ISSN 0269-9370

Kawasaki Y, Aoyagi Y, Abe Y, et al. (2009). Serum KL-6 levels as a biomarker of lung injury in respiratory syncytial virus bronchiolitis. *J Med Virol*, Vol. 81, pp. 2104-2108, ISSN 0146-6615

Kazanjian P, Armstrong W, Hossler PA *et al.* (2000). *Pneumocystis carinii* mutations are associated with duration of sulfa or sulfone prophylaxis exposure in AIDS patients. *J Infect Dis*, Vol. 182, pp. 551–557, ISSN 0022-1899

Kazanjian P, Armstrong W, Hossler P.A, et al. (2001). *Pneumocystis carinii* cytochrome b mutations are associated with atovaquone exposure in patients with AIDS. *J Infect Dis*, Vol. 183, pp. 819-822, ISSN 0022-1899

Kelly, MN. & Shellito, JE. (2010). Current understanding of *Pneumocystis* immunology. *Future Microbiol*, Vol.5, pp. 43-65, ISSN 1746-0913

Kovacs JA, Ng VL, Masur H *et al.* (1988). Diagnosis of *Pneumocystis carinii* pneumonia: improved detection in sputum with use of monoclonal antibodies. *N Engl J Med*, Vol. 318, pp. 589-593, ISSN 0028-4793

Krajicek. BJ., Limper, AH., & Thomas, CF. (2008). Advances in the biology, pathogenesis and identification of *Pneumocystis* pneumonia. *Curr Opin Pulm Med.* 2008; Vol. 14, pp. 228-234, ISSN 1070-5287

Krajicek, BJ., Thomas, CFJr. & Limper, AH. (2009). *Pneumocystis* pneumonia: current concepts in pathogenesis, diagnosis, and treatment. *Clin Chest Med*, Vol.30; pp. 265-278, ISSN 0272-5231

Kutty G, Hernandez-Novoa B, Czapiga M, Kovacs JA. (2008). *Pneumocystis* encodes a functional S-adenosylmethionine synthetase gene. *Eukaryot Cell*, Vol. 7, pp. 258–267, ISSN 1535-9786

Langford CA, Talar-Williams C, Barron KS, Sneller MC. (2003). Use of cyclophosphamide-induction methotrexate-maintenance regimen for the treatment of Wegener's granulomatosis: extended follow-up and rate of relapse. *Am J Med*, Vol. 114, pp. 463–469,ISSN 0002-9343

Larsen HH, Masur H, Kovacs JA *et al.* (2002). Development and evaluation of a quantitative, touchdown, real-time PCR assay for diagnosing *Pneumocystis carinii* pneumonia. *J Clin Microbiol*, Vol. 40, pp. 490–494, ISSN 0095-1137

Larsen HH, Masur H, Kovacs JA. (2004). Current regimens for treatment and prophylaxis of *Pneumocystis jiroveci* pneumonia. In: *Pneumocystis carinii Pneumonia, 3rd edition*, Walzer PD, Cushion MT (eds.), Marcel Dekker, Inc., New York, 505-538, ISBN 0-8247-5451-4

Limper, AH., Hoyte, JS. & Standing, JE.. (1997). The role of alveolar macrophages in *Pneumocystis carinii* degradation and clearance from the lung. *J Clin Invest*, Vol.99, pp. 2110-2107, ISSN 0021-9738

Lopez Bernaldo de Quiros JC, Miro JM, Peña JM, et al. (2001). A randomized trial of the discontinuation of primary and secondary prophylaxis against *Pneumocystis carinii* pneumonia after highly active antiretroviral therapy in patients with HIV infection. *N Engl J Med*, Vol. 344, pp. 159-167, ISSN 0028-4793

Lu, JJ. & Lee CH. (2008). *Pneumocystis* pneumonia. *J Formos Med Assoc*, Vol.107, pp. 830-842, ISSN 0929-6646

Medina I, Mills J, Leoung G, et al. (1990). Oral therapy for *Pneumocystis carinii* pneumonia in the acquired immunodeficiency syndrome: a controlled trial of trimethoprim-sulfamethoxazole versus trimethoprim-dapsone. *N. Engl. J. Med*, Vol. 323, pp. 776-782, ISSN 0028-4793

Medrano FJ, Montes-Cano M, Conde M, et al. (2005). *Pneumocystis jirovecii* in general population. *Emerg Infect Dis*, Vol. 11, pp. 245-250, ISSN 1080-6059

Miller RF, Le Noury J, Corbett EL, Felton JM, De Cock KM. (1996). Pneumocystis carinii infection: current treatment and prevention. J Antimicrob Chemother. Vol. 37, Suppl B, pp. 33-53, ISSN 0305-7453

Miller RF, Wakefield AE. (1999). *Pneumocystis carinii* genotypes and severity of pneumonia. *Lancet*, Vol. 353, pp. 2039-2040, ISSN 0140-6736

Miller RF, Ambrose HE, Wakefield AE. (2001). *Pneumocystis carinii* f. sp. hominis DNA in immunocompetent health care workers in contact with patients with *P. carinii* pneumonia. *J Clin Microbiol*, Vol. 39, pp. 3877-3882, ISSN 0095-1137

Mofenson LM, Brady MT, Danner SP, et al. (2009). Guidelines for the Prevention and Treatment of Opportunistic Infections among HIV-exposed and HIV-infected children: recommendations from CDC, the National Institutes of Health, the HIV Medicine Association of the Infectious Diseases Society of America, the Pediatric Infectious Diseases Society, and the American Academy of Pediatrics. *MMWR Recomm Rep*, Vol. 58 (RR-11), pp. 1-166, ISSN 1057-5987

Montes-Cano MA, Chabe M, Fontillon-Alberdi M, de La Horra C, Respaldiza N, Medrano FJ, et al. (2009). Vertical transmission of *Pneumocystis jirovecii* in humans. *Emerg Infect Dis*, Vol. 15, pp. 125-127, ISSN 1080-6059

Mori S, Polatino S, & Estrada-Y-Martin RM. (2009). *Pneumocystis*-associated organizing pneumonia as a manifestation of immune reconstitution inflammatory syndrome in an HIV-infected individual with a normal CD4+ T-cell count following antiretroviral therapy. *Int J STD AIDS*; Vol. 20. pp. 662-665, ISSN 0956-4624

Morris A, Beard CB, Huang L. (2002). Update on the epidemiology and transmission of *Pneumocystis* carinii. *Microbes Infect*, Vol. 4, pp. 95-103, ISSN 1286-4579

Morris A, Wei K, Afshar K, Huang L. (2008). Epidemiology and clinical significance of *Pneumocystis* colonization. *J Infect Dis*, Vol. 97, pp. 10-17, ISSN 0022-1899

Nahimana A, Rabodonirina M, Bille J, Francioli P, Hauser PM. (2004). Mutations of *Pneumocystis jirovecii* dihydrofolate reductase associated with failure of prophylaxis. *Antimicrob Agents Chemother*, Vol. 48, pp. 4301-4305, ISSN 0066-4804

Nakamura H, Tateyama M, Tasato D *et al.* (2009). Clinical utility of serum beta-D-glucan and KL-6 levels in *Pneumocystis jirovecii* pneumonia. *Intern Med*, Vol. 48, pp. 195-202, ISSN 1349-7235

Nevez G, Chabé M, Rabodonirina M *et al.* (2008). Nosocomial *Pneumocystis jirovecii* infections. *Parasite*, Vol. 15, pp. 359-365, ISSN 1776-1042

Ng VL, Yajko DM, Hadley WK. (1997). Extrapulmonary pneumocystosis. *Clin Microbiol Rev*, Vol. 10, pp. 401-418, ISSN 0893-8512

Nyamande, K., Lalloo, UG., & Vawda, F. (2007). Comparison of plain chest radiography and high-resolution CT in human immunodeficiency virus infected patients with community-acquired pneumonia: a sub-Saharan Africa study. *Br J Radiol*, 2007; Vol. 80, pp. 302-306, ISSN 0007-1285

Olsson M, Elvin K, Löfdahl S, Linder E. (1993). Detection of *Pneumocystis carinii* DNA in sputum and bronchoalveolar lavage samples by polymerase chain reaction. *J Clin Microbiol*, Vol. 31, pp. 221-226, ISSN 0095-1137

Olsson M, Eriksson BM, Elvin K, Strandberg M, Wahlgren M. (2001). Genotypes of clustered cases of *Pneumocystis carinii* pneumonia. *Scand J Infect Dis*, Vol. 33, pp. 285-289, ISSN 0036-5548

Podzamczer D, Salazar A, Jimenez J, et al. (1995). Intermittent trimethoprim-sulfamethoxazole compared with dapsone-pyrimethamine for the simultaneous primary prophylaxis of *Pneumocystis* pneumonia and toxoplasmosis in patients infected with HIV. *Ann Intern Med*, Vol. 122, pp. 755-761, ISSN 0003-4819

Pontón J. (2009). Utilidad de los marcadores biológicos en el diagnóstico de la candidiasis invasora. *Rev Iberoam Micol*, Vol. 26, pp. 8-14, ISSN 1130-1406

Powles MA, Liberator P, Anderson J, et al. (1998). Efficacy of MK-991 (L- 743,872), a semisynthetic Pneumocandin, in murine models of *Pneumocystis carinii*. *Antimicrob Agents Chemother*, Vol. 42, pp. 1985-1989, ISSN 0066-4804

Prevost, MC., Escamilla, R., Aliouat, EM., et al. (1998) Pneumocystosis pathophysiology. *FEMS Immunol Med Microbiol*, Vol. 28, pp. 123-128, ISSN 0928-8244

Richards CG, Wakefield AE, Mitchell CD. (1994). Detection of *Pneumocystis* DNA in nasopharyngeal aspirates of leukaemic infants with pneumonia. *Arch Dis Child*, Vol. 71, pp. 254–255, ISSN 1743-0585

Sato H, Callister ME, Mumby S, et al. (2004). KL-6 levels are elevated in plasma from patients with acute respiratory distress syndrome. *Eur Respir J*, Vol. 23, pp. 142-145, ISSN 0903-1936

Schliep, TC., Yarrish, RL. (1999). *Pneumocystis carinii* pneumonia. *Semin Respir Infect*, 1999; Vol. 14, pp. 333-343, ISSN 0882-0546

Sepkowitz., KA., Telzak, EE., & Gold, JW, et al. (1991). Pneumothorax in AIDS. *Ann Intern Med*, 1991; Vol. 114, pp. 455-459, ISSN 0003-4819

Short CE, Gilleece YC, Fisher MJ, Churchill DR. (2009). Trimetrexate and folinic acid: a valuable salvage option for *Pneumocystis jirovecii* pneumonia. *AIDS*, Vol. 23, pp. 1287-1290, ISSN 0269-9370

Sukoh N, Yamamoto H, Kikuchi E, et al. (2001). A case of severe Legionella pneumonia monitored with serum SP-A, SP-D, and KL-6. *Nihon Kokyuki Gakkai Zasshi*, Vol. 39, pp. 126-130, ISSN 0301-1542

Rabodonirina M, Vanhems P, Couray-Targe S, et al. (2004). Molecular evidence of interhuman transmission of *Pneumocystis* pneumonia among renal transplant recipients hospitalized with HIV-infected patients. *Emerg Infect Dis*, Vol. 10, pp. 1766-1773, ISSN 1080-6059

Respaldiza N, Medrano FJ, Medrano AC, Varela JM, de la Horra C, Montes-Cano M, et al. (2004). High seroprevalence of *Pneumocystis* infection in Spanish children. *Clin Microbiol Infect*, Vol. 10, pp. 1029-1031, ISSN 1198-743X

Respaldiza N, Montes-Cano MA, Friaza V, et al. (2006). Usefulness of oropharyngeal washings for identifying *Pneumocystis jirovecii* carriers. *J Eukaryot Microbiol*, Vol. 53, (Suppl 1), pp. 100-101, ISSN 1066-5234

Rivero L, de la Horra C, Montes-Cano MA, Rodríguez-Herrera A, Respaldiza N, Friaza V, et al. (2008). *Pneumocystis jirovecii* transmission from immunocompetent carriers to infant. *Emerg Infect Dis*, Vol. 14, pp. 1116-1118, ISSN 1080-6059

Roblot, F. (2005). Management of *Pneumocystis* pneumonia in patients with inflammatory disorders. *Expert Rev Anti Infect. Ther*, Vol. 3, pp. 435-444, ISSN 1478-7210

Rodriguez, M., Fishman, JA. (2004). Prevention of infection due to *Pneumocystis* spp. in human immunodeficiency virus-negative immunocompromised patients. *Clin Microbiol Rev*, 2004; Vol. 17, pp. 770-82, ISSN1098-6618

Sattler FR, Frame P, Davis R, et al. (1994). Trimetrexate with leucovorin versus trimethoprim-sulfamethoxazole for moderate to severe episodes of *Pneumocystis carinii* pneumonia in patients with AIDS: a prospective, controlled multicenter investigation of the AIDS Clinical Trials Group Protocol 029/031. *J Infect Dis*, Vol. 170, pp. 165-172, ISSN 0022-1899

Skelly M, Hoffman J, Fabbri M, Holzman RS, Clarkson AB Jr, Merali S. (2003). S-adenosylmethionine concentrations in diagnosis of *Pneumocystis carinii* pneumonia. *Lancet*, Vol. 361, pp. 1267–1268, ISSN 0140-6736.

Skelly MJ, Holzman RS, Merali S. (2008). S-adenosylmethionine levels in the diagnosis of *Pneumocystis carinii* pneumonia in patients with HIV infection. *Clin Infect* Dis, Vol. 46, pp. 467–471, ISSN 1058-4838

Stein CR, Poole C, Kazanjian P, Meshnick SR. (2004). Sulfa use, Dihydropteroate sythase mutations, and *Pneumocystis jirovecii* pneumonia. *Emerg Infect Dis*, Vol. 10, pp. 1760-1765, ISSN 1080-6059

Steele, C., Shellito, JE. & Kolls, JK. (2005). Immunity against the opportunistic fungal pathogen *Pneumocystis*. *Medical Mycology*, Vol. 43; pp. 1-19, ISSN 1369-3786

Stringer SL, Stringer JR, Blase MA, Walzer PD, Cushion MT. (1989). *Pneumocystis carinii*: sequence from ribosomal RNA implies a close relationship with fungi. *Exp Parasitol*, Vol. 68, pp. 450-456, ISSN 0014-4894

Tamburrini E, Mencarini P, Visconti E, et al. (1998). Potential impact of *Pneumocystis* genetic diversity on the molecular detection of the parasite in human hosts. *FEMS Immunol Med Microbiol*, Vol. 22, pp. 37-49, ISSN 0928-8244

Tasaka S, Hasegawa N, Kobayashi S, et al. (2007). Serum indicators for the diagnosis of pneumocystis pneumonia. *Chest*, Vol. 131, pp. 1173-1180, ISSN 0012-3692

Teramoto S, Sawaki D, Okada S, Ouchi Y. (2000). Markedly increased plasma (1-->3)-beta-D-glucan is a diagnostic and therapeutic indicator of *Pneumocystis carinii* pneumonia in a non-AIDS patient. *J Med Microbiol*, Vol. 49, pp. 393-394, ISSN 0022-2615

Thomas, CF., Limper, AH. (2004). *Pneumocystis* pneumonia. *N Engl J Med*,. 2004; Vol. 350, pp :2487-2498. ISSN 0028-4793

Thomas CF Jr, Limper AH. (2007). Current insights into the biology and pathogenesis of *Pneumocystis* pneumonia. *Nat Rev Microbiol*, Vol. 5, pp. 298-308, ISSN 1740-1526

Toma E, Thorne A, Singer J, et al. (1998). Clindamycin with primaquine vs. Trimethoprim-sulfamethoxazole therapy for mild and moderately severe *Pneumocystis carinii* pneumonia in patients with AIDS: a multicenter, double-blind, randomized trial. *Clin Infect Dis*, Vol. 27, pp. 524-30, ISSN 1058-4838

Totet A, Pautard JC, Raccurt C, Roux P, Nevez G. (2003). Genotypes at the internal transcribed spacers of the nuclear rRNA operon of *Pneumocystis jirovecii* in nonimmunosuppressed infants without severe pneumonia. *J Clin Microbiol*, Vol. 41, pp. 1173-1180, ISSN 0095-1137

Tsolaki AG, Miller RF, Wakefield AE. (1999). Oropharyngeal samples for genotyping and monitoring response to treatment in AIDS patients with *Pneumocystis carinii* pneumonia. *J. Med. Microbiol*, Vol. 48, pp. 897-905, ISSN 0022-2615

van Hal SJ, Gilgado F, Doyle T *et al.* (2009). Clinical significance and phylogenetic relationship of novel Australian *Pneumocystis jirovecii* genotypes. *J Clin Microbiol*, Vol. 47; pp. 1818-1823, ISSN 0095-1137

Vassallo, R., Kottom, TJ., Standing, JE. et al. (2001). Vitronectin and fibronectin function as glucan binding proteins augmenting macrophage responses to *Pneumocystis carinii*. *Am J Respir Cell Mol Biol*, Vol.25, pp. 203-211, ISSN1044-1549

Vidal S, de la Horra C, Martín J, *et al.* (2006). *Pneumocystis jirovecii* colonisation in patients with interstitial lung disease. *Clin Microbiol Infect*, Vol. 12, pp. 231-235, ISSN 1058-4838

Utili R, Durante-Mangoni E, Basilico C, Mattei A, Ragone E, Grossi P. (2007). Efficacy of caspofungin addition to trimethoprim-sulfamethoxazole treatment for severe

Pneumocystis pneumonia in solid organ transplant recipients. *Transplantation*, Vol. 84, pp. 685-688, ISSN 0041-1345

Vargas SL, Ponce CA, Gigliotti F, et al. (2000). Transmission of Pneumocystis carinii DNA from a patient with *P. carinii* pneumonia to immunocompetent contact health care workers. *J Clin Microbiol*, Vol. 38, pp. 1536-1538, ISSN 0095-1137

Wakefield AE, Pixley FJ, Banerji S *et al.* (1990). Detection of *Pneumocystis carinii* with DNA amplification. *Lancet*, Vol. 336, pp. 451–453, ISSN 0140-6736

Wakefield AE. (1996). DNA sequences identical to *Pneumocystis carinii* f. sp. carinii and *Pneumocystis carinii* f. sp. hominis in samples of air spora. *J Clin Microbiol*, Vol. 34, pp. 1754-1759, ISSN 0095-1137

Walzer, PD. (1993). *Pneumocystis carinii*: recent advances in basic biology and their clinical application. *AIDS*, Vol.7, pp. 1293-1305, ISSN 0269-9370

Walzer PD. (2004). Immunological Features of *Pneumocystis* Infection in Humans. In: *Pneumocystis carinii Pneumonia, 3rd edition*, Walzer PD, Cushion MT (eds.), Marcel Dekker, Inc., New York, 451-477, ISBN 0-8247-5451-4

Wang P, Huang L, Davis JL *et al.* (2008). A hydrophilic-interaction chromatography tandem mass spectrometry method for quantitation of serum s-adenosylmethionine in patients infected with human immunodeficiency virus. *Clin Chim Acta*, Vol. 396, pp. 86-88, ISSN 0009-8981

Wazir, JF., Ansari, NA. (2004). *Pneumocystis carinii* infection. Update and review. *Arch Pathol Lab Med*, 2004; Vol. 128, pp. 1023-1027, ISSN 0003-9985

Wislez M, Bergot E, Antoine M, et al. (2001). Acute respiratory failure following HAART introduction in patients treated for *Pneumocystis carinii* pneumonia. *Am J Respir Crit Care Med*, Vol. 164, pp. 847-851, ISSN 1073-449X

Wright, TW., Gigliotti, F., Finkelstein, JN., et al. (1999). Immune-mediated inflammation directly impairs pulmonary function, contributing to the pathogenesis of *Pneumocystis carinii* pneumonia. *J Clin Invest*, Vol.104, pp. 1307-1317, ISSN 0021-9738

Wright, TW., Johnston, CJ., Harmsen, AG. et al. (1999). Chemokine gene expression during *Pneumocystis carinii*-driven pulmonary inflammation. *Infect Immun*, Vol.67, pp. 3452-3460, ISSN 0019-9567

Wright, TW., Notter, RH., Wang, Z., et al. (2001). Pulmonary inflammation disrupts surfactant function during *Pneumocystis carinii* pneumonia. *Infect Immun*, Vol.69, pp. 758-764, ISSN 0019-9567

Wright, TW., Pryhuber, GS., Chess, PR., et al. (2004). TNF receptor signalling contributes to chemokine secretion, inflammation, and respiratory deficits during *Pneumocystis* pneumonia. *J Immunol*, Vol.172, pp. 2511-2521, ISSN 0022-1767

Wu AK, Cheng VC, Tang BS, et al. (2004). The unmasking of *Pneumocystis jiroveci* pneumonia during reversal of immunosuppression: case reports and literature review. *BMC Infect Dis*, Vol.4, pp.57, ISSN 1471-2334

Zolopa A, Andersen J, Powderly W, et al. (2009). Early antiretroviral therapy reduces AIDS progression/death in individuals with acute opportunistic infections: a multicenter randomized strategy trial. *PLoS One*, Vol. 4, pp. e5575, ISSN 1932-6203

2

Poverty, Parasitosis and HIV/AIDS - Major Health Concerns in Tanzania

Kennedy Daniel Mwambete and Mary Justin-Temu
Muhimbili University of Health and Allied Sciences,
Tanzania

1. Introduction

Poverty, parasitosis and HIV/AIDS are closely interlinked and co-circulate in many populations. HIV/AIDS, parasitic infections like malaria and other opportunistic infections, and in a few are by far the commonest causes of ill-health and death in the poorest countries of the world, that happen to be in the tropics and temperate countries in Africa, Asia, and South America. Parasitic infections remain an important cause of morbidity and mortality in developing countries especially among HIV-infected persons.

There are indications that HIV-1 (the most prevalent in Tanzania) interacts significantly with many other parasitic infections within individual hosts, but the population-level impacts of co-infection are not well-characterized. Among those parasitic opportunistic infections, *Cryptosporidum parvum, Isospora belli, Cyclospora cayetanensis* and *Microspordia* species frequent causes of diarrhea. Likewise, *Pneumocystis jiroveci* pneumonia and *Candida* species infections have been implicated in life threatening fungal infections among people living with HIV/AIDS.

In this chapter, poverty is defined as a state of having little or no money and few or no material possessions. Poverty can be caused by unemployment, low education, deprivation and homelessness. Lack of health facilities and low-cost healthy foods, along with public space for physical activities, may be among the factors that contribute to poor health and even higher risk of death due to curable diseases among patients who live in poverty.

HIV/AIDS deepens poverty and increases inequalities at every level, household, community, regional and sectoral. The HIV/AIDS epidemic undermines efforts at poverty reduction, income and asset distribution, productivity and economic growth resulting in reverse progress of development targets. Certainly, there is relationship between poverty and the development of epidemics of communicable diseases and at the same time epidemic diseases, like any illness, have the potential to increase poverty.

The impact of HIV/AIDS and poverty on children has different dimensions that include children being deprived of education to care for sick adults, thus compromising their basic right to education, placing the household at further long-term risk for poverty that may take decades to reverse. Illiteracy and/or lack of skills also appear to influence vulnerability to HIV infection. A correlation between educational qualifications and HIV infection exists, which indicates that people with formal educational qualifications acquire economic independence and threfore do not engage in risky behaviors as compared to those without it.

Financial constrains or budgetary deficits in government expenditure on health in Tanzania, like most African countries translate into an increase in a number of untreated disease conditions, including sexually transmitted diseases that are known to facilitate the rapid transmission of HIV. HIV/AIDS appears to interact strongly with poverty and has increased the depth of vulnerability of the affected families/households because of being in needs (caring ill relatives, death and decreased manpower to seek for daily bread). The relation between poverty and HIV/AIDS is bidirectional. However, there is conceptual confusion about the nature of the relationship, probably because of lack of rigorous scientific researches on the links between poverty, HIV/AIDS and parasitosis.

There is strong evidence that socio-economic and gender inequalities exacerbate the spread of HIV while AIDS-related diseases and death increases these inequalities, a potentially vicious cycle. Poverty per se may not be the most important factor conditioning the risk of being exposed to HIV, but undoubtedly, it is the poor in these countries, and especially poor women, who are suffering the most with the subsequent impacts of AIDS. Given that malnutrition is a function of poverty, there is thus a good reason to assume that poverty helped to hasten the spread of HIV in sub-Saharan Africa.

However, when examining HIV vulnerability at the level of households and communities, the evidence appears to be mixed. Since the richer and better educated are likely to have better access to reproductive health care, condom use is generally low in Africa and other resources-limited countries. It is also postulated that poverty is placing individuals from poor households at greater risk of exposure to HIV through the economically-driven adoption of risky behaviors. Moreover, poverty and food insecurity (malnutrition) seem to increase sexual risk taking, particularly among women who may engage in transactional sex to procure food for themselves and their children.

Consequently, combating malnutrition, including worm infestation, requires more than providing treatment. It requires multisector approaches to address the broader causes such as poor water and sanitation provision and lack of food security. The approaches should also focus on HIV/AIDS control involving but not be limited to mainstreaming of HIV implications into the policy and practice of many sectors.

Although HIV prevalence has fallen in Tanzania over the past decade, thousands of people become infected with HIV every year and 86,000 Tanzanians died from AIDS in 2009 alone. While the poor are undoubtedly hit harder by the downstream impacts of AIDS, in a variety of ways, their chances of being exposed to HIV in the first place are not necessarily greater than wealthier individuals or households. Poverty, in a nutshell includes illiteracy, parasitosis/diseases, food insecurity plus HIV/AIDS are the major problem currently facing Tanzanians. Therefore, a joint effort is urgently required to combat them in their totality, with that approach, the victory is evident.

2. Poverty, parasitosis and HIV/AIDS

2.1 HIV/AIDS
2.1.1 A brief history and Trends of HIV and AIDS in Tanzania

The first cases of AIDS were reported in the Kagera region (north western of Tanzania) in 1983 and by 1987 every region in the country had reported AIDS cases. In 1985, the government set up the National AIDS Control Programme (NACP) to coordinate the response and established AIDS coordinators in each district in the country, Tanzania Commission for AIDS (TACAIDS). In order to confront the growing epidemic, the NACP developed a medium term plan for the period 1987-1991 which was then followed by two more medium term plans covering 1992-1996 and 1998-2002. These plans had three main aims: the decentralization of the health sector responses, reducing HIV transmission and relieving the social consequences of HIV/AIDS through care and assistance. However, according to Tanzania's first National Multisectoral Framework (2003-2007) the three medium term plans did not halt the spread of HIV. By the time the third medium term plan came into being HIV prevalence had reached 8 percent.

A national policy, which had been under development since 1991, was finalized in 2001, following the declaration of 'war' on HIV/AIDS by former His Excellency President Mkapa. TACAIDS was then established in 2002 to coordinate the multisectoral response, bringing together all stakeholders including government, business and civil societies to provide strategic guidance to HIV/AIDS programmes, projects and interventions.

A study published in 2005, using evidence drawn from the past 20 years exposed some findings which challenged some widely held assumptions about the effects of HIV and AIDS. The study found that generally the highest prevalence of HIV was found amongst the well off individuals/households, particularly affecting rich women, as opposed to poorer and rural households (Shelton et al., 2005). The findings pointed out that wealthier people tend to have the resources which lead to greater and more frequent mobility and expose them to wider sexual networks, encouraging multiple and concurrent relationships. But it was also observed that the wealthier people tend to have greater access to HIV medications that prolong their lives and are more likely to live in urban areas, which have the highest prevalence.

However, HIV prevalence gap between poor urban groups and poorer rural communities is slowly closing. A 2008 study found that knowledge of sexually transmitted infections (STI) was 'alarmingly low' in rural Tanzania and associated with low condom use and HIV infection. Reduced prevalence has mainly been noted among the most educated (those who attended secondary school) while among those with no formal education, prevalence has not decreased and the number of new infections has risen (Hargreaves et al., 2010). Because access to health care and knowledge of HIV and AIDS is typically lower in rural areas. This led to adoption of more aggressive measures towards educating the rural people on preventive efforts and thus further spread of the epidemic.

In a nut shell, some contextual factors shaping the HIV/AIDS epidemic in the country include:

- Poverty and transactional sex with increasing numbers of commercial sex workers
- Men's irresponsible sexual behaviour due to cultural patterns of virility
- Social, economic and political gender inequalities including violence against women
- Substance abuse such as alcohol consumption
- Local cultural practices e.g. widow cleansing
- Mobility in all its forms which leads to separation of spouses and increased establishment of temporary sexual relationships
- Lack of male circumcision

2.1.2 Immigration and rural-urban migration of people

HIV infection is unevenly distributed across geographic area, gender, age, groups and social economic classes in the country. The prevalence rates of HIV/AIDS range from less than 1%

to more than 15% in certain regions. Nevertheless, the epidemic has struck more the most economically active group of adults, those aged 15-45, which is also the productive age-group of individuals. Population movement is common in Tanzania, especially among the youths (18-45 years old). Growth and/or expansion of the mining sector and education have led to greater urbanization and mobility between rural and urban areas. This created an avenue for young and sexually active persons to interact socially and forming 'high risk sexual networks', which include sex workers, women at truck stops and miners, whom most of them are HIV seropositive.

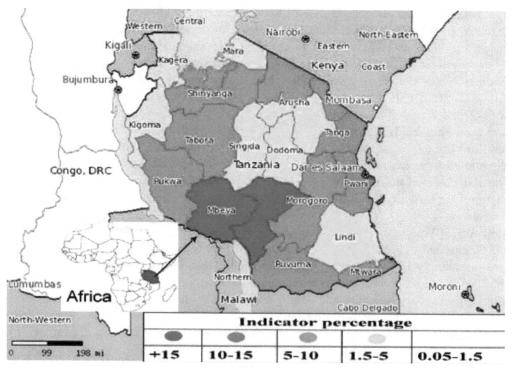

Fig. 1. Prevalence of HIV/AIDS among adults in Tanzania

Tanzania is also well known for its hospitality. Since the era of the Former President Late Mwalimu Nyerere, founder of the nation, our country has been hosting a myriad of refugees from all over the continent, who definitely had established close ties with citizens. This relationship could also have brought some "exogenous and detrimental effects".

2.1.3 Dependence on foreign aids on combating HIV infections and stigma

On the other hand, Tanzania's coastal trade as well as its border with eight countries exposes its vulnerable populations to HIV. In border and lake areas, 1 in 5 people are HIV positive. A study conducted by International Organization of Migration in 2010, revealed that transport workers, fishermen, border personnel, and seafarers were more likely to have multiple sexual partners and less likely to use condoms than the general population. Worse still, access to treatment and prevention initiatives in these areas was also minimal; underlining the regional variation in access to HIV services.

About only 8 years ago, the National Policy on HIV/AIDS recognized antiretroviral therapy as a right for all people living with HIV, at a time when no Tanzanians were receiving antiretroviral treatment. In 2003, the William J. Clinton Foundation and a group of Tanzanian experts created a Care and Treatment Plan (2003-2008), which was then adopted by the Tanzanian Government. The five-year plan proposed the roll out of antiretroviral therapy aiming at providing antiretroviral drugs free of charge to all people living with HIV by 2008. However, by 2004, only about 0.5% of those with advanced HIV were receiving treatment. Presumably, one of the major reasons is the Tanzanian HIV/AIDS response being heavily dependent on foreign funding sources. Because about 95% of the funding for HIV/AIDS programmes comes from foreign donors of whom more than two thirds is from the Global Fund and the U.S. President's Emergency Plan for AIDS Relief (PEPFAR). HIV/AIDS funding makes up one third of all aid coming to Tanzania.

Discrimination leads to an unwillingness to take an HIV test and to disclose results to family, friends or sexual partners. One study conducted in Dar es Salaam in 2005, found that only half of HIV positive respondents had disclosed their status to intimate partners. Time lapse from receiving results to disclosing them was 2.5 years for men and 4 years for women. Stigma, specifically fear of abandonment, job or property loss and violence were reasons for this delay. Contradictory perceptions exist among Tanzanians in respect of contracting STI, some believe that is a symbol of being sexually active and potent while other think it is ungodly and is a shame. However, when it comes to seeking for medical attentions, both groups find it uneasy. Such mixed notions ascribe to fear and hesitancy to disclose their status thus that increasing the chance of transmitting the STI, HIV inclusive to a partner, by avoidance of preventative measures and thus delay of timely of treatment (Mshana et al., 2006; Roura, 2009). In most regions/communities lack of knowledge about HIV/AIDS is a major cause of stigma and discrimination. Four out of ten women and a third of men surveyed in the 2007-2009 HIV and Malaria Indicator Survey reported that they would not buy fresh vegetables from a shopkeeper who has HIV, and half of all women and 40% of men said they would feel it necessary to keep it a secret if a family member was infected with HIV.

2.2 Poverty and HIV/AIDS
2.2.1 Economy overview
Tanzania is one of the world's poorest economies in terms of per capita income, however, Tanzania average 7% gross domestic product (GDP) growth per year between 2000 and 2010 on strong gold production and tourism. The economy depends heavily on agriculture, which accounts for more than one-fourth of GDP, provides 85% of exports, and employs about 60% of the work force. The World Bank, the IMF, and bilateral donors have provided funds to rehabilitate Tanzania's aging economic infrastructure, including rail and port infrastructure that are important trade links for inland countries.

"Hunger is the first obstacle to ending poverty. Hungry is poverty. A person who is always hungry is always poor. We can talk about the eradication of poverty all we want. We can never achieve it, if we don't first end hunger. The hungry live in rural areas and urban slums, in refugee camps and on farming homesteads. Wherever they are, hungry families live in the grey area between crisis and normality. Their poverty keeps them vulnerable to hunger. And hunger keeps them poor. Investments in infrastructure need to place more emphasis on ensuring that the assets truly are for the poor like community-based ponds, woodlots, roads and the like. Yet physical infrastructure alone cannot lead to less poverty or better food security. A bridge may make the local market half an hour away rather than half a day. But when you have no education, poor health, and no energy, all the opportunities the market holds are beyond your reach," Statement by the Executive Director World Food Programme.

Therefore, defining poverty is a great challenge to researchers because of its complex nature. Poverty is the state of having little or no money and few or no material possessions. Poverty can be caused by unemployment, low education, deprivation and homelessness. Lack of local health clinics and low-cost healthy foods, along with public space for physical activities, may be among the factors that contribute to poor health and even higher risk of death due to curable diseases among patients who live in poverty. East Africans are some of the poorest people in the world ranking in this order: Kenya-Uganda-Tanzania. Therefore, Tanzania being one of the poorest countries, her citizens face several socio-economic problems, especially for unemployed, elders and orphans. The World Bank defines poverty as "the inability to attain a minimum standard of living" and produced a "universal poverty line", which was "consumption-based" and comprised of two elements: "the expenditure necessary to buy a minimum standard of nutrition and other basic necessities and a further amount that varies from country to country, reflecting the cost of participating in everyday life of society. The World Bank uses this definition largely for inter-country comparisons, and is not necessarily depicting what happens in households.

Poverty is also about more than income and economics. There are many types of poverty:

- Service poverty, where people are unable to access or are not provided with services such as health and education;
- Resource poverty, where though they have sufficient incomes people are unable to access resources because they may be poor in terms of their rights, representation or governance.

However, for reasons of space and scope of this theme, we focus on types of poverty outlined above centering on income and social capital, which seem to apply in Tanzania.

2.2.2 Decomposition changes in poverty

Most of the tools used in the analysis of poverty can be similarly used for the analysis of inequality. One could draw a profile of inequality, which would look at the extent of inequality among certain groups of households. This informs on the 'homogeneity' of the various groups, an important element to take into account when designing interventions. Gini-coefficient of inequality: This is the most commonly used measure of inequality. The coefficient varies between 0, which reflects complete equality and 1, which indicates complete inequality (one person has all the income or consumption, all others have none). Using 1993 as a baseline for Tanzania, **Table 1** below shows how per capita growth rates and changes in inequality would translate into changes in poverty over a 20-year period. With a zero real per capita growth rate and no change of inequality, the poverty rate would

Poverty rate with	1993	2005	2015
0 % growth , no growth in Gini	50	50	50
1.5% growth, no change in Gini	50	35	18
1.5% growth, Gini reduction by 0.5%/year	50	30	3
3.0% growth, no change in Gini	50	25	5

Table 1. Poverty, Inequity, and Growth in Tanzania.

remain unchanged. A 1.5 percent sustained per capita growth rate with no change in the distribution of income (all household get a 1.5 percent income gain per year) would yield a substantial reduction in poverty. If inequality were to improve at the same time, the poverty reduction would be greatly accelerated, even with a similar growth level.

Equally, the impact of economic growth can be analyzed by various ways viz. by comparing inequality between different groups, by decomposing inequality to assess the major contributors to inequality, by analyzing inequality, growth and poverty and their relationship and finally, by decomposing changes in inequality over time as shown in **Table 1**.

Therefore, it is occasionally feasible to elucidate how much of the observed changes in poverty over time can be attributed to changes in distribution and to changes in mean income or consumption. For example, lower poverty could result either from a general increase in the income of all households (without change in the income distribution) or from a decrease in inequality (redistribution from the rich to the poor without change in mean income or consumption). A change in poverty can always be decomposed into a growth component, a redistribution component, and a 'residual' component. An example can be taken from rural Tanzania, which experienced a decrease in poverty but an increase in inequality. Decomposing changes in poverty incidence (headcount) and depth (poverty gap) reveals that while the poor benefited from growth over the period, the rich captured a much greater share of economic improvement. In fact, if the distribution of income hadn't changed, the reduction in poverty incidence would have been much larger and the poverty gap would have also decreased. **Table 2** below presents the results of the analysis and show that, using a high poverty line, the head count would have decreased by 38% and the poverty gap by 24%. The changes in distribution (and interaction factors) resulted in a decrease in the head count of only 14% and in the poverty gap of only 2%.

Poverty line	Growth component	Redistribution component	Residual	Total change in poverty
		Head count index		
High	-38.5	11.8	12.6	-14.1
Low	-34.4	16.7	5.7	-12.0
		Poverty gap index		
High	-23.7	20.5	1.6	-1.6
Low	-19.0	22.9	-1.9	2.0

Table 2. Decomposition in changes in Poverty in Rural Tanzania (1983-1991). Source (Ferreira, 1996)

Tanzania suffers widespread and severe poverty, with nearly 60% of the population living on less than $2 per day and an estimated 20% living on less than $1 per day. As a result, Tanzania is ranked 164th out of 177 countries in the U.N. Human Development Index. As it also suffers a heavy disease burden, Tanzania exemplifies the intimate link between poverty and health. Lacking funds and infrastructure lead to difficulties in accessing primary health care for more than two-thirds of the population, with 39.9% lacking the money needed for treatment and 37.6% unable to travel the necessary distance for treatment.

Consequently, HIV/AIDS may deepen poverty and exacerbates inequalities at every level, household, community, regional and sectoral. The epidemic undermines efforts at poverty reduction, income and asset distribution, productivity and economic growth. HIV/AIDS has reversed progress towards international development goals because of the influence it has on all development targets. There is an undoubted relationship between poverty and the development of epidemics of communicable diseases and at the same time epidemic diseases, like any illness, have the potential to increase poverty.

It has been suggested that illness and poverty affect household resources and income, as consequence of rising costs of medical care/treatment, and an increased need for nutritious foods. When adults/parents are stricken by HIV/AIDS or any other illness, with the progression of the illness, the demand for care also rises. Children are often withdrawn from schools to care for sick adults, compromising their basic right to education. The deprivation of education could place the household at further long-term risk for poverty, lack of skills and disempowerment. Consequently, this results in a cycle of household impoverishment that may take decades to reverse. Illiteracy and/or lack of skills also appear to influence vulnerability to HIV infection. One previous study in South Africa found that those with tertiary educational qualifications had lower rates of HIV infection than those with only school level qualifications. This implies that people with the necessary educational qualifications, thus acquiring economic independence for survival do not engage in risky behaviors than those with limited education.

Financial constrains or budgetary deficits in government expenditure on health in most African countries translate into an increase in a number of untreated STIs that are known to facilitate the rapid transmission of HIV. This could have serious long-term health implications resulting from the rapid spread of HIV. Apparently, HIV/AIDS appears to interact strongly with poverty and has increased the depth of vulnerability of those households already vulnerable to shocks. HIV/AIDS has acted to intensify the disadvantages imposed on the poor households and communities. HIV/AIDS leads to financial, resource and income impoverishment as households become poorer as a result of the illness and death of members, and in many cases it is the income-earning adults who are lost. Ultimately the high cost of care and burials leave heavy burden on the already overburdened households, orphans and dependants, people living with HIV/AIDS (PLHAs) and vulnerability to HIV infection (Ngalula et al., 2002). Therefore the 'poverty factor' at the household level has to be addressed simultaneously with the National efforts to combat the HIV/AIDS epidemic.

However, the impact is more than financial. Illness and death leads to an erosion of social capital and socially reproductive forces. In other words, the term social capital refers to the effort that goes into the reproduction of social and economic infrastructures. Therefore, at the social level, there are variety of relationships such as physical infrastructures, beliefs about trust, rituals of bargaining and price setting, mechanisms for regulating weights and measures, means of resolving disputes, and repeated activities which ensure that all these things continue to exist. These are not only matters of economic activity but also the maintenance and development of institutions, the reinforcement of community daily activities that also become negatively affected as consequence of the HIV/AIDS. Ultimately, the human capital loss has serious social and economic development in all sectors and at all levels. Hence, raising living standards of households and communities over the long-run through productivity-enhancing investments in agricultural technology generation and diffusion, improved crop marketing systems, basic education, infrastructure, and governance could improve their ability to withstand the social and economic stresses caused by HIV/AIDS.

It is now recognized that poverty significantly influences the spread and impact of HIV/AIDS. In many ways it creates vulnerability to HIV infection, causes rapid progression of the infection in the individual due to malnutrition and limits access to social and health care services. Poverty causes impoverishment as it leads to death of the economically active segments of the society and bread winners leading to reduction in income or production. Impacts of HIV/AIDS in most developing countries, Tanzania inclusive, have been visualized with poor resolution microscopes and thus studies of the effects of AIDS on households and most focus on economic impacts of death rather than illness. These show a distorted image. In Northern Tanzania (Kagera), a study conducted by the World Bank with Tanzanian co-investigators found that households stricken by deaths of their beloved ones especially adults, spent more on medical care and number of working time was significantly reduced. Similarly, it was revealed that even in well off families/households (for African standards) 29% of non-orphaned children were stunted while 50% of orphaned children were wasted. In poorer households 39% of non-orphaned children were stunted while 51% of orphaned children were wasted. These figures point to the effects on all children of growing up in a poor society.

Most African countries were performing poorly even before HIV/AIDS began to spread, largely due to their government's start-stop approach to economic reform. With the HIV/AIDS epidemic now at full force, these countries can only begin counteracting the effects of the epidemic if they undertake far more dramatic restructuring than they were prepared to previously. However, HIV/AIDS has worsened the situation as school-going age children born from HIV victimized families suffer both long-and short term consequences. Some of the effects are poor physical conditions, compromised immune systems and mental functioning is negatively affected by stunted growth, which is their long term effect. Hence, it may affect the ability of children to benefit from education and to function socially and economically later in their lives. Usually, orphans are unlikely to have proper schooling as the death of a parent or both parents in a family reduces a child's school attendance or just being unable to pay for schooling. This may automatically force the child to engage into "adults' duties". Sick adults may have reduced expectations of the returns to investing in children's education, as they do not expect to live long enough to recoup the investment. When a child goes to another household after its parents' deaths, the obstacles become greater as the child is not their own, particularly when even their own children are not guaranteed with all basic needs: food, clothing and school fees. These are some of the results of poverty (under-resourcing of public education) as consequence of the HIV/AIDS epidemic. AIDS increases teacher deaths and they may be difficult to replace, particularly in deprived, rural or otherwise remote communities. On the other hand, teachers' illness can lead to pupils being untaught for extended periods and replacement is difficult while staff members are on sick leave.

Therefore, the relationship between HIV/AIDS and poverty is synergistic and symmetrical. HIV/AIDS impacts households on two main levels, namely the social and economic levels. On a social level, households have to deal with issues around stigmatization, social exclusion and disintegration of family structure and social support networks. On the economic level, households and the surviving members have to pay for medical costs and funeral expenses and, if the deceased was a breadwinner, there will be further financial impacts in a form of a loss of income. Thus HIV/AIDS can directly contribute to poverty.

As much as HIV/AIDS exacerbates poverty through morbidity and mortality of productive adults, poverty facilitates the transmission of HIV. In developing countries, especially those in Sub-Saharan region, HIV/AIDS is reaching a stage at which AIDS morbidity and mortality are increasing rapidly (Dorrington et al., 2001). Once adults are sick and some are bedridden, then the young and elderly are forced to care for them. The situation can exert unbearable pressure on households in their struggle for survival. Poor households are usually the worst hit and more vulnerable to the long-term effects of HIV/AIDS and poverty. In some regions of Tanzania, more than half of hospital beds are occupied by patients with HIV/AIDS related conditions. The treatment costs related to these admissions may lead to further impoverishment especially at household level. Poverty is associated with vulnerability to severe diseases like HIV, through its effects on delaying access to health care and inhibiting treatment adherence. The costs incurred while seeking diagnosis and treatment for HIV/AIDS are common causes of delays in accessing health care especially for the poor. To a certain extent, this forces some families to seek medical attentions from traditional healers, due to their easy accessibility and affordability. Poor households may not necessarily have the financial resources to seek help from health facilities, nor food security to enable members to adhere to their treatment. The lack of these resources is significant cause of the delays in accessing health services by poor households. Food security here is concerned with physical and economic access to food of sufficient quality and quantity. Food security is necessary, but by itself insufficient, for ensuring nutrition security. Nutrition security is achieved for a household when secure access to food is coupled with a sanitary environment, adequate health services, and adequate care to ensure a healthy life for all household members.

Poverty limits the options for treating infectious diseases like HIV. Infection with other STI is an important co-factor of HIV, and it provides a point of entry for HIV. Poor households become even more vulnerable when unable to raise the necessary funds to pay for treatment as they largely depend on the state to provide these services. Women in Tanzania also have severely limited access to education, employment, credit, and transportation. As a result, northern coastal women — married and unmarried, young and old — are increasingly turning to sex work, exposing them to a high risk of HIV infection. "We accept that it is now the female burden to provide for our children," says a woman from Mkwaja village. "We risk dying from AIDS for the sake of our children". The true scope of HIV prevalence in the coastal region is not known because of low diagnostic and testing rates. (Fifty-eight percent of all Tanzanian adults living with HIV/AIDS are women). A barmaid with a 3-years old baby in Mbeya says " I do sell myself in order to safeguard my child/daughter and guarantee that she has something to eat. If I don't do that right now, for sure she will die in my arms. Then what is the point seeing my kid dying or me dying in the next ten or so years?". Mbeya is one the two badly HIV/AIDS stricken regions in the country with prevalence rate of 15-20%; another region is Iringa. Mbeya has boarders with Malawi and Zambia. This kind of despair and total lack of hope of improving wellbeing at household, drive this woman and several other into "problem".

Contradictory evidences exist with regard to HIV vulnerability at the level of households and communities (Wojciki 2005; Giraldo, 1997). Early studies had demonstrated positive correlations between household economic resources, education, and HIV infection, as the epidemic progressed; however currently, this relationship is somehow slightly changing. Generally, in Tanzania and most African countries, relatively rich and better educated men and women have higher rates of partner change because they have greater personal autonomy and spatial mobility. The richer and better educated are likely to have better access to reproductive health care, condom use is generally low in Africa and other parts of the developing world. At a later stage, however, it has been argued that individuals with higher socioeconomic status tend to adopt safer sexual practices, once the effects of AIDS-related morbidity and mortality become more apparent. It is also postulated that poverty (possibly itself fuelled by AIDS) is placing individuals from poor households at greater risk of exposure to HIV via the economically-driven adoption of risky behaviors. Poverty and food insecurity are thought to increase sexual risk taking, particularly among women who may engage in transactional sex to procure food for themselves and their children.

For that reason, HIV/AIDS mortality can change the demographic structure of the household, reverse the roles of the members, exacerbate poverty, rob children of their parents thereby creating more orphans, infringe on the basic rights of the child in areas such as education, food, nutrition, health and others. Unless households are strengthened and empowered through focused interventions, poor households are likely to fall deeper into poverty for the generations to come. For PLHA and poor, it will be harder for them to sustainably access antiretroviral therapy, since some may not afford transport costs, regardless that they may be willing to go for the ART. But also some may be unable to afford to buy nutritious food, which is actually part and parcel of ART. At the household level, poverty will worsen the impacts of other livelihood stresses and shocks, and close down options for effectively dealing with hardships and challenges of life.

Therefore, food security is an important element for the survival of any household across the spectrum of wealth. Households affected by HIV and poor may find it difficult to maintain their food security. Both HIV and poverty exert tremendous pressure on the household's ability to provide for the basic needs like food. Let alone that poor nutrition is often linked with adverse outcomes in HIV/AIDS. Poor nutritional status is linked to vulnerability to progression from HIV infection to mortality. Poor nutrition weakens the body's defense against infection, and infection in turn weakens the efficiency of absorption of nutrients. Micronutrient deficiencies undermine the body's natural defenses against infections, thus contributing further to the vulnerability to HIV infection. Households experiencing food shortages as a result of poverty and effects of HIV/AIDS increase the chances of fast progression of HIV infection to AIDS and inevitable death of the ill person. Given that malnutrition is a function of poverty, therefore there is a substantial reason to assume that poverty helped hasten the spread of HIV in sub-Saharan Africa.

2.3 Poverty, malnutrition and HIV/AIDS

The term malnutrition was previously regarded as synonymous with undernutrition. This was before the emergence of the nutrition transition. Nowadays, a broader and more comprehensive definition of malnutrition is necessary since in actual sense, the term refers to the entire spectrum of deviant nutritional status, from short stature and below normal weight. There is considerable information describing the nutrition situation in different parts of Tanzania, based on spot surveys, child growth monitoring systems or research work. Most of this information is not nationally representative and is focused more on children under-fives than other population groups. Only scanty serial national information is available making it possible to discern trends over time in only a few indicators and in specific areas of the country. Tanzania's main problems of nutrition are similar to those of other countries in Sub-Saharan Africa. They are related to undernourishment, and these are protein-energy-deficiency (PED), iron deficiency anaemia (IDA), iodine deficiency disorders (IDD) and vitamin A deficiency (VAD).

Apart from these deficiency disorders, there are two nutrient excess disorders represented by fluorosis in the northern and north-western and central parts of mainland; and the problem of overweight, obesity and diet-related non-communicable diseases which seem to be increasing especially in the urban elite and business sections of the community emulating unhealthy food habits and lifestyles. Compared to Sub-Saharan Africa; Tanzania is just slightly better than the average of 30% for underweight. For developing countries, excluding China, Tanzania is worse off for stunting but better off in wasting and underweight. Since the young population depends on a small adult population to sustain the economy and to provide the resources needed for adequate food, care and health; malnutrition in adults is of serious consequence. In such a situation, malnutrition becomes both a result and a cause of poverty. Malnourished adults cannot respond well to the challenges of economic and even political reforms which need both physical and mental energy. Maternal malnutrition is of even more severe consequence, as malnourished women produce malnourished children who will grow into malnourished adults creating a vicious cycle.

The nutritional status of adults is anthropometrically measured by using the Body Mass Index (BMI) which is a number derived from dividing the subject's weight in kilograms by the square of the height in meters (W/H^2). The distribution of Body Mass Index (BMI) in a few regions surprisingly show that more than a third of adults have low BMIs with rural areas having higher prevalence rates of undesirable BMIs than urban areas. Nonetheless, economic and historical analysis, epidemiological evidence, and common sense indicate that widespread childhood malnutrition will undermine investments in health, education, and ultimately economic development. Investments in cost effective treatments combined with broader nutrition based interventions must get higher priority.

Demographics, food supply and epidemiological transitions determine the specific relevance of the malnutrition-infection interaction in individual circumstances. Until the advent of the AIDS pandemic, average life-expectancies were rising in Tanzania and everywhere in the world; this was largely as a consequence of a reduction in early deaths from infectious childhood diseases. Today, HIV/AIDS is a world-wide calamity, though its impact is heavily felt in Africa. All of the poverty-related poor health and poor health care factors that go into increased susceptibility to HIV also affect the speed with which it progresses to full-blown AIDS and to death by opportunistic infections (Barnett et al. 2001). In particular, poverty-related lack of access to medical treatment, either to reduce viral load or to prevent and treat opportunistic infections, results in a lower quality of life, more rapid development of AIDS, and more rapid demise for poor PLHA. For example, people infected with HIV, who also have latent tuberculosis, are 30-50 times more likely to develop active TB. Similarly, ten percent of HIV infected persons develop cryptococcal meningitis, a fungal infection which leads inexorably to an extremely painful death within 30 days unless treated with powerful fungicides.

Proper nutrition is required to ensure optimal health. Consumption of a wide variety of foods, with adequate vitamins and minerals intake, is the basis of a healthy diet. Nutritionists outline that no single nutrient is the key to good health, but that optimum nutrition is derived from eating a diverse diet, including a variety of fruits and vegetables. Because foods such as fruits and vegetables provide many more nutrients than vitamin supplements, food is the best source for acquiring vitamins and minerals.

2.3.1 Nutrition, immune system and infection/parasitosis

Nutrition (also called nourishment or aliment) is the provision, to living cells, tissues and organisms, of the materials necessary (in the form of food) to support life. Many common health problems can be prevented or alleviated with a healthy diet. One of the most innovative researches in the past 40 years is the increased knowledge on how the immune system operates; from a point of view of cellular biology and humoral responses, which formed the so-called immunobiology that encompasses other field of studies like the nutritional community (Maclean and Lucas, 2008). Recognizing the magnitude of nutritional problem in the country, the government established the Tanzania food and nutrition centre (TFNC) that deal with nutrition-related issues. Some of the main responsibilities of TFNC are:

- Reduction of all forms of malnutrition to acceptable levels
- Effective coordination of nutrition activities in the country
- Promote nutrition of the socio-economical deprived and nutritionally vulnerable groups

Tanzania, like other developing countries, her citizens faces a huge problem of malnutrition (undernutrition and/or over-nutrition), and this could greatly contribute to progression of HIV to AIDS. Until recently, obesity (overweight) was regarded as symbol of wealth and being healthy by majority of Tanzanians. Obese individuals demanded respect among the societies. On the other hand, skinny or slim persons were regarded as underfed/nourished, synonymous with being poor (unable to feed oneself adequately. With advent of HIV/AIDS, skinny 'slim" individuals were thought to be infected by HIV, from which the word "slim" was derived. However, when the government launched ART, and both slim and overweight individuals enrolled in the therapy, this perception has drastically changed. Though, the extent of knowledge between the urban and rural living people could still significantly differ. This to some extent is a product of illiteracy among the population. To date, overweight/over nutrition is not a major health concern to majority of Tanzanians.

Notwithstanding, over nutrition may result into accumulation/deposit of unused/excess of nutrients: excess of carbohydrates into fatty acids and proteins being converted to fatty acids and then stored as lipids as well. This kind of nutrients accumulation has detrimental effects to the body. The quantity and nature of lipids are important factors in the process of immune system modulation. Several mechanisms have been involved in the modulation of the immune system by fatty acids:

- Membrane fluidity,
- Production of lipid peroxides,
- Eicosanoid synthesis and
- Effect on gene regulation.

Speculations exist that fatty acid immuno-modulation occurs not only singly, but also as a collective action of these factors.

A change in phospholipids' fatty acid compositions due to dietary lipid manipulation is ascribable to alterations in the membrane fluidity. Fatty acids from dietary lipids can be incorporated into any of the different phospholipids within the plasma membrane and they are clearly altered by the availability of dietary lipids. The changes in fatty acid composition of this structure have great importance because of the alteration of plasma membrane characteristics. This fact may be attributed to changes produced in the activity of proteins associated with the membrane, which act as receptors, form ion channels or are related to enzymatic functions (Liu et al., 2003). Therefore, the changes in the expression of surface proteins may be due to a vertical displacement of the membrane proteins by lipid action. While the expression of surface molecules such as adhesion and major histocompatibility molecules from human monocytes are inhibited by eicosapentaenoic acid. Instead, a significant increase in the expression of human lymphocyte antigen (HLA) is observed in monocytes incubated with docosahexaenoic acid (Maclean and Lucas, 2008).

Fatty acids play a major role in the production of eicosanoids, because they are key determinants of membrane-bound enzyme and receptor expression. The influence of fatty acids on gene expression is not well understood. Nevertheless, fatty acids released from membrane phospholipids are important second messengers or substitute for the classical second messengers, such as inositide phospholipid or adenoside monophosphate cyclic (AMPc) signal transduction pathways. These messengers act in a reversible manner at a precise intracellular location for a very short time in order to amplify, attenuate or deviate a signal in a direct or indirect (by conversion from arachidonic acid to eicosanoids) pathway (Riemersma et al. 1998).

The human body is greatly affected by nutritional status that in turn has been associated with alteration of the immune responses. Several dietary fatty acids or free fatty acids are involved in the modulation of the immune system through mechanisms that modify the immune response (Franchin et al., 2000). The immune parameters susceptible to modification by fatty acids supplied in the diet or free fatty acids added into cellular cultures are lymphocyte proliferation, cytokine production, activity of natural killer (NK) cells, phagocytosis, and expression of markers in the surface of the cells (Calder, 1995; Kelley et al., 1999; Roitt et al., 2001). The immune system modulation induced by fatty acids depends on several biological and methodological factors, such as the type and concentration of fatty acids, cell types, species of experimental animals, serum used in the *ex vivo* or *in vitro* cultures and so on (De Pablo and Alvarez de Cienfuegos, 2000).

Therefore, it seems that because of immunomodulation role associated with fatty acids, in future they may be applied to the amelioration and prevention of diseases characterized by an over-activation of the immune system, such as inflammatory or autoimmune disorders. In addition to these applications, unsaturated fatty acids may be used to reduce the susceptibility against bacterial infections due to the possibility of several lipids playing important roles in the efficient elimination of different micro-organisms or reducing host resistance against an infectious process due to the immunosuppression promoted by dietary unsaturated fatty acids. However, it should be noted that immunosuppression promoted by different dietary lipids has to be balanced, because this process may lead to an impairment of host response and increase the risk of infections.

2.3.2 Protein-energy- malnutrition

Protein-energy-malnutrition (PEM) also known as protein-energy deficiency (PED) is generally a nutritional problem that results from varying proportions of protein and calorie deficiency in infants and young children of developing countries (Nnakwe, 1995). It is a global public health problem, affecting children from African, Asian, Latin American and Caribbean regions (de Onis et al., 2000; Bisai et al., 2010). PEM is directly or indirectly responsible for about half of the 10.8 million deaths per year in under five children in developing countries. In Tanzania, it is estimated that 60% of deaths, among children under 5 years of ages, are associated with undernutrition (Villamor et al., 2005). The major risk factors that can predispose a child to having PEM include poverty, lack of access to quality food, cultural and religious food customs, poor maternal education, inadequate breast feeding, and lack of quality healthcare. In addition to macronutrient deficiency, there is clinical and/or sub-clinical deficiency of micronutrients (Jahoor et al., 2008).

Recent researches show that HIV prevalence is highly correlated with falling calorie consumption, falling protein consumption, unequal distribution of income (inequity) and other variables conventionally associated with susceptibility to infectious disease, however transmitted. "The causal chain runs from macro-factors that result in poverty: through the community, the household, the individual and into the resilience of the individual's immune system. Work in cell biology has shown the mechanisms which connect malnutrition and parasite infestation; depressing both specific and non-specific immune responses by weakening epithelial integrity and the effectiveness of cells in the immune system. PEM, IDA, VAD, all of these poverty related conditions decrease resistance to disease in general and to HIV in particular.

Trace elements are required by human body for proper functioning but unlike most vitamins and minerals that our body needs, trace elements are needed only in extremely low quantities. The human body needs about 72 trace elements for normal functioning. There are seven essential trace elements described in human body chromium, copper, cobalt, iodine, selenium and zinc. Iron is an important dietary mineral and involves in various body functions. In humans, iron is an essential component of proteins involved in oxygen transport. It is also essential for the regulation of cell growth and differentiation. Iron is main component of hemoglobin a protein molecule that carries oxygen and plays critical role to the whole respiration process of the total iron in the body 60-70% is stored in hemoglobin. The body contains between 3.5 and 4.5% of iron 2/3 of which is present in hemoglobin (Pradeep et al., 2010).

The ubiquitous iron is an essential nutrient for most tissue cells and deficiency brings about recognizable deleterious results affecting many organs. The lymphoid apparatus is no exception. Iron deficiency with or without anemia is associated with partial atrophy of various lymphoid organs and alteration in many molecular and cellular immune functions. Iron and its binding protein have immunoregulatory properties and shifting of immunoregulatory balances by iron excess or deficiency may produce severe deleterious physiological effects. People with low levels of iron tend to have low resistance to infections. Anemia in HIV infected patients can have serious implication which varies from functional and quality of life decrement to an association with decreased progression and decreased survival. The prevalence of anaemia in HIV disease varies considerably ranging from 1.3-95%. Anaemia is more prevalent in HIV positive women, children and injected drug users. Human with advance HIV infection present some evidence of iron accumulation, which is manifested with an increased ferritin concentration (Pradeep et al., 2010).

Moreover, trace metal overload suppress immune function and increase the morbidity and mortality. If the iron overload becomes severe (usually when the amount of iron in the body exceeds 15 g) the condition is diagnosed as hemochromatosis. This is an inherited blood disorder that causes the blood to retain excessive amount of iron, which lead to serious health consequences such as cirrhosis of the liver (Bullen *et al.*, 1991). Irons stored in the body become depleted and hemoglobin synthesis is inhibited. Iron is central to physiology in general and required for particular steps of the HIV replication life-cycle in cells.

HIV infection has therefore been associated with disturbances in host iron metabolism. Advanced HIV/AIDS disease condition, anemia can coincide with increase ferritin and bone marrow iron content and the anemia is commonly unresponsive to iron supplementation (Strauss, 2004). Increased bone marrow iron is associated with shortened survival and increased opportunistic infections. Iron could be playing an important role in the interaction between host and virus. Host homeostasis adapt during deficiency, overload and infection to balance requirement against toxicity and availability to potential pathogens. Knowledge of these interactions is necessary to predict morbidity response to disturbance in host iron homeostasis (Pradeep et al., 2010). Because the progression of HIV infection towards its more advance stages is accompanied by increasing body iron stores there is urgent need for careful clinical studies to clarify the role of iron status on the course of HIV infection. Proper iron supplementation may provide sufficient iron to restore normal storage levels of iron and to replenish hemoglobin deficits thereby increase the survival of HIV sero-positives.

Nowadays it is well recognized that all infections have an adverse effect on nutritional status. However, the clinical and public health significance of the effect of a single infectious episode depends on the prior nutritional state of the individual. Recently, a clear synergistic relationship between nutrition and infection has been elucidated and thus most public health interventions for prevent infection focus on correction of malnutrition. With the ever increasing resistance of important pathogenic microorganisms to available chemotherapeutic agents, this area of study calls for further researches (Strauss, 2004; Villamor et al., 2005; Jahoor et al., 2008).

2.3.3 Impact of poverty on environment

The fact that HIV/AIDS affects people in their productive ages between ages 25 and 45 years, the poverty that the epidemic precipitates can have deleterious impacts on agricultural productivity and natural resources. These impacts can hit particularly hard in a country like Tanzania, where livelihoods are highly dependent on agriculture, mining and fishing. As men and women die or become too ill to work, family members are forced to find new ways to provide for their families. The loss of income from a male head-of-household puts additional burdens on his wife and children to find alternative sources of income, which can ultimately lead to more intense and less-sustainable resource use and extraction. Some regions in northern coastal Tanzania, such alternative practices often include unsustainable harvesting of forests and forest products such as wild foods and medicinal plants, which are then sold at local markets. Increased woodcutting to produce charcoal for sale is also common, especially when families face severe food shortages and must secure cash quickly to buy food. And the use of small-mesh nets for both marine and freshwater fishing has increased as widowed women and their children try desperately to make a living from declining shallow-water fish stocks.

Therefore, poverty and food insecurity increase sexual risk taking, particularly among women who may engage in transactional sex to procure food for themselves and their children. Women's economic dependence on their partners may also make it difficult for them to insist on safer sex like condom use. Several ethnographic studies have suggested that material poverty has increased the incidence of transactional sex. To some extent, this indicates that while the poor are undoubtedly hit harder by the downstream impacts of AIDS, in a variety of ways, their chances of being exposed to HIV in the first place are not necessarily greater than wealthier individuals or households. This brings a different school of thought that possibly poverty itself fuelled by AIDS, is placing individuals from poor households at greater risk of exposure to HIV via the economically-driven adoption of risky behaviors.

In Tanzania there are substantial urban-rural, regional and socio-economic divergences, which have driven youths to migrate to urban areas looking for jobs (better living) and some engaging themselves into risky activities like unsafe sex, prostitution and drug abuse just to mention a few. On the other hand, rural poor children are more likely than their urban counterparts to die, and when they survive, they are more likely to be malnourished as depicted in poverty and human development report (PHDR, 2005).

2.4 Parasitosis and HIV/AIDS

Since the first HIV/AIDS cases were described, a high prevalence of gastrointestinal alterations has been reported, especially diarrhea associated with parasitosis. This became more evident when the appearance of a syndrome named "Slim Disease", characterized by an intense weight loss accompanied by chronic diarrhea, prolonged fever and diffuse muscle weakness, was observed in Africa, especially in Uganda. However, the site and timing of the first reported cases suggest that the disease arose in Tanzania. Studies conducted in Tanzania, Uganda and other African countries have shown prevalence of 60 to 80% of parasitic organisms attributing to "Slim Disease", such as *Isospora spp., Cryptosporidium spp., Salmonella spp., Shigella spp.* and *Campylobacter* species, amounting to a prevalence of 60 to 80% (Tarimo et al., 1996; Brink et al., 2002). "Slim Disease" has been observed in advanced stages of HIV infection (Mhiri et al., 192). The expression "Wasting Syndrome" was adopted in substitution by WHO in 1987 on the basis of criteria laid down by the (Center for Disease Control [CDC, 1987]).

Opportunistic infections caused by intestinal parasites vary according to the geographical area and the endemic levels in each location. The progressive decline of immunological and mucous defense mechanisms predisposes patients to early, intermediary and late gastrointestinal manifestations of HIV infection. At later stages of the disease, the alterations in non-specific defense mechanisms in the production of immunoglobulin A and the reduction in local immune cell response also progress, thus increasing the susceptibility to a number of intestinal opportunistic pathogens, among which *Cryptosporidium parvum, Isospora belli* and Microsporidia species are the most prominent (Akinbo et al., 2010).

After the emergence of AIDS, these parasites, until then known solely in veterinary medicine, were no longer considered as commensal organisms and are nowadays recognized as opportunistic pathogens common to these patients. Infections by these agents constitute a major secondary aggravating factor of the disease, often responsible for worsening the general health conditions, due to manifestations of diarrhea which are difficult to control, sometimes resulting in the death of the patient. Thus, where as infections in the gastrointestinal tract play a critical role in AIDS pathogenesis and diarrheic diseases assume a prominent role, reaching a rate of up to 50% in developed countries, in developing countries there have been reports of incidence of up to 95%, as in Haiti and the African continent. Amongst the causes of diarrhea in developing countries, those of a parasitic origin are prominent in patients with HIV/AIDS (Akinbo et al., 2010).

The immune system can simplistically be divided into two components, namely, nonspecific immunity (skin, other mucosal barriers and soluble factors) and the adaptive immune system, which involve recognition of pathogens and subsequent production of antibodies as well as cell-mediated defense. The immune system is being challenged by the worldwide increment in immunological stressor agents of chemical, physical, biological, mental, and nutritional origin. However, the diversity and intensity of these risks or etiologic factors for HIV/AIDS vary from person to person, from group at risk to group at risk, from country to country, and from continent to continent. This is the principal reason why the frequency of AIDS is not homogeneous in all places and countries (Giraldo, 1998; Roitt et al., 2001).

The capabilities and possibilities of the immune system are neither infallible nor infinite. HIV/AIDS is the maximum state of deterioration that the human immune system can reach as result of HIV-infection. If the pathogenic process of AIDS is not stopped, eventually it will kill the person (Roitt et al., 2001). While the most important risk factor for HIV/AIDS in developed countries is the new epidemic of drugs abuse. The most important risk factor for

HIV/AIDS in underdeveloped countries is poverty, with all its consequences: malnutrition, unsanitary conditions, infections, parasites, and lack of hope for a better life, all of which have reached unprecedented high levels in the last few decades (Giraldo, 1998). Any component of the immune system can be functionally or genetically abnormal as a result of acquired, for instance through HIV infection, lymphomas, frequent use of high-dose steroids or other immune-suppressive medications) or congenital illnesses, with more than 120 congenital immunodeficiencies described to date that either affect humoral immunity or compromise T-cell function. Immunosuppression may also occur in malnourished persons, patients undergoing chemotherapy for malignancy, and those receiving immunosuppressive therapy. However, for parasitic infections, cell-mediated (T-cell) abnormalities predominate. Such persons tend to be susceptible to common pathogens with delayed clearance. With profound cell-mediated defects, reactivation of previously controlled pathogens may occur. Moreover, such individuals are at risk of infection by opportunistic "nonpathogenic" parasites (Cunningham and Fujinami, 2000). Nevertheless, with reconstitution of the cell-mediated immunity, the risk of parasitic infections reverts to that for a normal host.

The mechanisms, by which malnutrition, tuberculosis, STI, malaria, trypanosomiasis, schystosomiasis, leishmaniasis, systemic mycosis, as well as other infections and parasites weaken, destroy, and collapse the immune system will be briefly elucidated. These mechanisms should well understood for any attempt to design more effective interventions on the current occurrence of the HIV/AIDS epidemic in the poorest areas of the underdeveloped countries, where the poor have never before been so poor and so sick as they are now. Moreover, these poor countries, the levels of malnutrition, microbial and parasitic infections have reached very alarming levels (Cates, 1988).

Therefore, poverty, parasitosis and HIV/AIDS seem to be closely interlinked and co-circulate in many populations, particularly in underdeveloped countries. HIV/AIDS, parasitic infections like malaria and other opportunistic infections, and in a few are by far the commonest causes of ill-health and death in Tanzania and other poor countries of the world. Most of these countries happen to be in the tropics and temperate countries in Africa, Asia, and South America. Currently, parasitic infections are major health concerns attributed to high morbidity and mortality in developing countries especially among HIV-infected persons. Children aged 2 to 5 years are most at risk of severe morbidity (Chopra et al., 2006). Programs to prevent HIV transmission are unlikely to succeed unless they address the underlying causes of its spread. HIV prevention must be based on scientific evidence regarding cofactor conditions, not, as they currently are, on unproven assumptions about the primacy of behavioral factors. In addition to food security, deworming, schistosomiasis prevention and treatment, and malaria control programs should thus be integrated as critical components of a broad-based approach to HIV prevention.

2.4.1 Protozoan infections and HIV/AIDS

Malaria is caused by an intracellular protozoan transmitted via the bite of an infected female *Anopheles* mosquito. Malaria is not an opportunistic infection for HIV-infected people, but the effect of HIV infection on the natural history of malaria has not been completely defined. HIV infection and malaria coexist in regions where the health surveillance systems are poorly performing so that the magnitude of any interaction is difficult to determine. Nevertheless, the evidence of such interaction has recently grown and is still increasing (Nkuo-Akenji et al., 2008). The incidence of symptomatic malaria episodes, severe or uncomplicated, and the corresponding parasite density is higher in HIV infected individuals with low CD4 count (Atzori et al., 1993; Sherman, 1998).

In Tanzania, malaria is the major killer of children under 5 years of age. Prevalence rates of malaria among children between 6-59 months old vary according to geographic positions and socio-economic activities in a particular area. The highest rate has been observed around Lake Zone regions, Kagera region taking a lead with prevalence of 41.1% followed by Lindi (35.5%) while Zanzibar and Arusha have lowest rates of 0.8% and 0.4% respectively. Malaria is the cause of more mortality and morbidity in Tanzania than any other disease, in large part due to growing resistance to antimalarial drugs. It is estimated that over 1% of GDP is devoted to the disease, representing US$2.2 per capita, and 39% of total health expenditure nationally. Government facilities devote almost one-third of their resources to the disease.

Due to poor living conditions, the majority of Tanzanians suffer from malaria -a preventable disease that can have a serious negative impact on pregnant women and young children. Mothers who contract malaria during pregnancy run the risk of having low birth weight babies, maternal anemia, impaired fetal growth, spontaneous abortions, stillbirths, and premature babies. Recently, the country introduced an anti malaria campaign " Malaria Haikubaliki" a Swahili slogan that means "Malaria is unacceptable" - which involves all sectors of the society including entertainment, business, sport and religion sectors in the battle against malaria across the country. "Africans think that malaria is inevitable; that there is nothing they can do about it. We are going to prove this wrong. We can eliminate malaria deaths," said the Minister for Health and Social Welfare, Prof. David Mwakyusa. This initiative is of paramount importance because of the presumed potential interaction between malaria and HIV/AIDS.

Researchers have demonstrated a potential role for the dual infection in fueling the spread of HIV/AIDS and malaria in endemic regions (Whitworth et al., 2000; Abu-Raddad et al., 2006; Nkuo-Akenji et al., 2008). Besides a direct effect, HIV infection may indirectly influence the malaria burden by increasing the malaria parasite biomass and consequently the probability of drug resistant parasites emerging. Antimalarial drug resistance, particularly for *Plasmodium falciparum*, is considered a major contributor to the global resurgence of malaria observed over the last three decades and one of the greatest obstacles for an effective malaria control (Marsh, 1998). The basis of resistance lies in one or several genetic mutations in the parasite genome. Malaria parasites with such mutations when in contact with a given drug survive the treatment and eventually spread (Van Geertruyden et al., 2008). Evidences collected from four longitudinal population-based studies in rural Uganda and Malawi, where malaria is highly endemic showed odds ratios of symptomatic malaria in HIV infected compared to uninfected adults of 6.0, 3.4 and 1.2 for CD4 counts <200/µl, 200–499/µl and $\geq$ 500/µl, respectively, in Uganda (Whitworth et al., 2000). In Malawi, incidence rates of symptomatic malaria in HIV-1 infected adults varied with CD 4 count; compared to individuals with CD4 count of $\geq$ 500, the malaria incidence was 3 fold higher with a CD4 count of 200–499/µL and a 4.4-fold higher with a CD4 count<200/µL (Borkow et al., 2001; Graham et al., 2006).

Additionally, it is purported that HIV infection contributes to the emergence and spread of antimalarial drugs resistance by increasing drug exposure and drug pressure. HIV infection increases the probability of a malaria infection progressing to symptomatic illness and to a higher parasite density, increasing the probabilities of treatment and contact between the parasites and the drug (Nkuo-Akenji et al., 2008). This can be explained by the fact that,

HIV-infected patients with already low immunity suffer frequently of non-malaria-attributable acute fevers that may be misdiagnosed as malaria and treated with antimalarials. This phenomenon can justify the observed increase in the parasite biomass in HIV symptomatic patients and asymptomatic carriers alike. Besides contributing to the emergence and spread of antimalarials drug resistance, HIV infection may influence and modify its expected geographical pattern as consequence of and influence of various malaria control intervention by exposing large number of Plasmodium parasites to antimalarials. A way out for this is an easy access, prompt diagnosis and appropriate combination therapy that can alleviate or halt the emergence and spread of antimalarial drug resistance (Van Geertruyden et al., 2008).

A study conducted in a rural area of Malenga Makali (Tanzania) involving 300 sexually-active adults selected at random among patients, who were attending a dispensary because of diarrhoea of at least 2 weeks' duration, revealed potential associations between the patient's health (in terms of the WHO's clinical definition of AIDS), HIV-1 seroprevalence and malaria and other parasitic infections. Although malaria infection was more common in HIV-1 seropositives than in the seronegatives, the intensity of the *Plasmodium falciparum* infections, intestinal amoebiasis and giardiasis did not appear to be correlated with HIV infection. In contrast, intestinal infections with *Cryptosporidium parvum* and *Isospora belli* were virtually restricted to HIV seropositive individuals who had had diarrhoea for a relatively long time (Atzori et al., 1993). Similarly, it was noticed that maternal weight and low CD8+ cell counts were inversely associated with low body weight (LBW). While advanced-stage HIV disease, previous history of preterm birth, *Plasmodium falciparum* malaria, and any helmintic infection are associated with higher risk of LBW (Dreyfusset al., 2001). The intestinal parasites *Entamoeba histolytica* and *Strongyloides stercoralis* seemed to be predictors of LBW despite their low prevalence in the cohort. Moreover, the newborns' body mass index, midupper arm circumference, CD4 cell count <200 x 10^6 cells/L (200 cells/mm^3), primiparity, maternal literacy, and infant HIV infection at birth are significantly associated with birth weight in addition to risk factors associated with the LBW.

Cryptosporidiasis in AIDS patients usually causes chronic, bulky and intermittent diarrhea, with liquid non-bloody stools, accompanied by pain and abdominal colic, and a noticeable loss of weight can be observed. Asymptomatic cases are rarely described, occurring mostly in developing countries, Tanzania inclusive with patients showing milder. Cryptosporidium spp are common opportunistic parasites that cause chronic diarrhoea and wasting in HIV/AIDS patients with CD4+ T-cell counts <100 cells/µL and antimicrobial agents have limited efficacy in preventing or eradicating infections with it. Although studies assessing reduction in the incidence of cryptosporidiosis are lacking, diarrhoea due to cryptosporidia are known to resolve spontaneously with immune restoration among HIV/AIDS patients on antiretroviral therapy. Extra-intestinal manifestations have been clearly described in the literature, especially in the gall bladder, biliary ducts and pancreas, leading to conditions such as papillary stenosis, sclerosing cholangitis and calculous cholecystitis as well as chronic bronchitis (McGowan et al., 1997).

Isospora belli is a coccidian parasite that has a global distribution limited to mainly tropical regions in developing countries where it is endemic (especially Africa, the Middle East, and South America). The parasite invades the intestinal epithelium, where it completes its life cycle in the cytoplasm of the enterocyst. Unsporulated oocysts are excreted in feces and mature outside the host, where they develop into infective sporulated oocysts. Infection is then acquired through ingestion of these infective oocysts. Immunodeficiency was shown to increase the susceptibility to infection with *Isospora belli*, which accounted for up to 20% of cases of diarrhea in HV/AIDS patients. The lower prevalence of isosporiasis may be ascribed to the secondary prophylaxis for pneumocystosis through administration of sulfamethoxazole-trimethoprim during the course of HV/AIDS, since *Isospora belli* is sensitive to this chemotherapeutic agent.

The diarrheic condition is also noteworthy and is accompanied by fever, intestinal colic, anorexia, abdominal pain, loss of weight and peripheral eosinophilia. Isosporiasis can also show extraintestinal dissemination features, affecting the mesenteric, periaortic, mediastinal and tracheobronchial lymph nodes. It may also be related to biliary disease, causing manifestations of acalculous cholecystitis. Despite this high prevalence, classical protozoa such as *Giardia lamblia* and *Entamoeba histolytica* are less frequent as causes of severe illnesses in HIV-infected patients, when compared with *Isospora belli*and *Cryptosporidium parvum* and they are not considered as opportunistic infections in HV/AIDS. Amebiasis may present with invasive characteristics, but this has rarely been reported in the literature (Angarano et al., 1997).

Parasite infections especially malaria, and intestinal parasites undermine the nutritional status and compromise the immune system yet further, effectively exhausting it. These parasite infections are endemic in Tanzania, but the situation is made worse by inadequate health care and infrastructure, which actually by itself a function of poverty and low levels of development that leaves most parasite infections untreated.

2.4.2 Intestinal helminthic infections and HIV/AIDS

Neglected tropical diseases (NTDs) are a devastating burden for the people of Tanzania and are prevalent throughout the country. The country is endemic with all seven of the most common NTDs: schistosomiasis, lymphatic filariasis, onchocerciasis, trachoma, and the soil-transmitted helminths (hookworm, ascariasis, and trichuriasis). Such high prevalence rates of multiple NTDs increase the risk for co-infection with two or more diseases, a phenomenon that leads to more severe health consequences (Bundy et al., 2000; Luong et al., 2003).

Intestinal helminths are ubiquitous in low-income countries with prevalence of, for example 50–80% for ascariasis, trichuriasis and hookworm infections in many populations. Intestinal helminths induce immunological alterations that favor the progression from HIV seroconversion to AIDS. After HIV has spread to the systemic circulation its replication is limited by the fact that usually few activated lymphocytes and differentiated macrophages are present in the blood stream and that resting T cells and undifferentiated monocytes are not susceptible to HIV infection. However, in patients infected with intestinal helminths the number of activated T cells expressing human leucocyte antigen (HLA)-DR and HIV coreceptors is elevated. This is followed by HIV replication, preferentially in T-helper cells (Th cells) of Th2 and Th0 type clones. While Th2 cells are usually abundant in individuals infected with helminthes. Similarly, peripheral blood mononuclear cells of patients with helminthic infection are significantly more susceptible to infection with HIV than those of uninfected controls. Finally, elevated IL-4 levels, characteristic of the Th2 type of immune response in helminthic infections, down-regulate Th1 differentiation and function.

Therefore, parasitic infection could be a primary contributing factor to HIV/AIDS in Africa where men and women alike are at risk. Parasites are also endemic in people who are also at higher risk for HIV/AIDS, and most of these countries are underdevelopment/third world.

Activation of T cells, macrophages and other antigen presenting cells is necessary for HIV replication. This fact alone, may explain why lymphotropic and monocyte-tropic viruses originated in parasite endemic regions where suitable hosts reside. Indeed, Human T-lymphotropic virus-1 (TLV-1), HIV and Epstein-Barr virus (EBV). These are lymphotropic viruses that are found in close geographical relationship with parasite endemic regions. Women, especially in these developing countries of the world, are also prone to harbor chronic vaginal infections such as trichomoniasis, or have other predisposing vaginal factors for HIV/AIDS.

Among the helminthes in association with AIDS, there is no doubt that the most important pathogen is *Strongyloides stercoralis*, which is geohelminth presents its major effects in immunodepressed patients, leading to the dissemination of the infection. This occurs in transplanted patients, individuals presenting malnutrition and patients submitted to prolonged use of corticosteroids, suffering from leukemia, lymphomas or AIDS (Cimerman et al., 1998). In immunosuppressed patients, self-infestation is speeded up and a large number of larvae are released, causing the dissemination of the infection. Nevertheless, data from a single source published in 2010; show that in Tanzania the prevalence of helminthic infections in HIV-positive patients is around 8.2%, in comparison with 15.8% in non-HIV infected population (Mwambete et al., 2010). Hookworm (*Ancylostoma duodenale* and *Necator americanus*) infections being the most prevalent among HIV patients (17.1%) followed by *S. stercoralis* (3.3%). Although, there was no significant difference in respect of prevalence rates of helminthic infections between HIV-infected and non-infected patients; the study revealed direct correlation between CD4+ counts (HIV status) with helminthic infections among the HIV-infected patients. Nevertheless, helminthic infections are a grave health problem in Tanzania particularly among children from poor households as indicated in the Table 3 below (Mwambete and Kalison, 2006).

CD+4 counts	Helminthiasis (%)				
	Trichuris	Hookworm	Ascaris	None	Total
< 100	5(1.4)	2(0.6)	2(0.5)	14(3.8)	**23(6.4)**
101 - 200	50(13.7)	31(8.5)	35(9.6)	125(34.3)	**241(66.2)**
201 - 400	21(5.8)	6(1.6)	8(2.2)	31(8.5)	**66(18.2)**
401 - 500	7(1.9)	0(0.0)	1(0.3)	13(3.6)	**21(5.8)**
501 - 600	2(0.5)	0(0.0)	0(0.0)	4(1.1)	**6(1.6)**
601- 700	1(0.3)	0(0.0)	0(0.0)	6(1.6)	**7(1.9)**
Total	86(23.6)	39(10.7)	46(12.6)	193(53.0)	364

Table 3. Prevalence of helminthiasis in relation to HIV/AIDS status (CD+4 counts)

The other most common helminthes in Tanzania include *Ascaris lumbricoides*, *Trichuris trichura*, *Enterobius vermicularis* just naming a few. These are ubiquitous parasites in tropical and subtropical areas associated with causing diarrhea and hyperinfection syndrome in individuals with immunosuppressive disorders, including HIV/AIDS. Unfortunately, there are scant data or unavailable at all that relate and indicate the magnitude of the problem of parasitic infections among HIV-infected patients. A study conducted in rural Tanzania in 1995, revealed the prevalence rate of 81.8% (n= 287) of intestinal parasites in HIV-negative than in HIV-positive patients. The prevalence of *Ascaris lumbricoides* was higher in HIV-negative than in HIV-positive patients (p < 0.01; p < 0.04) (10.5% and 3.7% for *A. lumbricoides*). On the other hand, *Strongyloides stercoralis* prevalence was higher in HIV-positive than in HIV-negative patients (P < 0.01).

Schistosomiasis is another systemic helminthic infection, which is the second most prevalent tropical disease after malaria and affects approximately 200 million people in Africa, Asia, South America and other temperate regions. Severity of the infection largely depends on the intensity of infection, the *Schistosome* species involved, the topographic site affected by sequestered eggs and the immune responsiveness of the host. Urinary schistosomiasis is more prevalent in school-aged children than in adults. A prevalence of 57.9% was revealed in a study conducted in Kilosa (a semi-arid central district in Tanzania) among school–age children, which somehow is an indication of probably having even higher prevalence in lake areas (Mkopi et al., 2005; Clement et al., 2006).

In women, genital schistosomiasis occurs in about 60% of individuals infected with *Schistosoma haematobium*. Genital manifestations involve the vulva, vagina and the cervix as well as upper genital organs and result in pathology similar to that observed in some STIs. The cervix is the site predominantly affected, followed by the vagina and vulva. Thinning, erosion and ulceration of the epithelium is a typical clinical finding of genital schistosomiasis (Kjetland et al., 1996). This is important, as breaks in the integrity of the mucosal barrier, due to either trauma or sexually transmitted genital ulcer diseases are associated with an increased risk of HIV transmission (Mabey 2000).

Likewise, Schistosome eggs stimulate a complex array of cellular and humoral immune responses. Inflammations/granulomata form around eggs with a radius 5–10 times larger than the size of the egg. These granulomata are composed among others of activated lymphocytes, macrophages and epitheloid cells as well as some Lagerhan's giant cells, cell types known to express the CD4+ T cell receptor. In the wall of the bladder a considerable proportion of these granulomata ulcerate into the lumen. Similarly, in genital schistosomiasis egg-induced ulcerative lesions could be the port of entry for HIV. In the cervix, peri-oval granulomata are frequently formed near the basal layer of the epithelium. Within the egg granulomata, and also in adjacent areas, T cells, macrophages and Lagerhans cells abound (Helling-Giese et al., 1996). In mice, CD4+ T cells amount to 8–10% of all granuloma cells. The abundance of CD4 receptor-bearing cells within the confines of the granulomata and in adjacent areas make a rapid binding of virus after penetration through the friable and eroded epithelium of the cervix very likely. Therefore, genital schistosomiasis in males also points at an increased risk of HIV transmission. *Schistosoma haematobium* infection in males induces a chronic inflammation in the pelvic genitals, which looks like bacterial urethritis, accompanied with an increased viral shedding in the semen in HIV co-infected individuals.

Dar es Salaam, which is the largest commercial city, has an extensive drain network, mostly with inadequate water flow, making *Anopheles* and *Culex* larvae common. However, the importance of drains as larval habitats was previously unknown. The researchers analyzed detailed surveys of both mosquito habitats and drain conditions in the city; their findings suggest that simple but well-organized environmental management interventions, aimed to restore and maintain the functionality of drains, may help reduce mosquito-borne disease transmission. Lymphatic filariasis (LF) is a leading cause of disability due to parasitic infections in Tanzania. As of 2004, all districts were endemic with the disease, and prevalence rates reached up to 45%. Onchocerciasis (river blindness) has been documented in five regions and 15 districts throughout Tanzania, with an estimated 4 million people at risk for infection overall. In certain focal endemic areas, prevalence rates reach up to 64%.

Lymphatic filariasis is widely distributed in the tropics. It particularly occurs in areas with a high HIV prevalence such as sub-Saharan Africa and south-east Asia. There is no data available to show an impact of HIV infection on the prevalence or on the natural history of the disease. However, lymphatic filariasis is an example for a harmful interaction in the other direction. Replicative capacity of HIV is significantly enhanced in peripheral blood mononuclear cells from patients with untreated lymphatic filariasis. Consequently, untreated patients with lymphatic filariasis and co-infected with HIV could be at risk for rapid progression to AIDS once infected with HIV. Furthermore, the chronic manifestations of filariasis can have significant, and often very negative, social impacts. The chronic disabling manifestations of this disease, including lymphoedema of the limbs, breasts and external genitalia, have a profoundly detrimental effect on the quality of life of affected individuals.

The degree of social disability varies between cultural settings, but the degree of stigmatization appears to be directly correlated with the severity of visible disease (Evans et al., 1993). In conservative contexts, affected individuals avoid seeking treatment for fear of drawing attention to their condition. Failure to treat the disease results in recurrent acute febrile attacks and progressive damage to the lymphatic system. Without access to simple hygiene advice, sufferers are unable to prevent further progression of the outwardly visible complications of LF.

Women bear a double burden in societies where much of their role and identity is dependent upon marriage and the ability to give birth to children. Young unmarried women with LF may be forced to lead a reclusive existence in an attempt to hide their illness or because their limited marriage prospects make them a burden to their families. In Thailand and in West Africa there is a general perception that children born to a woman affected by LF will be similarly affected. Shame and anxiety related to difficulties in conceiving children are common for LF patients around the world (Evans et al., 1993). Young females with LF are considered poor marriage prospects because the disease's recurrent debilitating acute episodes limit their ability to perform paid and unpaid work. The costs associated with long-term health care as the disease progresses result in perceptions of these women as financial burdens.

2.4.3 Ectoparasite infections and HIV/AIDS

Epidermal parasitic skin diseases (EPSD) occur worldwide and have been known since ancient times. Despite the considerable burden caused by EPSD, this category of parasitic diseases has been widely neglected by the scientific community and health-care providers. This is illustrated by the fact that in the 2006 edition of The Communicable disease control handbook, a reference manual for public health interventions, only one EPSD (scabies) is mentioned (Fieldmeier and Heukelbach, 2009). Epidermal parasitic skin diseases fulfill the criteria defined by Ehrenberg and Ault (2005) for neglected diseases of neglected populations, but are not listed on national or international agendas concerning disease control priorities (Ehrenberg and Ault, 2005). This probably explains why efforts to control EPSD at the community level have very rarely been undertaken (Heukelbach et al., 2002).

Six EPSD are of particular importance: scabies, pediculosis (head lice, body lice and pubic lice infestation), tungiasis (sand flea disease) and hookworm-related cutaneous larva migrans. They are either prevalent in resource-poor settings or are associated with important morbidity. This chapter focuses on these diseases, summarize the existing knowledge on the epidemiology and the morbidity in resource-poor settings and focus on the interactions between EPSD and poverty. The distribution of EPSD is irregular, and incidence and prevalence vary in relation to area and population studied. A study in a resource-poor community in urban Bangladesh, for example, showed that virtually all children aged less than 6 years developed scabies within a period of 12 months (Stanton et al., 1987). In a rural village in Tanzania, the overall prevalence is 6% and in rural India 13%, while in Australian Aboriginal communities the prevalence in this age group approached 50% (Sharma et al., 1984; Currie and Carapetis, 2000). Situation is even worse in displaced communities, where of 5-9-year-olds children in Sierra Leone, 86% are infested with *Sarcoptes scabiei*.

Poverty influences the epidemiology of EPSD in several ways because it creates animal reservoirs, ensures ongoing transmission, facilitates atypical ways of spreading the infectious agent and increases the chances of exposure. This results in an extraordinarily high prevalence and intensity of infestation and significant morbidity of EPSD. Again, stigma, lack of access to health care and hesitancy in seeking health care are the reasons why EPSD frequently progress untreated.

Inequality and neglect seem to be the major driving forces that keep the disease burden at an intolerably high level. Health-care stakeholders and political decision-makers must acknowledge that EPSD are debilitating and merit much more attention from health professionals than hitherto given. The ongoing uncontrolled urbanization in Tanzania and other developing countries makes it likely that EPSD will remain the overriding parasitic diseases for people living in extreme poverty and remain indicators of neglect by societies and particularly public health policies.

3. Conclusion

There are plenty of ways to help prevent HIV/AIDS by changing the biological and economic context in which the epidemic is spreading. Behavioral interventions are necessary, but their effectiveness is often a matter of faith more than documented results. So far, neither preaching abstinence nor handing out condoms has had an appreciable impact on the epidemic because sexual behavior is not the most important difference between high-prevalence and low-prevalence populations. Governments can change customs regulations or deliver safe water supplies and multivitamins more easily than they can chase down every person having unprotected sex. It is not a coincidence that the countries with the highest rates of HIV have serious environmental, economic, and bureaucratic problems. Most of the worst affected countries like Tanzania have problems of border-breach, ineffective parasitic infections control programmes, risky environment for HIV infection that all together is HIV/AIDS related.

Researchers have shown that there is a common immunopathogenetic basis for the detrimental interaction between HIV and pathogens biologically as different as for example, plasmodia and helminthes. Chronic immune activation by parasitic infection could be one of the several causes of T cells depletion in HIV infection and could considerably contribute to the progression of HIV disease. Infection with intestinal helminthes, parasitic organisms living in a compartment aside of the systemic immune system, induces a status of chronic immune activation. The prolonged and enhanced immune activation is even more prominent in systemic parasitic infections, whether protozoa or helminthes. Even before HIV infection supervenes, chronic immune activation induced by parasites is associated with several of the immunological features of HIV disease.

In principle, the fact that parasites preferentially activate a Th2 type of help, among other functions Th2 cells down-regulate the development of Th1 cells, inhibit macrophage activity and impair the cytotoxic T-lymphocyte response. They encourage entry of HIV through the CD4 receptors located on the Th2 cells surfaces. The early presence of IL-4 is the most potent stimulus for Th2 differentiation. The inducing effect of IL-4 dominates over other cytokines so that, if IL-4 levels reach a certain threshold, differentiation of the Th cell into the Th2 phenotype ensues, thus favoring proliferation of the HIV, and particularly because of the low levels of Th1 cells that are necessary for the containment of HIV infection via cell-mediated immunity, whereby intracellular pathogens like HIV could be removed.

In contrast to HIV infection, which in the tropics is mainly a sexually transmitted disease, parasitic infections usually abound in childhood and/or adolescence. Moreover, in endemic areas sensitization towards the respective antigens already occurs early during prenatal period (*in utero*) as mothers are likely to be infected with the parasites as well. Notwithstanding, exposure to antigens *in utero* results in generation of cytokine responses similar to those found in adults and the ability of primed T cells to react accordingly can persist into childhood. Such early exposure generate memory cells of Th2 type of help would be a considerable disadvantage when later in life the immune system of the affected individual encounters HIV. Consequently, not only is HIV infection acquired more easily but more rapid progression from asymptomatic HIV infection to AIDS disease.

Summarily, it seems evident that people living in the tropics not only face a health threat in view of still expanding HIV epidemic, they also have to fear that once infected with HIV this will alter the natural history of parasitic infections they are suffering from in an unfavorable way. Besides the parasites they harbor impair the immune response towards HIV. In this way makes rapid progression from HIV infection to AIDS rather likely. As the great majority of parasitic diseases can be treated and /or to some extent be prevented, it is now logical that the control of parasitic infections should be included as a tool in the combat of HIV infections.

Although HIV prevalence has fallen in Tanzania over the past decade, thousands of people become infected with HIV every year and 86,000 Tanzanians died from AIDS in 2009 alone. While the poor are undoubtedly hit harder by the downstream impacts of AIDS, in a variety of ways, their chances of being exposed to HIV in the first place are not necessarily greater than wealthier individuals or households. However, the poor are more prone to parasitic infections. Poverty (illiteracy, food insecurity, poor public services and inequality), parasitosis and HIV/AIDS are the major problem currently facing Tanzanians. Therefore, a joint effort is urgently required to combat them in their totality, with that approach, the victory is evident.

4. References

Abu-Raddad, LJ., Patnaik, P., and Kublin, JG. (2006). Dual infection with HIV and malaria fuels the spread of both diseases in sub-Saharan Africa. *Science* Vol. 314:1603-1606. ISSN: 113238

Akinbo, FO., Okaka, C E., and Omoregie, R. (2010). Prevalence of intestinal parasitic infections among HIV patients in Benin City, Nigeria. *Libyan J Med* Vol. 5: 5506. ISSN:1993-2820

Angarano, G., Maggi, P., Di Bari, MA., Larocca, AM., Congedo, P., Di Bari, C., Brandonisio, O., and Chiodo, F. (1997). Giardiasis in HIV: a possible role in patients with severe immune deficiency. *Eur J Epidemiol* Vol.13(4): 485-7. ISSN: 0393-2990

Atzori, C., Bruno, A., Chichino, G., Bernuzzi, AM., Gatti, S., Comolli G., and Scaglia, M. (1993). HIV-1 and parasitic infections in rural Tanzania. *Ann Trop Med Parasitol* 87:585-93. ISSN: 0003-4983

Barnett, T., Whiteside, A., and Desmond, C. (2001) "The Social and Economic Impact of HIV/AIDS in Poor Countries: a Review of Studies and Lessons" in *Progress in Development Studies* Vol. 1(2), pp. 151-170.ISSN:1464-9934

Bisai, S., Ghosh, T., and Bose, K. (2010). Prevalence of underweight, stunting and wasting among urban poor children aged 1- 5 years of West Bengal, India. *Int J Current Res* Vol. 6: 39-44. ISSN: 0975-833X

Borkow, G., Weisman, Z., Leng, Q., Stein, M., Kalinkovich, A., Wolday, D., Bentwich, Z. Helminths, human immunodeficiency virus and tuberculosis. *Scandinavian Journal of Infectious Diseases* 33, 568-571. PMID: 11525348. ISSN: 0036-5548

Brink, AK., Mahé, C., Watera, C., Lugada, E., Gilks, C., Whitworth, J., and French, N. (2002)."Diarrhea, CD4 counts and enteric infections in a community-based cohort of HIV-infected adults in Uganda." *J Infec* Vol. 45(2):99-106. PMID: 12217712. ISSN: 0163-4453

Bullen, JJ., Spalding, PB., Ward, CG., and Gutteridge, JMC. (1991). Hemochromatosis iron and septicemia caused by *Vibrio vulnificus*. *Arch Inter Med* Vol. 151: 1606-1609. ISSN 0022-2615. ISSN: 0300-5127

Bundy, D., Sher, A., and Michael, E. (2000). Good worms or bad worms: do worm infections affect the epidemiological patterns of other diseases? *Parasitology Today* Vol. 16:273-274. ISSN: 0169-4758

Calder, PC. (1995). Fatty acids, dietary lipids and lymphocyte functions. *Biochem Soc Trans* Vol. 23: 302-9. ISSN: 0300-5127

Cates, W Jr. (1988). The "Other STD's" Do They Really Matter? *JAMA* Vol. 259: 3606-36-08. ISSN: 0098-7484

CDC (1987). Revision of the CDC surveillance case definition for acquired immunodeficiency syndrome. *MMWR*. Vol. 36(Suppl 1):1S-15S. ISSN: 0149-2195

Chopra, M. (2006). Mass deworming in Ugandan children. *BMJ* Vol. 333 : 105. Doi: 10.1136/BMJ.333.7559.ISSN: 09598138

Cimerman, S., Cimerman, B., and Lew, SD. (1999). Enteric parasites and Aids. *Sao Paulo Med J* Vol.117 (6): 226-273. ISSN 1516-3180

Clements, AC., Lwambo, N., Blair, L., Nyandindi, U., Kaatano, G., Kinunghi, S., Webster, J., Fenwick, A., and Brooker, S. (2006). Bayesian spatial analysis and disease mapping: tools to enhance planning and implementation of a schistosomiasis control programme in Tanzania. *Trop Med Int Health* Vol. 11:490-503. ISSN:1360-2276

Cunningham, MW., Fujinami, RS. (2000). Effects of Microbes on the Immune System. Philadelphia: Lippincott Williams and Wilkins; 2000: 662. ISBN: 1555811949

Cunningham Rundles S, McNeeley DF and Moon A (2005) Mechanisms of nutrient modulation of the immune response. *J Allergy Clin Immunol* 115, 1119-1128. ISSN: 0091-6749

Currie, BJ., and Carapetis, JR. (2000). Skin infections and infestations in Aboriginal communities in northern Australia. *Australas J Dermatol*   Vol. 41:139-43. ISSN: OOO4 8380

De Onis, M., and Blössner, M. (2000). Prevalence and trends of overweight among preschool children in developing countries. *Am J Clin Nut Vol.* 72: 1032–9. Accesed on 21 February 2011, Available from: http://www.ajcn.org/content/72/4/1032.full.pdf. ISSN: 00029165

De Pablo, MA., and Alvarez de Cienfuegos, G. (2000). Modulatory effects of dietary lipids on immune system functions. *Immuno Cell Biol*   Vol. 78, 31–39. ISSN: 0818-9641 ISSN: 0002-9165

Dorrington, R., Bourne, R., Bradshaw, D., Laubscher, R. and Timaeus, IM. (2001). The impact of HIV/AIDS on adult mortality in South Africa. ISBN 1-919809-14-7.

Dreyfuss ML, Msamanga GI, Spiegelman D, Hunter DJ, Urassa EJN, Hertzmark E and Fawzi WW. Determinants of low birth weight among HIV-infected pregnant women in Tanzania. *Am J Clin Nutrition* Vol. 74(6): 814-826, December 2001. ISSN 0002-9165

Ehrenberg, JP., and Ault, SK. (2005). Neglected diseases of neglected populations: thinking to reshape the determinants of health in Latin America and the Caribbean. *BMC Public Health* Vol.5:119. ISSN: 1471-2458

Evans, DB., Gelband, H., and Vlassoff, C. (1993). Social and economic factors and the control of lymphatic filariasis: a review. *Acta Trop* Vol. 53: 1-26. ISSN: 0001-706X

Feldmeier, H., and Heukelbach, J. (2009). Epidermal parasitic skin diseases: a neglected category of poverty-associated plagues. *Bull World Health Organ* Vol.87 (2), Genebra. ISSN: 0042-9686

Ferreira, ML. (1996). In: Handbook on Poverty and Inequality. "Poverty and Inequality during Structural Adjustment in Rural Tanzania." Policy Research Working Paper No. 1641, World Bank, Washington, DC. ISBN: 9780821376133

Franchin, G., Zybarth, G., Dai, WW., Dubrovsky, L., Reiling, N., Schmidtmayerova, H., Bukrinsky, M., and Sherry, B. (2000). Lipopolysaccharide inhibits HIV-1 infection of monocyte- derived macrophages through direct and sustained down-regulation of CC chemokine receptor 5. *J Immunol* Vol. 164:2592–2601. ISSN: 0022-1767

Giraldo, RA. (1997). AIDS and Stressors III: A Proposal for the Natural History of AIDS. In: AIDS and Stressors, Medellín-Colombia. Impresos Begón. pp. 97-131. ISBN: 9589458033

Graham, SM., Taylor, TE., and Plowe, CV. (2006). Impact of HIV-associated immunosuppression on malaria infection and disease in Malawi. *J Infect Dis* Vol.193:872-878. ISSN: 00221899

Hargreaves, J. and Howes, LD. (2010). 'Changes in HIV prevalence among differently educated groups in Tanzania between 2003 and 2007. *AIDS* Vol. 24(5) 755-761. ISSN: 0269-9370

Helling-Giese, G., Sjaastad, A., Poggensee, G., Kjetland, E,. Richter, J., Chitsulo, L., Kumwenda, N., and Racz, P. (1996). Female genital schistosomiasis (FGS): relationship between gynecological and histopathological findings. *Acta Tropica* Vol.62: 257–267. ISSN: 0001-706X

Heukelbach, J., Mencke, N., and Feldmeier, H. (2002). Cutaneous larva migrans and tungiasis: the challenge to control zoonotic ectoparasitoses associated with poverty. *Trop Med Int Health* Vol. 7:907-10. ISSN:1360-2276

Jahoor, F., Badaloo, A., Reid, M., and Forrester, T. (2008). Protein metabolism in severe childhood malnutrition. *Ann Trop Paediatr* Vol. 28: 87-101. ISSN:0272-4936

Kelley, DS., Taylor, PC., Nelson, GJ., Branch LB., Taylor, PC., Rivera, YM., and Schmidt, PC. (1991). Docosahexaenoic acid ingestion inhibits natural killer cell activity and production of inflammatory mediators in young healthy men. *Lipids* Vol. 34: 317-24. ISSN: 0269-1205

Kjetland, EF., Poggensee, G., Helling-Giese, G., Richter, J., Sjaastad, A., Chitsulo, L., Kumwenda, N., Gundersen, SG., Krantz, I., and Feldmeier, H. (1996). Female genital schistosomiasis due to *Schistosoma haematobium* Clinical and parasitological findings in women in rural Malawi. *Acta Tropica* Vol.62: 239-255. ISSN: 0001-706X

Liu, Z., Wang, D., Xue, Q., Chen, J., Li, Y., Xiaoli, B., and Chang, L. (2003). Determination of Fatty Acid Levels in Erythrocyte Membranes of Patients with Chronic Fatigue Syndrome. *Nutritional Neuroscience* Vol.6 (6): 389–392. ISSN: 1028-415X

Luong, TV. (2003). De-worming school children and hygiene intervention. *Inter J Environ Health Res* Vol. 13: S153 – S159. ISSN 0960-3123

Mabey, D. (2000). Interaction between HIV infection and other sexually transmitted diseases. *Tropical Med Interl Health* Vol. 5 (Suppl.):A32–A36. ISSN:1360-2276

Maclean, WC. Jr and Lucas, A. (2008). Peadric nutrition: A distinct subspecialityIn: . In Duggan C, Watkins JB and Walker WA. Nutrition in peadiatric 4. Basic Science-Clinical applications. International Print-O-Pac Ltd. India. ISBN 978-1-55009-361-2

Marsh, K. (1998). Malaria disaster in Africa. *Lancet* Vol. 352:924. ISSN: 0140-6736

McGowan, I., Chalmers, A., Smith, GR., and Jewell, D. (1997). Advances in Mucosal Immunology. *Gastroenterol Clin North Am* Vol. 26:145-173. ISSN: 0889-8553

Mhiri, C., Bélec, L., Di Constanzo, B., Georges, A., and Gherardi, R. (1992). The slim disease in African patients with AIDS. *Trans R Soc Trop Med Hyg* Vol. 86:303-6. ISSN: 0035-9203

Mkopi, A., Urassa, H., Mapunjo, E., Mushi, F., and Mshinda, H. (2005). Impact of school health programme on urinary schistosomiasis control in school children in Kilosa, Tanzania. *Tanzania Health Research Bulletin* Vol.7. ISSN: 0035-9203

Mshana, GH., Wamoyi, J., Busza, J., Zaba, B., Changalucha, J., Kaluvya, S., and Urassa, M. (2006). 'Barriers to accessing antiretroviral therapy in Kisesa, Tanzania: a qualitative study of early rural referrals to the national program.' *AIDS Patient Care STDS* Vol. 20(9):649-57. ISSN: 1087-2914

Mwambete, KD., and Kalison, N. (2006). Prevalence of Intestinal Helminthic Infections Among Under fives and Knowledge on Helminthiases Among Mothers of Under fives in Dar es Salaam, Tanzania. *East Afr J Public Heath* Vol. 3(1):8-11. ISSN: 0856-8960.

Mwambete, KD., Justin-Temu, M., and Peter, S. (2010). Prevalence and management of intestinal helminthiasis among HIV-infected patients at MNH. *J Inter Asso Physicians AIDS Care* Vol. 9(3):150-156. ISSN: 1545-1097

Ngalula, J., Urassa, M., Mwaluko, G., Isingo, R. and Boerma, JT. (2002). Health service use and household expenditure during terminal illness due to AIDS in rural Tanzania. *Trop Med Int Health.* Vol. 7(10):873-7. ISSN:1360-2276

Nkuo-Akenji, T., Tevoufouet, EE., Nzang, F., Ngufor, N., and Fon, E. (2008). High prevalence of HIV and malaria co-infection in urban Douala, Cameroon. *African J AIDS Res* Vol. 7 (2):229 - 235 ISSN: 1608-5906

Nnakwe, N. (1995). The effect and causes protein-energy malnutrition in Nigerian children. *Nutr Res* Vol. 15:785-794. ISSN: 0300-9831

PHDR. (2005). Poverty and Human Development.Report-2005. The research and analysis working group. Published by Mkuki na Nyota Publisher. Dar es Salaam, Tanzania. ISBN 9987-686-72-9

Pradeep, MA., Thiruvalluvan, M,. Aarthy, K. and Mary Stella J. (2010). Determination of Iron Deficiency among Human Immunodeficiency Virus Sero Positives. *Am Medical J* Vol.1 (2): 77-79. ISSN 1949-0070

Riemersma, RA., Armstrong, R., Kelly, RW.,and Wilson, R. (1998). Essential oils and Eicosanoids-invited papers from the 4th International congress. AOCS Press. USA. ISBN: 0-935315-96-9.

Roitt, I., Brostoff J., and Male, D. (2001). Immunology. 6th Edtion. Mosby. London. ISBN: 0723432422.

Roura, M., Busza, J., Wringe, A., Mbata, D., Urassa, M., and Zaba, B. (2009). Barriers to sustaining antiretroviral treatment in Kisesa, Tanzania: a follow-up study to understand attrition from the antiretroviral program. *AIDS Patient Care STDS* Vol. 23(3):203-10. ISSN: 1087-2914

Scrimshaw, NS., and SanGiovanni, JP. (1997). Synergism of nutrition, infection and immunity: an overview. *Am J Clin Nutr* Vol. 66:464S–477S. Online ISSN: 1938-3207

Sharma, RS., Mishra, RS., Pal, D., Gupta, JP., Dutta, M., and Datta, KK. (1984). An epidemiological study of scabies in a rural community in India. *Ann Trop Med Parasitol Vol.*78:157-64. ISSN: 0003-4983

Shelton, JD., Cassell, M., and Adetunji, A. (2005). 'Is poverty or wealth at the root of HIV?'. *Lancet* Vol. 366 (9491): 1057-8. ISSN: 0140-6736

Sherman, IW. (1998). Malaria: Parasite biology, pathogenesis and protection. Washington DC. American Society of Microbioogy Press. ISBN:1-55581-131-0

Stanton, B., Khanam, S., Nazrul, H., Nurani, S., and Khair, T. (1987). Scabies in urban Bangladesh. *J Trop Med Hyg* Vol.90:219-26. ISSN: 0022-5304

Strauss, RG. (2004). Iron deficiency, infections and immune function: a reassessment. *Am J Clinical Nutrition* Vol. 79(3):516-521. ISSN: 0002-9165

Tarimo, DS., Killewo, JZ., Minjas, JN., and Msamanga, GI. (1996). Prevalence of intestinal parasites in adult patients with enteropathic AIDS in north-eastern Tanzania. *East Afr Med J* Vol.73(6):397-9. ISSN: 0012-835X

Van Geertruyden J, Menten J, Colebunders R, Korenromp E, and D'AlessandroU. (2008).The impact of HIV-1 on the malaria parasite biomass in adults in sub-Saharan Africa contributes to the emergence of antimalarials drug resistance. *Malaria Journal* Vol. 7:134-147. ISSN: 0043-3144

Villamor, E., Misegades, L., Fatak,i MR., Mbise, RL., and Fawzi, WW. (2005). "Child mortality in relation to HIV infection, nutritional status, and socio-economic background." *Inter J Epidemiol* Vol 34(1) 61-8. ISSN: 0300-5751

Wojciki, JM. (2005). Socio-economic status as a risk factor for HIV infection in women in East, Central and Southern Africa: a systematic review. *J Biosocial Sci* Vol. 37:1-36. ISSN: 0021-9320

3

The Impact Water, Sanitation and Hygiene Infrastructures has on People Living with HIV and AIDS in Zimbabwe

Natasha Potgieter[1], Tendayi B. Mpofu[1] and Tobias G. Barnard[2]
[1]Department of Microbiology, University of Venda,
[2]Water and Health Research Unit, University of Johannesburg,
South Africa

1. Introduction

Acquired Immune Deficiency Syndrome (AIDS) emerged in the 1980s as the most terrifying epidemic of modern times. AIDS as a disease is caused by a virus called the Human Immunodeficiency Virus (HIV). The total number of people living with HIV worldwide in 2009 was 33.3 million (UNAIDS, 2009). Sub-Saharan Africa continues to be the hardest hit by the global HIV and AIDS epidemic with an estimated 22.5 million infected people in 2009. AIDS was first reported in Zimbabwe in 1985 and by the beginning of the 1990s, around 10% of the adult population were thought to be infected with HIV (UNAIDS 2005). The estimated adult HIV prevalence rate (aged 15-49) during 2009 in Zimbabwe was reported to be 14.3% (UNICEF webpage).

Presently very little data is available on how water, sanitation and hygiene infrastructures are affecting the lives of people living with HIV and AIDS (PLWHA) in Zimbabwe. Literature has identified a series of linkages between water, sanitation and hygiene and HIV and AIDS (USAID/WSP, 2007). According to UNICEF (2005), a hygienic environment, clean water and adequate sanitation are key factors in preventing opportunistic infections associated with HIV and AIDS, and in the quality of life of people living with the disease. PLWHA are more susceptible to water-related diseases than healthy individuals, and they become sicker from these infections than people with healthy immune systems (UNICEF, 2005).

The urban areas of the Bulawayo metropolitan province of Zimbabwe consist primarily of high-density sub-urban areas and peri-urban settlements with municipal treated water supplies. Some peri-urban areas have unprotected water sources (rivers) and limited or totally inadequate sanitation. Although communal taps serve most peri-urban settlements, critical water shortages force these communities to rely on water from boreholes, unprotected wells and rivers for domestic use. Most of these households use pit latrines and some use the bush. Households in the rural areas mainly rely on boreholes as water sources, with a few households having piped water supply from Zimbabwe National Water Authority (ZINWA). This made the Bulawayo metropolitan the ideal study area to obtain representative data about the possible impact water, sanitation and hygiene infrastructures can have on the health of PLWHA in Zimbabwe.

Diarrhoeal diseases are the most common opportunistic infections experienced by PLWHA in Africa and elsewhere. Most of these diarrhoeal infections are either water borne or water washed. Patients with HIV infection or AIDS are commonly affected by gastrointestinal infections, with diarrhoea as the most common presentation (Janoff and Smith, 1988). Diarrhoea occurs in 30-60% of AIDS patients in developed countries and in about 90% of AIDS patients in developing countries (Framm and Soave, 1997). Enteric pathogens that cause diarrhoea include bacteria, parasites, fungi and viruses (Mitra et al., 2001). *Escherichia coli* (*E. coli*) are commonly used as an indicator of faecal pollution in water, indicating the possible presence of other bacterial pathogens that could have been shed into the water source.

Although *E. coli* is used as an indicator it also has the capability of contriburting to the diarrheal load in an area. Five classes of *E. coli* bacteria that cause diarrhoeal diseases are now recognised: enterotoxigenic *E. coli* (ETEC), enteroinvasive *E. coli* (EIEC), enterohaemorrhagic *E. coli* (EHEC), enteropathogenic *E. coli* (EPEC) and enteroaggregative *E. coli* (EAEC). Each class falls within a serological subgroup and manifests distinct features in pathogenesis and subsequent diarrhoea (Todar, 2002). The importance of *E. coli,* both as an indicator organism and as a diarrhoeagenic pathogen is well documented. The aim of this study is therefore to determine the impact water, sanitation and hygiene infrastructures and their associated health risks facing people living with HIV and AIDS through detection of pathogenic *E. coli* in domestic drinking water and on sanitation facilities in the and around Bulawayo in Zimbabwe.

2. Materials and methods

2.1 Ethical consent
Registration of the project and ethical clearance was obtained from the University of Venda's Health, Safety and Research Ethics Committee. The Medical Research Council of Zimbabwe and the City of Bulawayo, through the Director of Health Services provided the necessary authority to proceed with the study.
Staff at Opportunistic Infections Clinics (OICs) was used to identify the HIV and AIDS patients and only those that volunteered and signed consent forms were included in the study. The consent forms were translated into the vernacular language of the patient.

2.2 Data collection using questionnaires
Structured questionnaires were used to obtain information regarding household demographics, water sources used, water collection practices; time spent collecting water, water storage practices, costs involved in water and sanitation services, hygiene practices associated with sanitation and the level of hygiene understanding in each household.

2.3 Study area
The Bulawayo metropolitan in Zimbabwe was chosen as the study site for the project. A total of 414 households with individuals living with HIV and AIDS from high density sub-urban areas (n=150 households), peri-urban areas (n=121 households) and rural villages (n=142 households) in and around Bulawayo were included in this study.

2.4 Sample collection
Samples were collected aseptically from household water storage containers in sterile 1 litre plastic bottles and transported on ice to the laboratory for further analysis. Toilet seats were

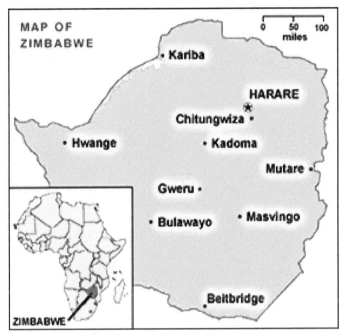

Fig. 1. Map of Zimbabwe showing the location of the study area

swabbed using sterile methods and the swab placed into sterile containers with 100 ml phosphate buffered saline (pH 7.4) (PBS) and transported on ice to the laboratory for further analysis. Hands of 20% of the people living with HIV and AIDS in each of the three areas included in the study, were swabbed and the swabs placed into sterile containers with 100 ml PBS and transported on ice to the laboratory for further analysis.

2.5 Determination of total coliform bacteria and *Escherichia coli*

Total coliforms and *E. coli* were detected using the Colilert® Quanti-Tray/2000 System manufactured by IDEXX and supplied by DEHTEQ. Appropriate dilutions of the samples were made according to the procedures described by the manufacturers (IDEXX). The trays were incubated at 35°C for 18 to 22 hours and the positive (yellow and fluorescing) wells and *E. coli* bacteria were counted and converted into the most probable number of total coliforms and *E. coli* present in samples, using tables and formulae provided by the manufacturer. Included in the experiment were positive and negative controls (distilled water, *E. coli*, *Klebsiella* and *Pseudomonas*).

Selection of potential *E. coli* bacteria was made of fluorescing wells that could clearly be counted as the actual indicator in the selective growth media. The contents of positively identified *E. coli* wells were collected using 1 ml syringes and kept in clearly marked cryotubes at -70°C. A multiplex PCR method was performed according to Omar et al., (2010). The five diarrhoeagenic strains of *E. coli* and a commensal *E. coli* strain that were employed in the study are shown in Table 1.

All strains were obtained from the South African National Health Laboratory Services (NHLS) (2010), and stored at -70°C in a mixture of Plate Count Agar (PCA) with 10% (v/v) glycerol. The strains were routinely cultured on PCA and incubated under aerobic conditions at 37°C. Liquid cultures of the bacteria were obtained by inoculating 5 ml Luria-

Bacterial strain	Reference number	Genes targeted
Enterotoxigenic *Escherichia coli* (ETEC)	H10407	*Mdh, Lt, St*
Enteropathogenic *E. coli* (EPEC)	B170	*Mdh, eaeA*
Enteroaggregative *E. coli* (EAEC)	3591-178	*Mdh, Eagg*
Enterohaemorrhagic *E. coli* (EHEC)	C4193-1	*Mdh, eaeA, stx1, stx2*
Enteroinvasive *E. coli* (EIEC)	C316-58	*Mdh, Ial*
Commensal *E. Coli*	Field isolate, API20E confirmed	*Mdh*

Table 1. Bacterial strains used for the experimental work

Bertani (LB) media in test tubes for 16 hours while rotating at 200 rpm at 37°C. Genomic DNA isolation was performed on 2ml of each sample using an adapted protocol as described in Omar et al., (2010). All buffers used, were prepared as described by Omar et al (2010).

2.6 DNA extraction and multiplex polymerase chain reactions (PCR)
The samples were centrifuged at 12,000xg for 2 minutes at room temperature to pellet any bacterial cells present. After removing the supernatant, each pellet was dissolved in 700 µl extraction buffer and left for 10 min at 37°C, after which 250 µl of 99% ethanol was added and thoroughly mixed. This was left for 10 minutes at 56°C, after which 40 µl celite suspension was added, mixed and left for 10 minutes with occasional mixing. Pellets were again collected by centrifugation at 12,000xg for 30 seconds at room temperature (the supernatant removed). The pellets were washed twice with 500 µl washing buffer. This was followed by two 70% (v/v) ethanol wash steps. The pellets were dried at 56°C for 10 minutes, mixed with 100 µl TE buffer (10 mM Tris-HCl, 1 mM EDTA, pH 8.0), heated for 10 minutes at 56°C and briefly centrifuged to pellet the celite. The DNA containing supernatant was removed and the elution repeated once as described. All PCR reactions were performed in BIORAD Mycycler™ Thermal cycler as described by Omar et al., (2010).
DNA was analysed on a horizontal agarose slab gel [1% (w/v)] with ethidium bromide (0.5µg/ml) in TAE buffer (40 mM Tris acetate; 2 mM EDTA, pH 8.3). Electrophoresis was done for one hour in an electrical field strength of 5.9 V.cm-1 gel and DNA was visualised with UV light (Gene Genius Bio Imaging system, Vacutec). The relative sizes of the DNA fragments were estimated by comparing their electrophoretic mobility with that of the standards run with the samples on each gel. Gene ruler (Fermentas) was used as standards.

2.7 Data analysis
The data from the questionnaires and microbiological data on commensal and pathogenic *E. coli* strains was coded and collated before being entered into an MS Excel spread sheet. The data was imported into the Stata Release 8.0 statistical software package for cleaning and editing. For categorical data, frequencies of occurrence of response were calculated. For numerical variables the data was summarised using the arithmetic, geometric and harmonic means and a corresponding 95% confidence interval. Testing was done at the 0.05 level of

significance. All statistical analyses were done by Professor Piet Bekker from the Medical Research Council Statistical Unit in Pretoria, South Africa.

3. Results and discussion

3.1 Age and gender distribution of study population

As indicated in Table 2, the average family size of the urban household was 5.2 people, with females constituting 57% and males 43% of the urban study population. There was an average of 2.2 males and 3 females in the urban households. The peri-urban household average family size was 4.7 people, with females being 54% and males 46% of the peri-urban study population. There was an average of 2.5 females and 2.2 males in the peri-urban households. In rural areas the average family size was 5.3 people; females formed 54% and males 46% of the household composition. There was an average of 2.9 females and 2.4 males in the rural household. The urban and rural family sizes were the same, with the peri-urban family size being slightly smaller, due to a number of single member families found in peri-urban areas. In all areas there were more females than males in the households; the peri-urban and rural household composition was the same, whilst the urban household composition had a larger difference between the female and male members of households.

In all areas the children aged between 5 years and 12 years were the largest age-group. There were significantly less men in the age group 41 to 50 years (15.5%) in rural areas compared to peri-urban (23.1%) and urban (25.3%) areas. This may be due to rural to urban migration of this age group in search of employment. In the age group 61 to 70 years there was a significantly higher percentage of males in rural areas (10.6%) compare to urban and peri-urban areas (3.3% in both areas). This again may be related to migrant work, with this age group having returned from urban areas where they had been working.

3.2 Age and gender distribution of PLWHA

Most of the PLWHA were in the age groups 31 to 40 years and 41 to 50 years. These results agree with household surveys in 28 sub-Saharan Africa which revealed that in all but five countries peak HIV prevalence occurs between the ages 30 and 34 for women and in the late 30s and early 40s or men (Macro International, 2008). These are the sexually active members of society and the results of this study showed that the HIV in Bulawayo could be predominantly sexually transmitted.

Of the one hundred and fifty PLWHA from urban areas one hundred and nine (73%) were female and forty-one (27%) were male. One of the participants was in the age group 16 to 22 years (0.7%); twelve were in the age group 21 to 30 years (8%); sixty-one were in the age group 31 to 40 years (40.7%); fifty-six were in the age group 41 to 50 years (37.3%); fifteen were in the age group 51 to 60 years (10%); three were in the age group 61 to 70 years (2%) and two were above 70 years of age (1.3%).

In peri-urban areas, twelve (9.3%) of the one hundred and twenty-two participants were in the age group 21 to 30 years; fifty-two (42.6%) were in the age group 31 to 40 years; forty-three (35.2%) were in the age group 41 to 50 years; eleven (9%) were in the age group 51 to 60 years and two (1.6%) were in each of the age groups 61 to 70 years and above seventy years of age.

Age in years	Urban Average family size = 5.2 Female = 57% Male = 43%			Peri-urban Average family size = 4.7 Female = 54% Male = 46%			Rural Average family size = 5.2 Female = 54% Male = 46%		
	F (n)	M (n)	Per age (%)	F (n)	M (n)	Per age (%)	F (n)	M (n)	Per age (%)
Infant 0-1	5	6	11 (2%)	10	6	16 (3%)	13	7	20 (3%)
Toddler >1-5	31	40	71(9%)	27	24	51 (9%)	39	31	70 (9%)
Child >5-12	71	69	140 (18%)	65	67	132 (23%)	59	90	149 (20%)
Adolescent >12-16	60	40	100 (13%)	26	17	43 (8%)	34	36	70 (10%)
Adolescent >16-20	57	38	95 (12%)	21	25	46 (8%)	39	33	72 (10%)
Adult 21-30	58	43	101 (13%)	40	33	73 (13%)	50	43	93 (13%)
Adult 31-40	75	33	108 (14%)	49	38	87 (15%)	55	31	86 (12%)
Adult 41-50	50	38	88 (11%)	40	28	68 (12%)	46	22	68 (9%)
Adult 51-60	23	13	36 (5%)	11	12	23 (4%)	24	25	49 (7%)
Adult 61-70	13	5	18 (2%)	8	4	12 (2%)	15	15	30 (4%)
Adult >70	4	6	10 (1%)	8	7	15 (3%)	16	8	24 (3%)
Total	447	331	684 (100%)	305	261	566 (100%)	390	341	731 (100%)

Table 2. Demographics of study population

In rural areas, six (4.3%) of the one hundred and forty-two participants were in the age group 16 to 20 years; twenty-five (17.7%) were in the age group 21 to 30 years; forty-six (32.6%) were in the age group 31 to 40 years; thirty-nine (27.7%) were in the age group 41 to 50 years; twenty-one (14.9%) were in the age group 51 to 60 years and four (2.8%) were in the age group 61 to 70 years.

3.3 CD4 counts of PLWHA
The cells mostly affected by HIV when it infects humans are the CD4 cells. After having been affected for a long time the number of CD4 cells decreases indicating that the immune system is being weakened. Normal CD4 counts are usually between 500 and 1 600 (AIDS InfoNet , 2010). An HIV positive person with CD4 count of less than 200 is considered to have AIDS, and preventive therapy should be started even if the person has no symptoms

(Lab Test Online, 2009). Of late most health care providers begin antiretroviral therapy (ART) when the CD4 count goes below 350 (AIDS InfoNet, 2010).

The CD4 count results of all the 150 people living with HIV and AIDS in urban areas were obtained (Table 3). The geometric mean for the CD4 count results was 221. In peri-urban

HIV and CD4 count tests	Urban	Peri-urban	Rural
Where first HIV test was done	**n = 150**	**n = 121**	**n = 142**
New Start Centre	70 (46.7%)	59 (48.8%)	64 (45.1%)
Local clinic	49 (32.7%)	48 (39.7%)	51 (35.9%)
Hospital	26 (17.3%)	13 (10.7%)	27 (19.0%)
Private Doctor	1 (0.7%)	1 (0.8%)	0 (0%)
Other	4 (2.6%)	0 (0%)	0 (0%)
Where first CD4 count test was done	**n = 149**	**n = 121**	**n = 142**
Not done	0 (0%)	0 (0%)	1 (0.7%)
New Start Centre	8 (5.4%)	5 (4.1%)	7 (4.9%)
Local clinic	78 (52.4%)	49 (40.5%)	17 (12%)
Hospital	47 (31.5%)	20 (16.5%)	90 (63.4%)
Private Doctor	13 (8.7%)	0 (0%)	1 (0.7%)
Other	3 (2%)	47 (38.9%)	26 (18.3%)
Frequency of follow-up tests	**n = 150**	**n = 121**	**n = 133**
Not done	0 (0%)	3 (2.5%)	0 (0%)
Once a year	57 (38%)	16 (13.2%)	41 (30.8%)
Every 6 months	21 (14%)	5 (4.1%)	8 (6%)
Every 3 months	6 (4%)	3 (2.5%)	6 (4.5%)
Not done	43 (28.7%)	92 (76%)	77 (57.9%)
Other	23 (15.3%)	2 (1.7%)	1 (0.8%)
Last CD4 count test	**n = 149**	**n = 121**	**n = 114**
Not done	2 (1.34%)	47 (38.84%)	0 (0%)
Within last month	38 (25.5%)	72 (59.5%)	21 (18.4%)
>1 month, <3 months	13 (8.7%)	13 (10.7%)	23 (20.2%)
3 to 6 months	10 (6.7%)	4 (3.3%)	13 (11.4%)
6 to 12 months	32 (21.5%)	14 (11.6%)	24 (21.1%)
>12 months	56 (37.6%)	18 (14.9%)	33 (28.9%)

Table 3. Details of places of testing and or frequency for HIV and CD4 tests

areas 119 PLWHA out of 121 in the study had their CD4 count results recorded and the mean was 224. All the 141 PLWHA in rural areas had their CD4 count results obtained and the mean was 235. The mean CD4 count in all the areas was below the normal CD4 count of between 500 and 1 600, however it was above 200, at which one is said to have AIDS (AIDS InfoNet, 2010). PLWHA that had taken their first test for HIV at a New Start Centre were 47% in urban areas, 49% in peri-urban and 45% in rural areas. Those that were first tested for HIV at their local clinic were 33% in urban areas, compared to 40% in peri-urban areas and 36% in rural areas. Those that had their first test for HIV done at a hospital were 17% in urban areas, 11% in peri-urban areas and 19% in rural areas. The rest (3% in urban areas and 1% in peri-urban areas) had been first tested for HIV at a private doctor or some other testing facility.

The first CD4 count tests were done at the local clinic for 52% of PLWHA in urban areas, 41% of those in peri-urban areas and 12% of those in rural areas. Those that had the first CD4 count test done at a hospital were 32% in urban areas, 17% in peri-urban areas and 63% in rural areas. CD4 tests done by private doctors were 9% in urban areas and 1% in rural areas. Some PLWHA (2% in urban areas, 39% in peri-urban areas and 18% in rural areas) had their first CD4 count test done as special request because they had been commenced on treatment using the WHO staging without the CD4 count test.

After the initial CD4 count test getting a follow-up test was not easy, and most of the PLWHA had not had regular follow-up CD4 count tests. In urban areas 29% had not done a follow-up CD4 count test, compared to 76% in peri-urban areas and 58% in rural areas.

Those that had a CD4 count test done once every year were 38% in urban areas, 13% in peri-urban areas and 31% in rural areas. Those that had a follow-up test every 6 months were 14% in urban areas, 4% in peri-urban areas and 6% in rural areas. Those that a follow-up test every 3 months were 4% in urban areas, 2.5% in peri-urban areas and 6% in rural areas. In urban areas 15% had not had regular follow-up CD4 count tests, compared to 1% in peri-urban and rural areas.

3.4 Sanitation in study population

The Urban Councils Act and the municipal bylaws require all houses to have a flush toilet before being occupied. These provisions by and large complied with in the urban areas. Problems arose during periods of water unavailability when the households had to resort to pouring water to flush these toilets. Being situated in a water scarce region, Bulawayo needs a relook into the appropriate toilet technology for the city. A technology that would not be dependent on water would best suit the city. There is no specific policy on sanitation for peri-urban areas due to their semi-formal and in some cases informal nature. However, as in rural areas, the ventilated improved pit (VIP) latrine offers an appropriate option. The guidelines for rural sanitation recommend a VIP latrine for each household.

In urban areas 98% of the households had a water closet connected to a public sewer, the rest did not have toilet facilities and used the bush. In peri-urban areas 48% of the households had a VIP latrine, 2% had a water closet connected to a septic tank and 1% had a substandard pit latrine. The remaining 49% of the households had no toilet facilities and used the bush. In rural areas 66% of the households had VIP latrines, 15% had pit latrines with a slab and 4% had pit latrines without a slab. One household had a water closet connected to a septic tank. The remaining 14% of the households had no toilet facilities and used the bush.

Approximately 98% of households in the urban areas had access to improved sanitation; however, 49% of households in peri-urban areas and 34% in rural areas did not have access to an improved sanitation facility. The need for access to improved sanitation is critical for

HIV and AIDS patients. Nearby latrines are necessary for weak patients. In some patients, diarrhoea is chronic, further weakening them. In order for HIV infected people to remain healthy as long as possible and for people with AIDS to reduce their chances of getting diarrhoea, adequate sanitary facilities are of the utmost importance (Kamminga and Wegelin-Schuringa, 2003). The hygiene infrastructures were generally inadequate, especially with regards to hand washing facilities.

3.5 Water in study population
Zimbabwe does not have national standards for water accessibility; the SPHERE project recommended standard of 500m to a water point was therefore used (World Vision, 2006). Whenever water was available it was easily accessible from taps within the house (67%) or within the yard (33%) in urban areas. In peri-urban areas most of the households collected water from communal standpipes (70%) and boreholes (5%) to their homes over distances that varied from less than 500m to more than 2km. Up to 25% of the households collected water from unprotected wells or springs. Those that collected water from a water source more than 500m away from their homes were 9% of the households in peri-urban areas and 27.5% in rural areas. Table 4 summarises information on water availability. Travelling more than 500m to a water source is likely to be tedious especially to young children, the elderly and those weakened by illness. In peri-urban and rural areas containers of up to 25 litres were used to collect water and were mainly carried on the heads. This was a considerable strain especially for the vulnerable people. Whilst water sources were accessible to most households in all the three areas, the unavailability of water was a major constraint, especially in urban areas where 60% of the households reported that water was not always available. In peri-urban areas 36% of the households and 13% in rural areas said water was not always available. During the period August to September 2008, in urban areas and peri-urban areas supplied with municipal piped water was available only two days a week and in some cases only for a few hours. Some of these communities had gone for more than a month with intermittent water supplies. The intermittent water supply meant that even though water was piped to the house it had to be collected and stored for those periods when it was not available from the tap.

This resulted in increased water handling with a subsequent increase in opportunities for contamination (USAID, 2006). Unsanitary and inadequately protected water containers could contribute to the contamination of water at the point-of-use (Dunker, 2001). Inadequate storage conditions have been shown to result in the increase in the number of some microorganisms such as heterotrophic bacteria and total coliform bacteria over time (Reiff et al., 1996). Potable water is critical for PLWHA; they need it for taking antiretroviral (ARV) medication, bathing, washing soiled linen and clothing and for essential hygiene, which reduces exposure to opportunistic infections (WRC, 2005).

Various factors affected the availability of water in urban and peri-urban areas during different periods of the study. At one point the major supply dams had dried up resulting in water shortages. There was also a time when the municipality was reported to have run out of water treatment chemicals, and were unwilling to distribute water that had not been fully treated. In all the areas solving the water problems being experienced was taking quite long, with 39% in urban areas, 83% in peri-urban areas and 77% in rural areas having reported that it took more than a month to have the problems fixed. During these periods of water being unavailable from the usual sources 5% of households in urban areas collected water from unprotected wells, compared to 26.5% in urban areas and 10.5% in rural areas. Resorting to unsafe water sources puts the PLWHA at a risk of contracting water-borne diseases.

Water supplies	Urban % (n=150)	Peri-urban % (n=121)	Rural % (n =142)
Source			
Piped water into dwelling	66.67	0	2.82
Piped water to yard	32.67	0	11.97
Public tap/standpipe	0	70.25	23.94
Tubewell/borehole	0	4.96	50
Protected well	0	0	4.23
Unprotected dug well	0.67	23.97	6.34
Protected spring	0	0	0
Unprotected spring	0	0.83	0
Distance from home			
0 – 50m	99.33	23.97	21.83
>50 -100m	0	32.23	21.13
>100 – 200m	0.67	16.53	16.2
>200 – 300m	0	7.44	6.34
>300 - 400m	0	2.48	1.41
>400 – 500m	0	8.26	5.63
>500m – 1km	0	4.13	15.49
>1km – 2km	0	3.31	10.56
>2km	0	1.65	1.41
Time taken to water source and back			
<30 min	0.67	73.55	51.41
30 min – 1hr	0	16.53	27.46
>1hr	0	9.92	4.23
Water on premises	99.33	0	16.9
Frequency of unavailability			
	n=148	n=44	n=18
Always available	39.19	0	0
Everyday	5.41	11.36	38.89
Every other day	3.38	4.55	11.11
Twice a week	19.59	13.64	38.89
More than twice a week	25	47.73	5.56
Other	7.43	22.73	5.56
Time taken to fix problem			
	n=148	n=36	n=13
No problem	38.51	0	0
On the same day	8.11	2.78	0
1 day – 3 days	8.73	2.78	0
>3 days – 5 days	0	2.78	7.69
>5 days – 1 week	0	0	0
>1 week – 2 weeks	0	2.78	0
>2 weeks – 1 month	2.7	5.56	15.38
>1 month	39.19	83.33	76.92

Table 4. Details of sources of water supplies, water accessibility and availability

In urban areas under normal circumstances water was available on the premises and no collection times were applicable. However during periods of water shortages water had to be collected from alternative sources such as boreholes (31%) or water tankers supplied by the municipality (61%). During these time 79% of the respondents said they collected water in the morning, 23% at midday, 35% in the afternoon and 48% said they collected water in the evening.

In 3% of the households it was the responsibility of girls to collect water. Women were responsible for water collection in 30% of the household whilst men were responsible for water collection in 4% of the household. In 10% of the households women and girls were responsible for water collection. Women and boys collected water in 1% of the households and in another 1% it was women and children. The PLWHA collected water in 76% of the households. The main reasons why the PLWHA did not collect water were because they were too weak to do so (67%) or as men they did not consider it their chore (28%).

In peri-urban areas water was collected in the morning in 92% of the households, at midday in 6%, in the afternoon in 20% and in the evening in 36% of the households. Collection was done more than once a day in several households. Women were responsible for water collection in 42% of the households compared to 14% of the households where men were responsible. In 15% of the households women and girls were responsible for water collection. In 8% of the households all family members collected water. In 3% of the households it was women and children who collected water. Women and boys collected water in 2% of the households. The PLWHA collected water in 87% of the households. Where they did not collect water it was mainly because they were too weak to do so (56%) or they were ill at that moment (19%) or as men they did not consider water collection as their chore (19%).

In rural areas water was collected in the morning in 99% of the households, at midday in 17%, in the afternoon in 26% and in the evening in 45% of the households. In most households water was collected more than once a day. Women were responsible for collecting water in 54% of the households. In 10% of the households it was women and girls who collected water. Men were responsible for collecting water in 6% of the households. In 3% of the households all family members collected whilst in another 3% it was women and boys who collected water. Boys collected water in 2% of the households, and in another 2% of the household it was children who collected water. Women and children collected water in 1% of the households. In 81% of the households the PLWHA collected water. The reasons for not colleting water were that they were too weak to do so (46%) or they were ill at that moment (31%) or being men they did not consider it their chore to collect water. In all the areas more women than men were responsible for water collection, and 28% of men who did not collect water considered collecting water not to be one of their chores. This indicated that water collection to some extent remains a gender issue. Even though the majority of the PLWHA in all areas collected water, the fact that some did not do so because they were too weak to do so or they were ill at the time shows their vulnerability if water is not easily accessible.

In urban areas in 29% of the households water for drinking was boiled before it was consumed, compared to 18% in peri-urban areas and 17% in rural areas. The households where drinking water was disinfected with chlorine before consumption were 24% in urban areas, 21.5 in peri-urban areas and 23% in rural areas (Table 5). The disinfectant, in the form of *Aquatabs* (167mg sodium dichloroisocyanurate) was supplied either by the municipality or by some NGO supporting the PLWHA. Allowing the water to stand and settle was used by 8.3% of the peri-urban households, 4.9% of rural households and 0.7% of urban households.

Although the water was kept for long periods of time under sub-optimal conditions, the majority of households did not treat the water before consuming it. Water stored in the home tends to be more contaminated that water at the collection point, suggesting that substantial contamination takes place during transport, storage and use. Those households collecting water from communal supplies must, of necessity transport water to their homes and store it. Those households with water on the premises may have intermittent or poor quality water.

Proper handling and storage and household-level disinfection is therefore necessary to maintain the quality of water (USAID, 2006). It has been observed in a wide variety of settings that water quality improvements at the point-of-use are likely to have a positive impact on health at all levels of the water supply system (USAID, 2006). There are physical and chemical treatments available as interventions to improve the quality of water at the point of use (Sobsey, 2002).

Treatment method	Urban % (n=150)	Peri-urban % (n=121)	Rural % (n=142)
Boiling	29	18	17
Bleach/chlorine	24	21.5	23
Straining with cloth	4	0	0
Filter (sand, ceramic etc)	0	0	1.4
Solar disinfection	0	0	0
Stand and settle	0.7	8.3	4.9

Table 5. Domestic pre-treatment of drinking water

3.6 Total coliform and *Escherichia coli* counts

In urban areas 77% of the hands swabs from PLWHA were positive for total coliforms, compared to 83% and 72% in peri-urban and rural areas respectively. A total of 3% of the hand swabs in urban areas, 10% in peri-urban areas and 17% in rural areas were positive for *E. coli*. In 88% of the urban toilets, 83% of the peri-urban toilets and 73% of the rural toilets the toilet seat swabs were positive for total coliforms. *E. coli* was found in 41% of the urban, 58% of the peri-urban and 42% of the rural toilet seat swabs. The unsatisfactory cleaning of the toilets and the lack of use of disinfectants could be the reason for these results. Toilet seats can be classified as disease transfer points because they are regularly touched by the bare skin of more than one person. The spread of bacteria such as *E. coli* can not be controlled unless a disinfecting process is performed on these surfaces (CDC, 2008).

The results from the study indicated that the water collected from household storage containers was positive for total coliform bacteria in 93% of urban households, 98% of peri-urban households and 89% of rural households. The water samples positive for *E. coli* were 33% in urban areas, 67% in peri-urban and 41% in rural areas. The microbial quality of water did not meet the standards set out in the WHO guidelines which Zimbabwe uses. In all water intended for drinking, treated water entering the distribution system or treated water in the distribution system, total coliform bacteria and *E. coli* must not be detectable in any 100 ml sample (WHO, 2008). These results indicated contamination of the water from a faecal source, indicating indicating that the water might potentially be contaminated with pathogenic microorganisms. This is likely to expose the PLWHA to infection with diarrhoeal diseases and other opportunistic infections (Kamminga and Wegelin-Schuringa, 2003). The quality of drinking water is a well-recognised factor in the transmission route for infectious diarrhoea and other diseases (WHO, 2003).

Sample type	Urban	Peri-urban	Rural
	Number (%)	Number (%)	Number (%)
Hand swabs	24 (77%) n=31	25 (83%) n=30	21 (72%) n=29
Toilet seats	132 (88%) n=150	47 (83%) n=57	88 (73%) n=120
Water storage container	140 (93%) n=150	118 (98%) n=121	127 (89%) n=142

Table 6. Total coliform counts given as colony forming units per 100 ml (cfu/100 ml)

Sample type	Urban	Peri-urban	Rural
	Number (%)	Number (%)	Number (%)
Hand swabs	1 (3%) n=31	3 (10%) n=30	5 (17%) n=29
Toilet seats	61 (41%) n=150	33 (58%) n=57	50 (42%) n=120
Water storage container	50 (33%) n=150	81 (67%) n=121	58 (41%) n=142

Table 7. *E. coli* counts given as colony forming units per 100 ml (cfu/100 ml)

Contamination of water at household levels has been shown to be a risk factor in the transmission of the Hepatitis E virus (DREF, 2008). More than half of the hospital beds in the developing countries are estimated to be occupied by patients suffering from ailments associated with water of poor quality (UNDP, 2006). Improving the quality of water at household level would go a long way in addressing diarrhoeal diseases, particularly amongst PLWHA. The storage conditions and the unhygienic maintenance of containers could have contributed to the poor results.

3.7 Prevalence of pathogenic *Escherichia coli* strains

The one *E. coli* positive sample found from the hand swab samples in urban areas and all three isolates from the peri-urban areas did not test positive for virulence genes virulence genes. In rural areas one of the three *E. coli* positive hand swab samples tested positive for atypical EPEC. The presence of atypical EPEC (which is more frequently isolated from diarrhoea cases than typical EPEC) on the hands of PLWHA indicates the potential risk of contracting diarrhoea.

In toilet seat samples, atypical EPEC was the most prevalent pathogenic *E. coli* strain found in urban areas at 25%, followed by typical EPEC at 24%. EAEC was also fairly prevalent at 18%, with ETEC following at 10%. Almost 83% of *E. coli* strains identified in urban areas were pathogenic, compared to 40% in peri-urban areas and 69% in rural areas. The higher presence of pathogenic *E. coli* strains in urban areas could contribute to higher diarrhoea prevalence.

In household water storage container samples from the urban areas, the most prevalent pathogenic strain was typical EPEC (25.5%), followed by atypical EPEC (11%), EAEC (9.1%), ETEC (0.8%), EHEC (1.8%) and EIEC (1.8%). The remaining 49% of the samples had commensal *E. coli*. In peri-urban water storage samples ETEC was 4.9%, atypical EPEC was 3.7% and EHEC was 2.5%. EAEC was the least prevalent at 1.2%. The rest of the *E. coli* positive samples (87.7%) only had commensal *E. coli* present. In rural areas the most prevalent pathogenic *E. coli* strain detected in water samples was EAEC (14%), followed by atypical EPEC and EHEC (5% each). ETEC was 3.4% and the least prevalent was EIEC at 1.7%.

E. coli from toilet seats could be transferred to water during storage and handling resulting in these poor results, especially with inadequate hand-washing after using the toilet. The presence of pathogenic strains of *E. coli* in water at household level indicated the risk that the PLWHA were exposed to diarrhoeagenic bacteria, reinforcing the need for appropriate household level water supply and storage. Most of the households in all the areas had to store water in their dwellings. In urban areas 99.3% of the households had water stored inside the house, 96% in peri-urban areas and 99.3% in rural areas also stored water inside the house. Those that stored water outside the house were 3.3% in urban areas, 9% in peri-urban areas and 2% in rural areas. A few households stored water both inside the house as well as outside the house. The same containers used for water collection were also used for storage. In most households in the urban and peri-urban areas the same room that was used for water storage was also used for various other uses such as sleeping, cooking and in some cases, even bathing. In general water was not adequately protected from contamination.

Though in most of the households water containers were found clean, both inside and outside of the container, quite a number of household containers were found with either loose particles of dirt inside (27% in urban areas, 40% in peri-urban areas and 43% in rural areas) or with a biofilm (3% in urban areas, 7% in peri-urban areas and 9% in rural areas). The external conditions of containers were found to be unsatisfactory in more than half of the households in all the three areas. In about half of the households in all areas (51% in urban areas, 54% in urban areas and 48% in rural areas) both wide-mouthed containers and those with screw-type mouths were used. In 41% of the urban households, 22% of the peri-urban households and 21% of the rural households, only containers with screw tops were used. Wide mouth bucket type containers were used in 8% of the urban households, 24% of the peri-urban households and 31% of the rural households.

The main water uses mentioned by the respondents in all the areas were cooking, drinking, bathing and laundry, dishwashing and cleaning. Some households in urban areas mentioned toilet flushing as a use whilst some peri-urban households mentioned drinking water for animals as a use. The largest volume of water was used for laundry in most households, however in most cases laundry was done only once or twice a week and in some rural households laundry was done at the water source. Bathing used the second largest amount of water in most of the households in all the areas.

The average total volume of water containers in each urban household was 95 litres. The average actual volume of water found in each household was 87 litres. The average volume used by each urban household was 127 litres per day. Considering that the average family size of an urban household was 5, the per capita per day volume of water used was 25.4 litres, which is satisfactory if the SPHERE project recommended volume of 15 litres per capita per day is used. Even if the average actual volume of water found in each household is used, the volume per capita per day of 17.4 litres is still above the SPHERE recommended standard.

In peri-urban areas the average total volume of water containers in each household was 79 litres and the average actual volume found was 61 litres. The average total volume of water used in each household was 121 litres. The per capita per day volume of water used was 25.7 litres. Based on the actual volume of water found in each household the per capita per day water available was 13 litres, which is below the SPHERE recommended volume.

Each rural household had an average total volume of containers of 70 litres. There was an average of 48 litres of water found in each household. According to the respondents, an

E. coli strain	Hand swab samples			Toilet seat samples			Water storage container samples		
	Urban	Peri-urban	Rural	Urban	Peri-urban	Rural	Urban	Peri-urban	Rural
Commensal E. coli	1 (100%)	3 (100%)	2 (40%)	13 (16.4%)	18 (60%)	16 (31.3%)	27 (49%)	71 (87.7%)	41 (70.7%)
Atypical Enteropathogenic E. coli	0 (0%)	0 (0%)	1 (20%)	19 (24.0%)	2 (6.6%)	7 (13.7%)	6 (11%)	3 (3.7%)	3 (5.2%)
Typical enteropathogenic E. coli (bfp and eae)	0 (0%)	0 (0%)	0 (0%)	20 (25.3%)	0 (0%)	0 (0%)	14 (25.5%)	0 (0%)	0 (0%)
Enterohaemorrhagic E. coli	0 (0%)	0 (0%)	0 (0%)	2 (2.5%)	0 (0%)	1 (1.9%)	1 (1.8%)	2 (2.5%)	3 (5.2%)
Enterotoxigenic E. coli	0 (0%)	0 (0%)	0 (0%)	8 (10.1%)	6 (20%)	3 (5.8%)	1 (1.8%)	4 (4.9%)	2 (3.4%)
Enteroaggregative E. coli	0 (0%)	0 (0%)	2 (40%)	14 (17.7%)	4 (13.3%)	22 (43.1%)	5 (9.1%)	1 (1.2%)	8 (13.8%)
Enteroinvasive E. coli	0 (0%)	0 (0%)	0 (0%)	3 (3.8%)	0 (0%)	2 (3.9%)	1 (1.8%)	0 (0%)	1 (1.7%)

Table 8. Pathogenic E. coli strains detected in hand swabs, toilet seat and water storage container samples

average of 157 litres of water was used in each house every day. Based on this, the per capita per day volume of water used is 30 litres, however based on the average volume of water found in each household, the figure drops to 9.2 litres, far below the SPHERE project recommendation. The water volumes found in the rural house households were the lowest compared to the other areas.

In urban areas in 29% of the households water for drinking was boiled before it was consumed, compared to 18% in peri-urban areas and 17% in rural areas. The households where drinking water was disinfected with chlorine before consumption were 24% in urban areas, 21.5% in peri-urban areas and 23% in rural areas. The disinfectant, in the form of *Aquatabs* (167mg sodium dichloroisocyanurate) was supplied either by the municipality or by some NGO supporting the PLWHA. Allowing the water to stand and settle was used by 8.3% of the peri-urban households, 4.9% of rural households and 0.7% of urban households. Proper handling and storage and household-level disinfection is therefore necessary to maintain the quality of water (USAID, 2006). It has been observed in a wide variety of settings that water quality improvements at the point-of-use are likely to have a positive impact on health at all levels of the water supply system (USAID, 2006). There are physical and chemical treatments available as interventions to improve the quality of water at the point of use (Sobsey, 2002).

4. Conclusions

The presence of total coliforms and *E. coli* in water, toilet seat and hand swab samples was determined using the Colilert® Quanti-Tray/2000 System. Multiplex PCR was used to identify pathogenic strains of *E. coli*. The technique was found to be appropriate in detection of virulence genes to identify various pathogenic *E. coli* strains from water, sanitation and hygiene samples. The presence of total coliforms and *E. coli* in household samples, especially in water samples and hand swabs indicated the potential risk of enteric diseases that the PLWHA are exposed to. Pathogenic *E. coli* strains found in household samples indicated the risks to which PLWHA are exposed to, more so in view of their compromised immune status.

There is therefore need for hygiene education at the household level on the importance of household water storage to prevent contamination. Appropriate household water treatment systems, such as filters or disinfectants are needed, especially in households where there are PLWHA, to ensure that the water is safe for human consumption. The presence of total coliforms in hand swabs was indicative of inadequate hand washing, especially non-use of soap and disinfectants. This increases the potential of faecal-oral transmission of enteric pathogens. Hygiene education on appropriate and effective hand washing needs to be reinforced in all the communities. Adequate cleaning and disinfection of toilets seats, which can be disease transfer points, is needed to reduce the potential of disease transmission.

5. References

AIDS infoNet (2010). AIDS InfoNet Fact Sheet Number 124; CD4 CELL TESTS http://www.aidsinfonet.org/ (accessed 2010-06-02)

CDC (2008) Guideline for Disinfection and Sterilization in Healthcare Facilities, 2008 http://www.cdc.gov/hicpac/pdf/guidelines/Disinfection_Nov_2008.pdf (accessed 2010/06/02)

DREF (2008). Uganda: Hepatitis E Virus (HEV). DREF operation n o MDGRUG009. International Federation of Red Cross and Red Crescent Societies.

Dunker L (2001) The KAP tool for Hygiene. A manual on: knowledge, attitudes and practices in rural areas of South Africa. Water Research Commission Report TT144/00. Water Research Commission, Pretoria, South Africa.

Framm SR and Soave R. (1997). Agents of diarrhea. *Med Clin North Am* 1997; *81:* 427-47.

Janoff EN and Smith PD. (1998) Prospectives on gastrointestinal infections in AIDS. *Gastroenterology Clinics of North America* 1988; *17:* 451-63.

Kamminga E and Wegelin/Schuringa M. (2003) HIV/AIDS and water, sanitation and hygiene. Thematic Overview Paper. Delft: IRC International Water and Sanitation Centre. http://www.irc.nl/page.php/111

Mitra AK, Hernandez CD, Hernandez CA and Siddiq Z. (2001) Management of diarrhea in HIV infected patients. *International Journal of STD & AIDS* 2001; *12:* 630/9.

Omar KB, Potgieter N and Barnard TG (2010) Development of a rapid screening method for the detection of pathogenic Escherichia coli using a combination of Colilert ® Quanti/Trays/2000 and PCR. *Water Science & Technology: Water Supply.* 10.1: 7/13.

Reiff F M, Roses M, Venczel L, Quick R and Witt VM (1996) Low cost safe water for the world: A practical interim solution. *Journal of Public Health Policy* 17, 398-408

Sobsey MD (2002) Managing water in the home: Accelerated health gains from improved water supply. World Health Organization Sustainable Development and Healthy Environments. World Health Organization, Geneva. WHO/SDE/WSH/02.07.

Todar K (2002) Pathogenic *E. coli.* University of Wisconsin/Madison Department of Bacteriology, USA

UNDP (2006) Sharing Innovative Experiences; Examples of Successful Experiences in Providing Safe Drinking Water, United Nations Development Programme, New York, USA

UNICEF (2009). UNICEF – Children and HIV and AIDS – Statistics.http;//www.unicef.org. Accessed March 2011

UNAIDS (2005) Evidence for HIV decline in Zimbabwe: A comprehensive review of the epidemiological data. November 2005.

UNICEF (2005) Water, Sanitation and Hygiene: Common water and sanitation-related diseases. http://www.unicef.org/wash/index_wes_related.html (accessed 2010-03-23)

USAID (2006) Environmental Health, Technical Areas, Hygiene Improvement for Diarrhoeal Disease Prevention, Point-of-use (POU) Water Quality, November 2006.

USAID/WSP (2007) Analysis of Research on the Effects of Improved Water, Sanitation, and Hygiene on the Health of People Living with HIV and AIDS and Programmatic Implications; Prepared by the USAID /Hygiene Improvement Project with the Water and Sanitation Program/World Bank. October 2007.

World Vision (2006) Zimbabwe Emergency Water and Sanitation Program (ZEWSP) Baseline Survey Report: Mangwe, Gwanda and Beitbridge District (Matabeleland South Province)

WHO (2003) Domestic Water Quantity, Service Level and Health. World Health Organisation, Geneva, Switzerland

WHO (2008) Guidelines for Drinking/water Quality THIRD EDITION INCORPORATING
    THE FIRST AND SECOND ADDENDA Volume 1 Recommendations; ISBN 978 92
    4 154761 1; World Health Organisation, Switzerland
WRC (2005). Human rights project workbook 2. WRC report TT 296/07. Water Research
    Commission, Pretoria, South Africa.

4

Toxoplasmosis in HIV/AIDS Patients - A Living Legacy

Veeranoot Nissapatorn
University of Malaya
Malaysia

1. Introduction

The coccidian *Toxoplasma gondii* (*T. gondii*) is a ubiquitous, intracellular, protozoan parasite that causes toxoplasmosis, a cosmopolitan zoonotic disease. *Toxoplasma* infections are reported in approximately half of the world's population but most are asymptomatic. *T. gondii* may serve as one factor that can enhance the immunodeficiency found after HIV-1 infections. Co-infection with other pathogens in humans infected with HIV-1 may enhance the progression of the disease to AIDS (Lin & Bowman, 1992). In concurrence with HIV infection, cerebral toxoplasmosis (CT) occurs primarily due to reactivation of latent *Toxoplasma* infection and is one of the most frequent opportunistic infections, particularly in patients with full-blown AIDS. CT is the most common clinical presentation of toxoplasmosis (Luft & Remington, 1992), and is one of the most frequent causes of focal intracerebral lesions that complicates AIDS (Nissapatorn et al, 2004). CT is undoubtedly a serious life-threatening disease but it is treatable when there is a timely diagnosis and prompt treatment, and there are no other concurrent co-infections. When HIV-infected patients develop CT this poses many diagnostic and therapeutic challenges for clinicians (Israelski & Remington, 1992), particularly in developing countries where the infrastructure is limited but the number of patients infected with HIV is increasing. This chapter focuses on the clinico-epidemiological aspects of toxoplasmosis in HIV/AIDS patients at the time of transition to treatment with highly active anti-retroviral therapy (HAART). The course of toxoplasmosis in HIV/AIDS patients should be able to provide us with a better understanding of the clinical scenario and future management of this so-called "enigmatic parasite" of the tropics.

2. Pathogenesis - from source to host defense mechanism

2.1 Morphology

T. gondii is a coccidian, that is ubiquitous and an obligate intracellular parasite with a complex life cycle and felids are the definitive hosts. There are three infectious stages of *T. gondii* in the environment. Tachyzoites (or endozoites), crescent to oval in shape, are seen in an active infection. They can be transmitted through the placenta from mother to fetus, by blood transfusion, or by organ transplantation. Tissue cysts, containing thousands of bradyzoites, the terminal life cycle stage, are transmitted by eating infected meat or organs, and may persist life-long in an intermediate host. In this stage, they are associated with latent infections, but reactivation occurs in persons who lose their immunity. Bradyzoites (or cystozoites) are less susceptible to chemotherapy and the presence of this infective stage in host tissues is of clinical significance, particularly in immunosuppressed individuals. The oocyst stage, is excreted in the cat's feces, and this most tolerant form of *T. gondii*, is ubiquitous in nature, is highly resistant to disinfectants and environmental influences, as well as playing a key role in transmission through the fecal-oral route.

2.1.1 Life cycle and transmission

The life cycle of *T. gondii* was described in 1970, before it was determined that members of the family Felidae, including domestic cats, were the definitive hosts and warm-blooded animals including most livestock and humans serve as intermediate hosts (Figure 1). In contrast to other protozoans, *T. gondii* is a parasite that can parasitize all mammals. *T. gondii* has a large host range; this parasite can be found throughout the world. *T. gondii* is a common infection in humans; it becomes more important in the field of veterinary and medical infectious diseases. *T. gondii* is a potential organism causing a serious public health hazard due to infected meat-producing animals and a severe economic loss to the livestock owners. *T. gondii* can be transmitted (Figure 2) through one of the following routes (Tenter et al, 2000; Derouin et al, 2008).

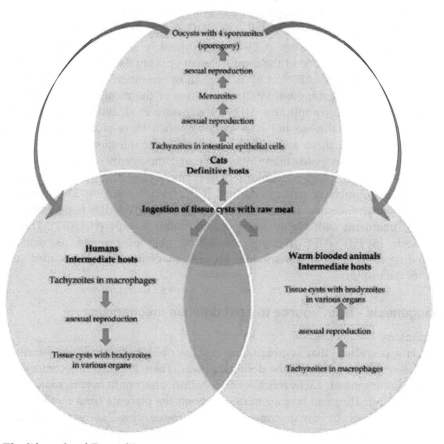

Fig. 1. The life cycle of *T. gondii*.

In the definitive hosts, infection with *T. gondii* occurs following not only ingestion of tissue cysts in under-cooked meat but also after ingesting the rapidly-multiplying tachyzoite forms or the oocysts shed in feces. The cyst wall of *T. gondii* is dissolved by the proteolytic enzymes of both stomach and small intestine, releasing the slowly-multiplying bradyzoite form. The asexual cycle begins after the invasion of *T. gondii* into the epithelial cells of the small intestine. While, the sexual cycle is very specific and occurs only in the gut epithelial cells of feline species. The oocyst forms are produced by gamete fusion and are then shed in the feces of the definitive hosts. These oocysts are highly infective to other definitive and intermediate hosts once they are in contact with a susceptible environment (Frenkel, 1973). The oocysts of *T. gondii* are less infective and pathogenic in the definitive host (cat) as compared with intermediate hosts (mice, pigs, humans) (Dubey, 1998).

In intermediate hosts, *T. gondii* undergoes two phases of asexual development. The infective stages (sporozoites or bradyzoites) transform into tachyzoites following *Toxoplasma* infection of the intestinal epithelial cells. In the first phase, tachyzoites multiply rapidly by repeated endodyogeny in an intracellular parasitophorous vacuole in many different types of host cells. The second phase develops from the tachyzoites of the last generation and results in tissue cysts (Tenter et al, 2000). Within the tissue cyst, bradyzoites multiply slowly by endodyogeny. Tissue cysts have a high affinity for neural and muscular tissues and are located mainly in the central nervous system (CNS), eye, skeletal and cardiac muscles as well as other visceral organs (Dubey et al, 1998). Tissue cysts break down periodically, with bradyzoites transforming into tachyzoites that reinvade host cells and again transform to bradyzoites within new tissue cysts (Dubey, 1998).

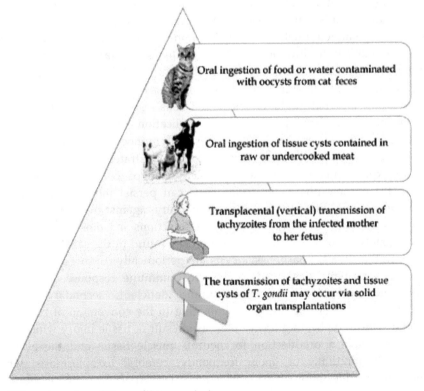

Fig. 2. The different routes of *T. gondii* transmission.

2.1.2 *T. gondii* antigens, host defense mechanisms and cerebral toxoplasmosis

In patients with AIDS, tissue cysts rupture and the released bradyzoites may multiply locally and spread to other organs. Infected patients may have serious complications or even death from symptomatic toxoplasmosis. The pathology of *Toxoplasma* infection is due to the invasion process initiating the lytic cycle that consequently leads to cell and tissue destruction. In the host cell cytoplasm, *T. gondii* induces the formation of a parasitophorous vacuole that contains secretions of both parasite and host proteins that normally promote phagosome maturation, , and thereby prevent lysosome fusion (Dubey et al, 1998; Carruthers, 2002). Despite this rapid, dynamic and significant process, there are very few secretory proteins that have so far been discovered (Zhou et al, 2005). These proteins (antigens) are essential components for low-grade stimulation that boosts the immune system. These antigens have been shown to stimulate antibody production as well as a T-cell response (Carruthers, 2002).

T. gondii excretory/secretory antigens (ESAs) represent the majority of the circulating antigens in host sera of patients with acute toxoplasmosis (Pereira-Chioccola et al, 2009). ESAs include the tachyzoite, sporozoite and encysted bradyzoite stages (Tilley et al, 1997). The secretions by the bradyzoite cysts maintain a long-lasting immunity to *T. gondii* (Cesbron-Delauw & Capron, 1993). The ESAs released by tachyzoites are highly immunogenic (Prigione et al, 2000; Carruthers, 2002) and may induce either antibody dependent or cell mediated immunity (Costa-Silva et al, 2008). Anti-ESA antibodies develop in high titers when circulating blood tachyzoites are present in AIDS-associated CT patients (Meira et al, 2008). *Toxoplasma* infection results in pathological changes such as inflammation and is usually followed by necrosis. This parasitic infection also induces strong type 1 polarized innate and adaptive immune responses. It is known that the host defense mechanism to infection with *T. gondii* is mediated by production of pro-inflammatory cytokines, including IL-12, IFN-γ and TNF-α (Suzuki et al, 1989). The important sources of IFN-γ in response to *Toxoplasma* infection are CD4-T lymphocytes, CD8-T lymphocytes, natural killer cells and T cells responding to IL-12 (Yap et al, 2000). These major mechanisms prevent rapid replication of tachyzoites and subsequent pathological changes (Denkers, 2003). Of these, T lymphocytes are a crucial source of IFN-γ during the first 2-3 weeks after infection, as demonstrated in antibody-mediated T-cell depletion experiments that resulted in reactivation of *Toxoplasma* infection (Denkers, 2003). In the chronic phase, the tissue cysts can persist indefinitely in the brain and muscle, developing lifelong protective immunity against re-infection (Dubey, 1998; Montoya & Liesenfeld, 2004). There are re-infections in some cases because slightly different genotypes of *T. gondii* strains have been found in the same patients (Ferreira et al, 2008). In the clinical phase, tissue cysts are periodically ruptured, but the bradyzoites released are normally destroyed by the host immune response. At the time when asymptomatic individuals become immune deficient, secondary reactivation of latent/chronic infection may occur, culminating in the conversion of bradyzoites to the active and rapidly replicating tachyzoites, as a result of tissue injury which is often fatal. As the cysts have a predilection for neural, muscle tissue and the eye, most cases reactivate chorioretinitis or, more frequently, cerebral toxoplasmosis, which is the predominant manifestation in patients with AIDS. Apart from these mechanisms, the development of cerebral toxoplasmosis has recently been studied and shown to have a significant correlation with the HLA genes (class I and class II) in HIV-infected patients. The MHC is one of the most polymorphic genetic systems in humans and controls the adaptive immune response by class I (HLA-A, HLA-B, HLA-Cw) and class II (HLA-DRB1, HLA-DQB1, HLA-DPB1) against both intra-and extracellular microorganisms as well as it being correlated with infection susceptibility or resistance. Class I HLA-B35 antigen was associated with retinochoroiditis (Veronese Rodrigues et al, 2004). Class I HLA-B8 and class II HLA-DRB1*17 antigens were associated with cerebral toxoplasmosis (Castro Figueiredo et al, 2000). The presence of class II HLA-DQB1*0402 and DRB1*08 alleles (Habegger de Sorrentino et al, 2005) and the HLA-DR52 haplotype represent risk factors to the development of cerebral toxoplasmosis, whereas the HLA-DR53 haplotype was associated with resistance to *Toxoplasma* infection (Pereira-Chioccola et al, 2009).

Among patients with AIDS, CT is a multifocal process that occurs spontaneously. The use of the highly sensitive technique of magnetic resonance imaging (MRI) reveals that >80% of patients will have multiple lesions (Ciricillo & Rosenblum, 1990). With this technique, the percentages are probably an underestimation of the multifocal pathological process that may be occurring as they will be below its resolution. The spontaneous and simultaneous development of multifocal brain lesions strongly indicates that although CT arises because of reactivation of a latent infection, the multiple areas of the brain that are involved are likely a result of the hematogenous spread of the parasite, and involvement of the brain is due to the particular proclivity of *T. gondii* for causing disease in the CNS (Luft & Remington, 1992). The latter is likely due to the fact that the brain is an immunologically original site rather than an actual site of the organism. This supposition is further supported by the observation that patients who relapse after receiving an adequate course of therapy often develop new lesions in areas of the brain previously free of infection (Leport et al, 1989).

3. Epidemiology - from source to gene

The high rates of latent *Toxoplasma* infection (41.9–72%) were reported in South America and in approximately half of the studies (≥ 40%) from the Asian continent. In North America, however, the rate of *Toxoplasma* infection was low. Surprisingly, only 8 of the 50 studies were conducted on HIV-infected pregnant women and 2 of those studies, interestingly, reported a very high seroprevalence of toxoplasmosis of 53.7% in Thailand and 72% in Brazil. Latent toxoplasmosis is still prevalent as an infection that coexists with HIV infection. The level of anti-*Toxoplasma* (IgG) antibodies was, interestingly, unaffected by either antiretroviral drugs or therapeutic regimes/prophylaxis used for toxoplasmosis in these patients (Machala et al, 2009). Supporting these epidemiological studies, screening for *Toxoplasma* infection should be included in routine investigations in order to monitor primary infections even though it is not very common in such patients. It may also prevent secondary reactivation of latent infections, especially in HIV-infected patients with limited resource settings where the majority are unable to access primary chemoprophylaxis and/or antiretroviral therapy.

How do the plausible risk factors play their roles in association with *Toxoplasma* infection in HIV-infected patients? Age and race/ethnicity, among other demographic characteristics, were shown to have a positive interaction with this parasite. A study from the United States demonstrated that *Toxoplasma* prevalence rates reported in HIV-infected women aged ≥ 50 years were significantly higher compared to those who were younger (Falusi et al, 2002). This was dissimilar to a study from Malaysia which reported that HIV-infected patients in the younger age group had higher *Toxoplasma* seroprevalence rates than the older age group although it was not statistically significant (Nissapatorn et al, 2001). Based on these findings, *Toxoplasma* infection is acquired irrespective of age, and preventive measures are needed to curb the prevalence rate especially in areas where the parasite is highly endemic. The study by Falusi and colleagues in 2001 further pointed out that those women born outside the U.S. were more likely to have higher rates of latent toxoplasmosis although race did not affect *Toxoplasma* seroprevalence between black and white women in that country (Falusi et al, 2002). In a country like Malaysia, a higher rate of *Toxoplasma* infection was more likely to be found among Malays, the predominant ethnic group in this region compared to others including Chinese and Indian (Nissapatorn et al, 2007). Traditionally, Malays keep cats as pets, which could explain this association. Based on these studies, demographic characteristics certainly make significant contributions to the epidemiological surveillance of *Toxoplasma* infection in a given population, such as HIV/AIDS patients.

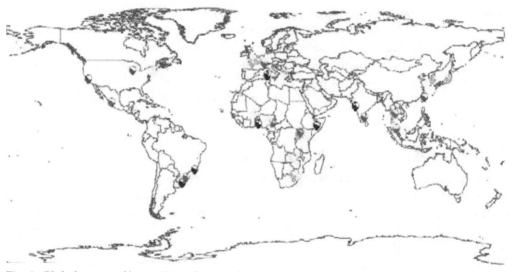

Fig. 3. Global status of latent *Toxoplasma* infection in HIV-infected patients.

Dark red equals prevalence above 60%, light red equals 40-60%, yellow 20-40%, blue 10-20% and green equals prevalence <10%. White equals absence of data. (Courtesy of Dr. Rattanasinchaiboon O and Dr Phumkokrux S, Bangkok, Thailand.)

There are not many studies on how the T-cell response could affect *Toxoplasma*-seropositive patients. It has been recognized that T-helper (CD4) cells, among several types of T-cell responses, are involved in *Toxoplasma* infection by stimulating T-cytotoxic cells which are then able to lyse tachyzoites directly and participate in the activation of B-cells which then go on to produce antibodies against *Toxoplasma* (Ho-Yen, 1992.). An earlier study showed that there is a greater likelihood of problems with *Toxoplasma* infection in situations in which there is a reduction of T-cell function (Pendry et al, 1990). Supporting this literature, a U.S.

study demonstrated a significant association between CD4 counts of 200-499 cells/mm^3 and *Toxoplasma*-seropositivity in patients (Falusi et al, 2002). The authors were unable to provide an explanation for this association except that patients with low CD4 counts were more likely to be foreign born. So far, similar findings have not been reported from previous studies (Nissapatorn et al, 2001; Nissapatorn et al, 2002). Looking at other possible risk factors such as a history of close contact with cats, consumption of contaminated meat, and receiving blood transfusions from *Toxoplasma*-seropositive patients, there was however no significant association found from studies reported earlier (Wallace et al, 1993; Nissapatorn et al, 2001; Nissapatorn et al, 2002). This possibly explains that these patients had been constantly exposed to *Toxoplasma* infections (with no definite time frame) before acquiring HIV infection. The other reason is that patients acquired *Toxoplasma* infection from other sources such as eating raw vegetables or drinking contaminated water, risk factors that were not included in these studies. However, primary behavioral practice such as avoiding close contact with cats, consumption of clean and properly cooked foods is necessary and advisable for HIV-infected patients regardless of *Toxoplasma* serostatus. Interestingly, patients with *Toxoplasma*-seropositivity were more likely to develop CT and tended to be patients receiving HAART (Nissapatorn et al, 2007). From this observation, primary chemoprophylaxis or antiretroviral drugs including HAART (if available) should be instituted to these patients after clinical evaluation.

Apart from the host immune status, the genotype of the infecting parasites may influence the course of disease (Lindström et al, 2006). Genetic analyses have shown that the vast majority of all *T. gondii*-strains typed to date fall into one of three clonal lineages, type I, II, and III (Howe & Sibley, 1995), which differ in virulence but do not show clear host or geographic boundaries (Lindström et al, 2006). Studies from different parts of the world have produced similar findings in which the genotyping of the SAG2-locus revealed that the type II allele was the most disease-causing strain (reactivation of chronic infections) found in immunocompromised individuals (Dardé et al, 1992; Howe and Sibley, 1995; Howe et al, 1997; Fuentes et al, 2001; Lindström et al, 2006; Ajzenberg et al, 2009).

This high prevalence of type II strains in human toxoplasmosis may simply reflect the source of the strains that led to human infections (Howe et al, 1997). Also, the low level of gamma interferon and other factors related to the immune system in these patients might increase the possibility of reactivation of the infective forms of the parasite by developing bradyzoites and increasing the formation of cysts in the brain (Gross et al, 1997). During this same period, a few studies have reported on uncommon type I strains (Khan et al, 2005), type I/III (Genot et al, 2007), and a high rate of genetic polymorphism (Ferreira et al, 2008) in *T. gondii* strains isolated from immunocompromised patients. Despite these differences, genotyping studies could serve as an important mile-stone for improving the diagnosis and management of human toxoplasmosis, in addition, for the development of novel drugs and vaccines. Surprisingly, genotyping studies on *T. gondii* strains have not been reported from HIV-infected patients in the Asian continent even though there are a number of these patients, in endemic areas for latent *Toxoplasma* infections (Subsai et al, 2006; Nissapatorn et al, 2007), and cases of clinical toxoplasmosis detected in AIDS patients (Subsai et al, 2006; Lian et al, 2007). Future studies are recommended to elucidate the distribution of genotypes and to establish any correlations between genotyping of *T. gondii* strains and human toxoplasmosis in Asian HIV patients.

Based on these findings, it certainly poses a question as to whether there is an association between genotyping of *T. gondii* strains and human toxoplasmosis. One study interestingly indicates that the type of infecting parasitic strain does not predominantly influence the pathogenesis of toxoplasmosis in immunocompromised patients and fully support the need for specific prophylaxis in patients infected by *T. gondii*, regardless of the strain genotype (Honoré et al, 2000). In addition, other host factors are more involved than parasite factors in patients' resistance or susceptibility to toxoplasmosis in immunocompromised hosts (Ajzenberg et al, 2009).

A total of 50 studies have been reported from different parts of the world including Asia, Europe, North America, South America and Africa (Table 1). The varying seroprevalence of toxoplasmosis (latent/chronic infection) interestingly showed low to high rates of infection being >60% (9 studies), 40-60%, (12 studies), 20-40% (21 studies), 10-20% (3 studies), and <10% (5 studies).

Study (Ref)	City, Country	No. of HIV/AIDS patients	Seroprevalence in %
Asia			
Wongkamchai et al, 1995	Bangkok, Thailand	40	42.5
Meisheri et al, 1997	Bombay, India	89	67.8
Yoong and Cheong, 1997	Kuala Lumpur, Malaysia	49	59.0
Chintana et al, 1998	Bangkok, Thailand	253 (pregnancy)	21.1
Sukthana et al, 2000	Bangkok, Thailand	190	23.2
Oh et al, 1999	Seoul, South Korea	173	4.0
Nissapatorn et al, 2001	Bangkok, Thailand	183	22.4
Shivaprakash et al, 2001	Pondicherry, India	216	11.5 (IgM)
Wanachiwanawin et al, 2001	Bangkok, Thailand	838 (pregnancy)	53.7
Shamilah et al, 2001	Kuala Lumpur, Malaysia	729	31.3
Nissapatorn et al, 2002	Kuala Lumpur, Malaysia	100	21.0
Nissapatorn et al, 2003	Kuala Lumpur, Malaysia	406	51.2
Nissapatorn et al, 2004	Kuala Lumpur, Malaysia	505	44.8
Hung et al, 2005	Taipei, Taiwan	844	10.2
Nissapatorn et al, 2005	Kuala Lumpur, Malaysia	162	35.8 and 14.8 (IgM)
Naito et al, 2007	Tokyo, Japan	56	5.40
Nissapatorn et al, 2007	Kuala Lumpur, Malaysia	693	43.85
Nissapatorn et al, [In print]	Songkhla, Thailand	300	36.3
Europe			
Holliman, 1990	London, UK	500	26.6 and 1.4 (IgM)
Sykora et al, 1992	Prague, Czechoslovakia	67	29.8

Study (Ref)	City, Country	No. of HIV/AIDS patients	Seroprevalence in %
Zufferey et al, 1993	Lausanne, Switzerland	715	50.0
Oksenhendler et al, 1994	Villejuif, France	499	25.4
Raffi et al, 1997	Nantes cedex, France	186	97
Bossi et al, 1998	Paris, France	399	97
Letillois et al, 1995	Grenoble, France	37	64.9
Reiter-Owona et al, 1998	Bon, Germany	183	33.3 (in 1987) and 36.6 (in 1995)
Millogo et al, 2000	Burkina Faso, France	1,828	25.4
Machala et al, 2009	Prague, Czech Republic	626	33.2
North America			
Grant et al, 1990	New York, USA	411	32.0
Israelski et al, 1993	California, USA	1,073	11.0
Minkoff et al, 1997	Brooklyn, USA	138	20.2
Ruiz et al, 1997	Rhode Island, USA	169 (pregnancy)	22.0
Falusi et al, 2002	Chicago, USA	1,975	15.1
South America			
Wainstein et al, 1993	RS, Brazil	516	65 and 49 (CSF)
Galván Ramirez et al, 1997	Universidad de Guadalajara, Mexico	92	50.0 and 1.0 (IgM)
Cruz et al, 2007	RJ, Brazil	767 (pregnancy)	74.0
Lago et al, 2009	Rio Grande do Sul, Brazil	168 (pregnancy)	72.0
Africa			
Brindle et al, 1991	Kenya, Nairobi	94	22
Zumla et al, 1991	Zambia and Uganda	373 (186-Uganda and 187-Zambia)	34 (Ugandan) and 4 (Zambian)
Woldemichael et al, 1998	Addis Ababa, Ethiopia	127	74.2
Maïga et al, 2001	Bamako, Mali	?	22.6 and 60
Uneke et al, 2005	Jos, Nigeria	219	38.8
Lindström et al, 2006	Kampala, Uganda	130	54
Hari et al, 2007	Johannesburg, South Africa	307	8
Ouermi et al, 2009	Burkina faso, agadougou	138 (pregnancy)	31.9 and 3.6 (IgM)
Akanmu et al, 2010	Lagos, Nigeria	380	54
Sitoe et al, 2010	Maputo, Mozambique	58 (pregnancy)	31.3
Oshinaike et al, 2010	Lagos, Idi Araba, Nigeria	83	85.5

Table 1. Summary of studies on seroprevalence of toxoplasmosis in HIV-infected patients.

4. Toxoplasmosis - from epidemiology to clinical implication

4.1 Congenital toxoplasmosis

Seven of the 50 studies were conducted on HIV-infected pregnant women, 2 reported a high seroprevalence, 53.7% in Thailand (Wanachiwanawin et al, 2001) and 74% in Brazil (Cruz et al, 2007). Considering these epidemiological studies (Table 1), geographical location, environment, socio-economic, clinical and diagnostic methods are among the factors that can pin point the differences of *Toxoplasma* infections between these affected areas. Latent toxoplasmosis is still prevalent and coexists with HIV infections. The level of anti-*Toxoplasma* (IgG) antibodies does not appear to be affected by antiretroviral drugs or therapeutic regimes/prophylaxis used to treat toxoplasmosis in these patients (Machala et al, 2009). Given the results of these epidemiological studies, screening for *Toxoplasma* serostatus should be carried out among HIV-infected women in the prenatal period even though it is not a common practice. It may also prevent secondary reactivation of latent toxoplasmosis during pregnancy, especially among HIV-infected women in limited resource settings where the majority of these patients are unable to access primary chemoprophylaxis and/or antiretroviral therapy.

In HIV-infected pregnant women, a secondary reactivation of chronic *Toxoplasma* infection may occur during pregnancy particularly in those who are severely immunocompromised. There are cases of cerebral toxoplasmosis reported in HIV-infected pregnant women and congenital toxoplasmosis in the fetus of these infected mothers but it is found only at a low incidence (Dunn et al, 1997). A case of CT was earlier reported in an HIV-infected pregnant woman who responded well with a standard regimen of pyrimethamine and sulfadiazine, with a normal fetal outcome (Hedriana et al, 1993). Another case of CT was confirmed in an HIV-infected pregnant woman during the puerperium with her CD4 count being < 200 cells/cumm (Biedermann et al, 1995). A prophylactic treatment was recommended to prevent maternal reactivation and congenital transmission of toxoplasmosis in such a case. In recent years, an HIV-infected pregnant woman with CT who was at risk for transmitting HIV (low CD4 and high viral load) and *Toxoplasma* infections to her fetus; she responded well to anti-*Toxoplasma* therapy and HAART (Nogueira et al, 2002). In this case, the combined *Toxoplasma* therapy (pyrimethamine and sulfadiazine) and HAART were benefitial not only to the mother but also prevented transmission to the fetus. Despite this evidence of success in most cases, there have been reports of poor outcomes when an HIV-infected mother has CT during pregnancy, with vertical transmission of one or both infections to the fetus and an increase of morbidity and mortality in the mother (Mitchell et al, 1990; O'Riordan & Farkas, 1998; Fernandes et al, 2009). Maternal-fetal transmission of toxoplasmosis due to reactivation of chronic infection during pregnancy occurs in mothers with a very low CD4 cell counts (Minkoff et al, 1997) or in the presence of other immunological disorders (Montoya & Liesenfeld, 2004). A case of severe congenital toxoplasmosis was reported from an HIV-infected mother with moderate immunosuppression as a result of reactivation (Bachmeyer et al, 2006). This indicates that a routine screening for not only children from HIV-infected mothers should be used to detect congenital toxoplasmosis but also in pregnant women to confirm an early diagnosis of a reactivation of a chronic *Toxoplasma* infection. The first case of congenital toxoplasmosis was reported in Brazil, this was from an HIV-infected mother with a high titer of IgG but negative for IgM antibodies (Cruz et al, 2007). This highlights the special attention needed for analysis of maternal titers of anti-*Toxoplasma* antibody during HIV prenatal care. Two years later, a contrasting study reported a case of congenital toxoplasmosis in an HIV-infected pregnant woman with a low titer of IgG to *T. gondii* and a negative result for IgM antibodies (Lago et al, 2009). It is important to keep this in mind that a high titer for IgG antibody is fairly common in HIV-infected mothers. This phenomenon is not significantly associated with an increased risk of congenitally acquired toxoplasmosis during pregnancy. Compliance to antiretroviral therapy is a medical challenge which led to a rare case of congenital toxoplasmosis from a severely immunosuppressed HIV-infected woman as a result of reactivation (Fernandes et al, 2009). Under this circumstance, prophylaxis is required in addition for strict adherence to therapy in pregnant women infected with HIV. The most recent cases of congenital toxoplasmosis were reported from HIV-infected mothers who had a high titer for IgG and were negative for IgM antibodies (Azevedo et al, 2010). Due to the increasing number of HIV- infected women in childbearing age worldwide, the possibility of maternal-fetal transmission from mothers infected with chronic *Toxoplasma* infection is more likely to occur and may have a huge impact on public health perspectives, especially in those endemic areas with *Toxoplasma* infection. It is surprising that there has been no reported case of clinically confirmed congenital toxoplasmosis or CT in HIV-infected pregnant women from Asian countries. In fact, HIV infection is fast growing in this region compared to other parts of the world. This could be explained either because of the overall low prevalence of toxoplasmosis in HIV-infected women or those cases of toxoplasmosis are under-reporting. Therefore, clinicians should be more aware of this parasitic infection to establish an early diagnosis and better management in both qualities of care and treatment among HIV-infected pregnant women in this continent. To conclude, HIV and *Toxoplasma* infections are common in developing countries with resource limited settings, it is therefore imperative that drugs related to both infections are easily accessible particularly for pregnant women living in low-socio-economic conditions. Due to the effectiveness of anti-*Toxoplasma* therapy and increasing global availability of HAART in HIV-infected pregnant women, the incidence of congenital toxoplasmosis should decline or even disappear.

4.2 Cerebral toxoplasmosis

Neurological complications of AIDS patients are often due to opportunistic infections (OIs) in the central nervous system (CNS). Toxoplasmosis is one of the most common CNS-OIs and causes high rates of morbidity and mortality in patients with advanced HIV infection. With the advent of the HIV pandemic, epidemiological studies have shown CT to be one of the most common OIs in AIDS patients and the most commonly reported CNS-OIs on 5 continents: Asia (India, Malaysia and Thailand), Europe (France, United Kingdom and Germany), North America (USA), South America (Brazil and Mexico), and recently from South Africa (Amogne et al, 2006; Oshinaike et al, 2010). The incidence of CT varies according to geographical locations and the prevalence of *Toxoplasma* infections in the general population. Other factors such as the mode of transmission, gender, ethnicity, severe immunodeficiency, and differences in genotypes of *T. gondii* isolates are also found to influence the occurrence of CT (Richards et al, 1995; Khan et al, 2005). In the pre-HAART era, ~25% of AIDS patients from France had CT compared to ~10% in some cities from the USA (Dal Pan & McArthur, 1996). The rate of CT was found to vary from between 16-40%

in the USA and UK, ~60% in Spain, 50-80% in Brazil, 75-90% in France (Pereira-Chioccola et al, 2009), and <20% in Asian countries including India (Sharma et al, 2004), Malaysia (Nissapatorn et al, 2003-2007), or Thailand (Anekthananon et al, 2004; Subsai et al, 2004). CT is frequently diagnosed in adults but rarely occurs in children with AIDS; the infection accounted for 0.86% of AIDS-defining illnesses (Richards et al, 1995) or <1.0 per 100 person years (Dankner et al, 2001; Gupta et al, 2009). CT is the most common cause of focal intracerebral lesion(s) in patients with AIDS. More than 95% of CT is caused by the reactivation of latent (chronic) *Toxoplasma* infection as a result of the progressive loss of cellular immunity in AIDS patients (Luft & Remington, 1988). In clinical practice, the incidence of CT patients is related both to *Toxoplasma* IgG seropositivity and the CD4 cell count. The risk of developing CT among seropositive patients with AIDS was 27 times that of seronegative ones (Oksenhendler et al, 1994). AIDS patients who are *Toxoplasma* seropositive, have CD4 count of <100 cells/cumm, and failure to receive prophylaxis are among the identified risk of developing CT (Luft and Remington, 1992; Nascimento et al, 2001; Nissapatorn et al, 2004). The clinical presentations of CT depend on the number of lesions and location. Headache, hemiparesis and seizure (Nissapatorn et al, 2004; Vidal et al, 2005a) are among the most common neurological presentations found in CT patients. Other clinical manifestations include disarthria, movement disorders, memory and cognitive impairments and neuropsychiatric abnormalities. These neurological deficits remain in surviving patients even after good clinical response to therapy (Hoffmann et al, 2007). More than 50% of CT patients may have focal neurological findings. CT is a life-threatening but treatable condition provided there is early diagnosis and treatment. CT can be prevented by primary behavioral practices in avoiding acquisition of *Toxoplasma* infection such as consumption of well cooked meat, avoiding close contact with stray cats, contaminated soil and/or water, and receiving unscreened blood transfusions. Compliance to both therapeutic regimens for treatment and prophylaxis of toxoplasmosis is an imperative to prevent relapse of CT in areas where HAART is not fully accessible for people living with HIV/AIDS. This ultimately reduces the number of hospital admissions as well as the mounting medical care cost of AIDS-associated CT patients, particularly in limited resource settings.

There are atypical/unusual clinical manifestations reported in AIDS-associated CT patients. Ventriculitis and obstructive hydrocephalus, characteristics of congenital toxoplasmosis, are rarely seen in adult AIDS-associated CT. Ventriculitis has so far been reported in nine adult AIDS patients (Cota et al, 2008), accompanied by hydrocephalus, occurred as the primary manifestations of toxoplasmosis or as complications of a preexisting, recognized cerebral toxoplasmosis. In addition, hydrocephalus without mass lesions was the only abnormal finding from a computed tomography (CAT) scan in an adult AIDS patient (Nolla-Salas et al, 1987). It is very rare for patients with CT to present as a neuropsychiatric illness with an acute psychosis followed by a rapid mental and somatic decline, however one case has been reported in a patient with AIDS (Ilniczky et al, 2006). Extrapyramidal movement disorders are one of the atypical clinical manifestations reported in AIDS patients. Toxoplasmosis is one of the main underlying opportunistic infections and causes movement disorders in AIDS patients. These movement disorders are becoming well known and increasingly recognized as a potential neurological complication in AIDS patients (Tse et al, 2004). In hyperkinetic movements, holmes (also known as rubral or midbrain tremor) tremor is the earliest reported symptom of CT and might present with other focal neurological signs that indicates a midbrain localization (Koppel & Daws, 1980). The appearance of hemichorea-hemiballism is considered as a pathognomonic of CT and is most commonly associated with a subthalamic abscess (Navia et al, 1986; Maggi et al, 1996). The presence of hemichorea-hemiballism in CT patients is low (7.4% of cases) compared to the pathological studies which show 50% of *Toxoplasma* abscesses occur in the basal ganglia (Navia et al, 1986; Maggi et al, 1996). Generalized chorea may occur as a result of bilateral abscesses of toxoplasmosis (Gallo et al, 1996). Myoclonus, is generalized and elicited by sudden auditory stimuli that resembles a startled response, has also been described in AIDS-associated CT patients (Maher et al, 1997). A case of focal dystonia of the left arm and hand has been reported in an AIDS patient due to the right lenticular nucleus and thalamic abscesses of toxoplasmosis (Tolge & Factor, 1991). A few cases with parkinsonian features, hypokinetic movement disorders, due to toxoplasmosis were also described in patients with AIDS (Carrazana et al, 1989; Murakami et al, 2000). Movement disorders in AIDS patients and particularly in countries with a high prevalence of toxoplasmosis, should indicate the possibility of CT (Noël et al, 1992). In AIDS patients, opportunistic infections may affect endocrine organs. Diabetes insipidus (DI) is uncommon but has also been reported in relation to CT. Imaging studies may demonstrate pathological situations and assist in the diagnosis (Brändle et al, 1995). A case of CT with massive intracerebral hemorrhage leading to a fatal vehicular crash was also reported in a patient with AIDS (Gyori & Hyma, 1998). Cerebellar toxoplasmosis is another infrequent complication of HIV/AIDS that should prompt a high index of clinical suspicion and early institution for presumptive therapy in poor resource settings (Emeka et al, 2010). These unusual neurological presentations of AIDS patients associated toxoplasmosis have rarely been reported in Asia (Chaddha et al, 1999; Nissapatorn et al, 2004; Subsai et al, 2006; Nissapatorn et al, 2007).

4.3 Extracerebral toxoplasmosis
Overall, the prevalence of extracerebral toxoplasmosis (ECT) in patients with AIDS is estimated to be 1.5%-2% (Rabaud et al, 1994) which is far less common than CNS toxoplasmosis. Ocular toxoplasmosis (OT) is the most common form of ECT associated with CT, being detected in 50% of ECT in AIDS patients and has the best prognosis (Rabaud et al, 1994; Zajdenweber et al, 2005). OT, in contrast to intracranial disease, is uncommon in patients with AIDS (Lamichhane et al, 2010). However, OT is a serious eye problem in HIV-infected patients, especially in developing countries (Chakraborty, 1999). OT is an important disorder and may be the first manifestation of life-threatening intracranial or disseminated *T. gondii* infections. Accurate diagnosis may allow early referral to a neurologist and infectious diseases specialist (Holland et al, 1988). Generally, OT tends to cause retinochoroidal scars with less retinal pigment epithelium hyperplasia (Arevalo et al, 1997). It has no association between the ocular findings and a positive titer of toxoplasmosis (Mansour, 1990.). However, the presence of IgM antibodies may support this diagnosis, although antibody levels in AIDS patients may not reflect the magnitude of the disease (Gagliuso et al, 1990). OT was first reported in 2 of 34 AIDS patients with a 'cotton wool' spot as one of the most common retinal manifestations (Schuman & Friedman, 1983). It is also characterized by several features, including single or multifocal retinal lesions in one or both eyes or massive areas of retinal necrosis. These lesions that are not associated with a pre-existing retinochoroidal scar indicate a manifestation of acquired rather than congenital

disease (Gagliuso et al, 1990). A unique pattern of bilateral retinitis due to OT was observed in a patient in the late stages of AIDS in which the recognition of this pattern is important for providing the appropriate treatment of an immunosuppressed patient (Berger et al, 1993). Toxoplasmosis should therefore be considered in the differential diagnosis in an AIDS patient with necrotizing retinitis (Moorthy et al, 1993). There have been few studies reported on toxoplasmosis as being one of the most common causes of neuro-ophthalmological disorders in neurologically symptomatic HIV-infected patients such as palsy involving the sixth and third cranial nerves (Mwanza et al, 2004). Thus, clinicians should be more aware of this pathogen to avoid consequences, such as damaging visual pathways leading to visual impairment or blindness in these patients. With more affordable and accessibility of HAART, the prevalence of ocular toxoplasmosis will decline over time.

Toxoplasmosis is known to cause widely disseminated and extracerebral disease which is less common and more difficult to diagnose in AIDS patients. *Toxoplasma*-induced cystitis or pseudoneoplastic bullous cystitis is rarely detected in these patients. The diagnosis may be difficult because this condition is associated with misleading radiologic and endoscopic findings (Welker et al, 1994). With these studies, the diagnosis was eventually confirmed by the presence of *Toxoplasma* cysts on histopathological examination of bladder biopsies (Hofman et al, 1993). Therefore, disseminated toxoplasmosis should be considered in the differential diagnosis of AIDS patients with culture-negative cystitis (Welker et al, 1994). For unclear reasons, gastrointestinal involvement is exceedingly rare and occurs only in the context of severe immunosuppression and disseminated disease (Merzianu et al, 2005). Gastric toxoplasmosis has been reported in AIDS patients. It presents as diarrheoa and other nonspecific GI symptoms. Biopsy shows the presence of *Toxoplasma* trophozoites in the forms of tachyzoites, bradyzoites, and pseudocysts which are mandatory for definite diagnosis. It responds well to anti-*Toxoplasma* therapy (Alpert et al, 1996; Merzianu et al, 2005). It is of interest, that disseminated toxoplasmosis with sepsis has also been found in AIDS patients and should be considered in patients with sepsis of unknown origin (Artigas et al, 1994). ECT has also been diagnosed in the heart (Guerot et al, 1995; Chimenti et al, 2007), lung (Touboul et al, 1986; Kovari et al, 2010), liver (Mastroianni et al, 1996), and spinal cord (Harris et al, 1990; Kung et al, 2011). ECT has a low incidence in AIDS patients. Many HIV-infected patients lack access to primary chemoprophylaxis and antiretroviral therapy, in limited resource settings hence, more cases are reported in this group.

5. Neuropathology of toxoplasmosis: from pre to HAART era

Toxoplasmosis is an important opportunistic infection, causing short-term and chronic mortality (Neuen-Jacob et al, 1993; Kumarasamy et al, 2010). Multifocal necrotizing encephalitis is the predominant neuropathological finding of CT in AIDS patients. Localization of multiple with ring enhancing lesions on neuroimaging in basal ganglia, frontoparietal cortex and thalamus suggests haematogenous spread. The predilection of *T. gondii* in the basal ganglia can result in a variety of movement disorders (Nath et al, 1993). The cerebral edema, encephalitic process and tissue destruction are significant and responsible for majority of neurological morbidity in HIV-infected patients presenting with focal brain lesion (Ammassari et al, 2000). Rupture of tissue cysts in AIDS- associated CT patients result in multiplication of bradyzoites into tachyzoites, which causes severe inflammatory reaction. Three morphological patterns of brain lesions in patients with CT are produced based on the stage of infection and degree of tissue reaction (Shankar et al, 2005): (i) In the acute stage (less than a few weeks duration): appearance of a necrotizing abscess or encephalitis seen as poorly circumscribed necrotic foci with variable degrees of haemorrhage, perifocal edema, acute and chronic inflammation, macrophage infiltration, with numerous *T. gondii* tachyzoites and encysted bradyzoites along the periphery. Also common are vascular thrombosis/fibrinoid necrosis of vessel walls, with polymorph infiltration, hypertrophy and the presence of tachyzoites in the hypertrophie arterial wall. (ii) A chronic lesion (weeks to months) : organized abscesses are found in CT cases treated for ≥ 2 weeks and seen as well circumscribed foci of central necrosis with a rim of congestion. In contrast to the acute phase, the central foci of an acellular necrosis is surrounded by a granulomatous reaction, with macrophages containing tightly packed lipid and haemosiderin, prominent hypertrophic occlusive arteritis with dense lymphocytic cuffing, and only a few organisms. (iii) Patients treated for ≥ 1 month show chronic abscesses in CT appear as small cystic cavities or linear orange-yellow scars and macrophages containing lipid and haemosiderin surrounded by a dense gliotic reaction. Calcification of vessels occurs and organisms are rarely found. In addition, a CAT scan can present as a diffuse, non-necrotizing, rapidly progressive encephalitis. The histological appearance seen as nodules of micrioglial cells with encysted bradyzoites and dispersed tachyzoites within the nodules.

Autopsy findings confirm the presence of the parasite and demonstration of *Toxoplasma* cysts is diagnostic of disseminated toxoplasmosis in AIDS patients (Holch et al, 1993). Despite the effectiveness of HAART, involvement of the brain in patients with AIDS remains a frequent autopsy finding (Masliah et al, 2000). AIDS-associated CT continues to be the major cause of mortality in the era of HAART (Rajagopalan et al, 2009; Kumarasamy et al, 2010). The expansion of earlier access to HAART could substantially reduce mortality, particularly in limited resource settings (Mzileni et al, 2008; Rajagopalan et al, 2009).

The seroprevalence of toxoplasmosis is generally high in HIV-infected patients and approximately 10% of CT is reported in AIDS patients. There has been no report of such neuropathological findings related to toxoplasmosis found in AIDS patients from Malaysia and its neighboring countries in the Southeast Asian region such as Thailand. This may be due to the fact it is not a common practice to conduct an autopsy in HIV/AIDS patients that could give the actual prevalence of AIDS-associated CT being underestimated. CT is one of the most common opportunistic infections of the CNS (Wadia et al, 2001; Nobre et al, 2003) as reported in an autopsy series conducted in India (Lanjewar et al, 1998a; Lanjewar et al, 1998b) and in other clinical settings (Petito et al, 1986; Souza et al, 2008). The majority of AIDS-related diseases diagnosed at autopsy had not been clinically diagnosed or suspected antemortem (Eza et al, 2006). The importance of an autopsy in evaluating clinical management and diagnosis (Eza et al, 2006) should be periodically done; particular in areas of high endemic toxoplasmosis where antiretroviral drugs, such as HAART, cannot be fully accessed.

There is scanty data about AIDS-associated neuropathological findings during the HAART era in Asia and Sub-Sahara Africa. This is mainly due to delayed introduction of these agents to these regions. It is expected that more autopsy studies will be carried out in this part of the world in the near future. The incidence of toxoplasmosis in autopsy studies has declined since the introduction of HAART in various countries, such as the USA (Langford et al, 2003) and France (Vallat-Decouvelaere et al, 2003). These studies show that autopsy findings can be a valuable means for determining the range and relative frequency of infectious diseases in these patients (Lucas et al, 1993). In addition, this can potentially have an immediate impact on patient care by enabling appropriate interventions, based on the results obtained (Lucas et al, 1993).

6. Diagnostic approaches - from conventional to advanced technology

Among patients with AIDS, cerebral involvement is more common and more serious than extracerebral toxoplasmosis. The definitive diagnosis is crucial for CT patients by directly demonstrating the presence of the tachyzoite form of *T. gondii* in the cerebral tissues. The presumptive diagnosis for CT, including the clinical presentations, radio-imaging findings, molecular and sero-diagnosis for *Toxoplasma* infection, and good response to anti-*Toxoplasma* therapy are widely accepted in clinical practice. The favorable outcome of CT is the improvement of clinical and radiological features after 2 to 3 weeks of initiated empirical therapy. The clinical diagnosis is a dilemma due to CT mimics with other brain diseases making it difficult to diagnose. Differential diagnosis of AIDS-associated CT is extremely important and the local neuroepidemiology and the degree of immunosuppression in the host are two key factors involved (Vidal et al, 2008). Primary CNS lymphoma is the main differential diagnosis of CT reported from developed countries (Manzardo et al, 2005). While, focal forms of cerebral tuberculosis (tuberculoma and, less likely tuberculous brain abscess) allow for differential diagnosis of CT mainly in developing countries (Trujillo et al, 2005). Primary CNS lymphoma usually presents with a CD4 count of less than 50 cells/cumm, CT occurs below 100 cells/cumm, and cerebral TB is more frequently present with a CD4 count above 200 cells/cumm (Vidal et al, 2004a; Vidal et al, 2005a; Vidal et al, 2005b). In addition to these more common neurological diseases, the differential diagnosis of CT includes other opportunistic infections such as progressive multifocal leucoencephalopathy, herpes simplex encephalitis, and cryptococcal meningitis; AIDS-and non-AIDS-associated tumors such as metastases of disseminated lymphoma and glioblastoma multiforme, respectively; and vascular diseases. Overall, a rapid and accurate diagnosis of CT is necessary, as the earlier the treatment the better the clinical outcome and survival rate of these patients.

6.1 Radiological diagnosis

Radio-imaging findings, either by computed tomography (CAT scan) or magnetic resonance imaging (MRI), are useful tools for the presumptive or empirical diagnosis of CT. CT usually causes unifocal, and more frequently multifocal lesions, and less likely diffuse encephalitis. These findings are however not pathognomonic of CT. Radiological diagnosis (Vidal et al, 2005a) can be classified as typical findings of hypodense lesions with ring-enhancing and perilesional edema, are observed in ~80% of CT cases. A typical pattern of hypodense lesions found without contrast enhancing and with an expansive effect, CT patients without focal lesions and MRI demonstrating focal lesions, and diffuse cerebral encephalitis without visible focal lesions, are shown in ~20% of these cases. An unusual but highly suggestive image of patients with CT is the 'eccentric target sign', which is a small asymmetric nodule along the wall of the enhancing ring (Pereira-Chioccola et al, 2009). Figure 2 shows the main radiological features of AIDS-associated CT patients. A CAT scan seems to be a sensitive diagnostic method for patients with focal neurological deficits; however it may underestimate the minimal inflammatory responses seen during early disease (Gill et al, 1986).

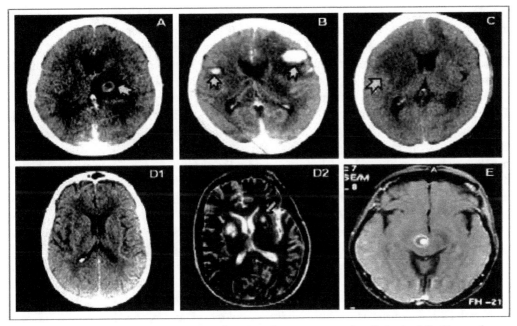

Fig. 4. Computed tomography images showing the spectrum of radiological findings of cerebral toxoplasmosis in HIV-infected patients.

Hypodense lesion with ring-enhancing and perilesional edema (A); nodular enhancing and perilesional edema (B); without contrast enhancing and with expansive effect (C). A CAT scan with contrast enhancement showed no abnormalities (D1) and corresponding T2-weighted MRI showed multiple basal ganglia focal lesions, with high-intensity signals (D2). T1-weighted MRI showed a ring-enhancing lesion with a small, enhancing asymmetric nodule along the wall of the lesion (E) ('the eccentric target sign'). The arrows show the abnormalities. (Courtesy of Dr. Pereira-Chioccola VL and Dr. Vidal JE, São Paulo, Brazil.)

MRI is recommended to be performed in patients with; neurological symptoms and positive serology to anti-*Toxoplasma* antibodies whose CAT scans show no or only a single abnormality, or persistent or worsening focal neurological deficits of disease if results of the initial procedure were negative (Luft & Remington, 1992). A CAT scan or MRI is useful for assessment of patients who had responded to initial empirical treatment. There may be a worsening of radiographic appearance in patients with a clinically improved condition before 3 weeks, and complete resolution of cerebral lesions seen on a CAT scan may vary from 3 week to 6 months after initiation of therapy (Luft & Remington, 1992). An evidence of either clinical or radiographic improvement within 3 weeks of initial therapy provides a confirmed diagnosis of patients with CT.

6.2 Serological diagnosis

Cerebral toxoplasmosis poses a diagnostic problem that relies on classical serological methods to detect anti-*Toxoplasma* immunoglobulins because clinical blood samples from patients with immunodeficiency can fail to produce sufficient titers of specific antibodies. Sero-evidence of *Toxoplasma* infection, independent of antibody levels, is generally seen in all patients before developing CT (Carme et al, 1988). Most CT patients have high titers of anti-*Toxoplasma* IgG antibodies with high IgG avidity that provides serological evidence of infection (Raffi et al, 1997; Vidal et al, 2005a), and this also supports a conclusion that this is the result of a secondary reaction of latent or chronic *Toxoplasma* infection (Dardé, 1996). Therefore, it is important to determine the *Toxoplasma* serostatus in all HIV-infected patients in order to define the population at risk for CT. At the onset of CT, significant rises in anti-*Toxoplasma* antibody titers are found in only a minority of these patients (Carme et al, 1988). The level of rising titers may occur before the onset of CT and it does not seem to predict the occurrence of CT. Anti-*Toxoplasma* IgM antibody, as measured by the indirect fluorescent or ELISA tests, is rarely found in CT patients (Luft & Remington, 1992). In cases of CT, a negative or low titer of serological results or even the absence of anti-*Toxoplasma* antibodies does not exclude positive diagnosis and the initiation of anti-*Toxoplasma* therapy should be immediately started without delay if clinical and radiological presentations are consistent with CT (Luft & Remington, 1992; Nissapatorn et al, 2004). A positive serology result seems to be even less useful in areas where there is a high prevalence of toxoplasmosis in the general population (Pereira-Chioccola et al, 2009). While, a negative result does have a high negative predictive value (Vidal et al, 2008) Determination of an increase of intrathecal anti-*Toxoplasma* IgG antibody production is normally characterized by the presence of *T. gondii* oligoclonal bands (OCBs) of IgG antibody in CT patients (Potasman et al, 1988). Immunological diagnosis using other clinical samples such as cerebrospinal fluid (CSF) is of limited use because of the sensitivity and specificity being only about 60-70% (Collazos, 2003). *T. gondii* excretory/secretory antigens (ESAs) are an excellent serological marker for the diagnosis of CT in AIDS patients (Pereira-Chioccola et al, 2009). ESAs are produced by *T. gondii* tachyzoites, the form responsible for disease dissemination, which plays an important role in stimulating humoral and cellular immunities in order to control *Toxoplasma* infection (Carruthers & Sibley, 1997; Cérède et al, 2005). Anti-ESA IgG antibodies are also present in CSF sample of AIDS patients with CT which can be determined by ESA-ELISA and immunoblot techniques and these samples are clearly distinguishable from AIDS patients who are *Toxoplasma* seropositive but with other brain diseases (Pereira-Chioccola et al, 2009).

6.3 Molecular diagnosis

Since the serological status is solely useful to recognize whether the patient is at risk for reactivation, the direct detection of *T. gondii* DNA in biological specimens by polymerase chain reaction (PCR) has provided a major breakthrough for the diagnosis of toxoplasmosis (Reischl et al, 2003). Over a period of two decades, these molecular methods based on PCR and specific genetic markers have been developed for routine use in assisting serology for the diagnosis of CT patients. PCR techniques are suitable for patients with AIDS because these methods do not depend on the host immune responses and allow for direct detection of *T. gondii* DNA from a variety of clinical samples. In addition, these methods are rapid, sensitive, specific, less time consuming, and can be used to replace invasive procedures such as stereotactic brain biopsy. The sensitivity and specificity of the PCR reactions depends on the types of reagents, protocols for DNA extraction, storage of clinical samples, and the timing between the start of a specific therapy and collection of clinical samples, which can make the interpretation of results difficult (Pereira-Chioccola et al, 2009). Among clinical/biological samples, blood and CSF are the most frequently used for the detection of *T. gondii* DNA in patients with CT. To yield a better result, clinical samples should be collected before or up until the first 3 days of anti-*Toxoplasma* therapy because the diagnostic sensitivity will be reduced after the first week of this specific treatment (Vidal et al, 2004b). In CSF samples, the varying sensitivity of the PCR technique ranges from 11.5% to 100% but a high specificity (96-100%) has been reported using CSF specimens (Novati et al, 1994; Dupon et al, 1995; Vidal et al, 2004b). The collection of CSF sample is invasive and is not recommended for patients with multiple brain lesions (Pereira-Chioccola et al, 2009). PCR in blood samples, as an alternative approach, has been reported with a wide range of sensitivities of between 16% and 86% (Dupouy-Camet et al, 1993; Dupon et al, 1995). A quantitative real-time PCR (qrtPCR), is a recent development among molecular methods, and accelerates the detection of *T. gondii* DNA in most positive samples and allows for amplification and simultaneous detection of DNA in 1 hour (Hierl et al, 2004). Its advantages over conventional and nested PCR include rapid, improved sensitivity, a broad dynamic range of targets, DNA quantitation and reduction of contamination. Despite these advantages, in some patients with low parasite load particularly in CSF samples; there is still the need for comparative results of both conventional nested and real-time quantitative PCR methods (Bretagne, 2003; Hierl et al, 2004; Apfalter et al, 2005). Future prospect on the diagnosis of patients with CT is more likely to rely on the development of molecular methods based on qrtPCR which provides quantitative results and is less time-consuming in preparation. However, this technique needs to have improved specificity and more importantly a reduction of the high cost of the necessary equipment.

6.4 Other diagnostic methods

There is a need for more specific or invasive approaches that will assist confirmation of the diagnosis of CT. Brain biopsy is generally reserved for those patients who present with a diagnostic dilemma or do not fulfill the criteria for presumptive treatment and for those patients who fail to improve clinically or radiologically over the succeeding 10-14 days after being empirically treated for toxoplasmosis initially so they do warrant a stereotactic brain biopsy (SBB) in order to institute specific and appropriate therapy (Luft & Remington, 1992). For patients with expansive brain lesions who fail to respond to empirical treatment initiated for CT within 14 days, SBB should be seriously considered relatively early in the course of treatment, with or without change in therapy (Pereira-Chioccola et al, 2009). Surprisingly, SBB is not commonly used for the diagnosis of CT or CT-associated other opportunistic CNS diseases in Asian countries (Yeo et al, 2000) compared to other settings where CT cases have been reported in patients with AIDS. Brain biopsies do not influence survival of CT patients (Sadler et al, 1998). SBB is an efficient, safe and important diagnostic procedure. In selected patients even expensive investigations should be undertaken before considering specific therapy and cost effective homecare (Armbruster et al, 1998). This procedure should be performed early during the patient's evolution in order to achieve a prompt and accurate diagnosis and to guide the therapeutic scheme for AIDS patients with FBL (Corti et al, 2008).

Recently, genotyping analysis of *T. gondii* strains isolated from clinical samples has been conducted in HIV-infected patients from different settings. However, it remains doubtful on how to ascertain the association between *T. gondii* strains and human toxoplasmosis since the majority of infected individuals are chronic and without any clinical symptoms, and it is difficult to isolate *T. gondii* strains from these patients. Therefore, a larger sample size should be carried out in human patients to identify specific *T. gondii* strains using high resolution typing methods such as multiplex nested PCR-RFLP which can genotype some DNA samples extracted directly from infected tissues. Serotyping of *T. gondii* strains has proved to be a promising tool using serum samples to overcome the diagnostic challenge (Kong et al, 2003; Peyron et al, 2006; Morisset et al, 2008; Sousa et al, 2008; Sousa et al, 2009). However, due to the limitation of serotyping it is not possible to differentiate type II from non-type II strains particularly in South America where there is a high diversity of *T. gondii* strain types. At present, this requires further developments of typing analyses to facilitate and be incorporated into the routine diagnosis of patients with CT.

7. Therapeutic approaches: from specific treatment to HAART

7.1 Anti-*Toxoplasma* therapy

One of the keys after diagnoses is how patients respond to the different therapeutic regimens used for treating this opportunistic disease. Most patients with CT respond well to anti-*Toxoplasma* agents as demonstrated by findings from studies in various settings. However, about 10% of CT cases died despite what was thought to be adequate treatment (Vidal et al, 2005a). There are few options other than anti-*Toxoplasma* regimens used as first-choice initial therapy; 6 weeks with sufadiazine (1.0-1.5 g per oral [PO] every 6 h) with pyrimethamine (100-200 mg PO loading dose, then 50 mg PO daily) and folinic acid (10-20 mg PO daily) that can reduce the hemato-toxicities related to pyrimethamine (Portegies et al, 2004). This standard combination has been successfully used in treating CT but has been associated with high toxicities such as Lyell's syndrome or Steven-Johnson syndrome (Katlama et al, 1996a; Torre et al, 1998). The other regimen is trimethoprim/sulfamethoxazole (Co-trimoxazole, 5/25 mg/kg PO or intravenous (IV) every 12 h for 4-6 weeks) (Canessa et al, 1992). This therapeutic regimen has been confirmed for its efficacy and safety in a single available randomized clinical trial (Canessa et al, 1992; Torre et al, 1998; Dedicoat & Livesley, 2006; Béraud et al, 2009). Several alternative therapies, principally used in patients who are intolerant to this combination, have been reported to be effective, including clindamycin and pyrimethamine or sulfadiazine (Katlama et al, 1996a; Tsai et al, 2002), clarithromycin and pyrimethamine (Fernandez-Martin et al, 1991), clindamycin and 5-fluoro-uracil (Dhiver et al, 1993), azithromycin and pyrimethamine (Saba et al, 1993; Jacobson et al, 2001), clindamycin and fansidar (Nissapatorn et al, 2004), sulfadoxine and pyrimethamine (Amogne et al, 2006), and atovaquone (Torres et al, 1997). There was no superior regimen among the three following combinations: pyrimethamine plus sulfadiazine, pyrimethamine plus clindamycin (Katlama et al, 1996a), and pyrimethamine plus sulfadiazine with Co-trimoxazole (Torre et al, 1998) that were reported in a recent review of comparative studies (Dedicoat & Livesley, 2006).

There is one case of toxoplasmosis resistant to standard combination therapy (pyrimethamine and sulfadiazine) that was improved with clindamycin and pyrimethamine (Huber et al, 1995). The other case was an AIDS patient with toxoplasmic myelopathy and myopathy resistant to standard anti-*Toxoplasma* therapy due to the possibility of immune reconstitution of the inflammatory syndrome, was reported (Kung et al, 2011). Another study suggested atovaquone as being effective in AIDS cases with resistant toxoplasmosis (Lafeuillade et al, 1993). This helps to identify drugs that are effective and may act synergistically (McFadden et al, 2001). Relapses of CT are frequently observed in AIDS patients non-compliant to therapy or prophylaxis, and in those who develop adverse drug effects (Luft & Remington, 1992; Nissapatorn et al, 2004; Béraud et al, 2009). There has been no evidence of treatment-induced resistance so far reported that have contributing to a relapse of CT. Few studies have arrived at a solution of how to prevent relapses. Pyrimethamine and sulfadoxine twice a week appears to give promising results for prevention of CT. Allergic reactions are usually mild and disappear on continuation, but may limit the value of this regimen (Ruf et al, 1993). Daily doses of pyrimethamine and sulfadiazine are more effective as maintenance therapy for preventing relapses of CT (4.4 compared to 19.5 per 100 patient-years; incidence rate ration, 4.36; p=0.024) than twice weekly administration (Podzamczer et al, 1995). Pyrimethamine and clindamycin has been shown to be a valuable alternative for treatment but is less effective, particularly for the long term prevention of relapses (Katlama et al, 1996a). Azithromycin and pyrimethamine have been used as alternative therapy, but maintenance with this combination or oral azithromycin alone is associated with relapses (Jacobson et al, 2001).

Atovaquone is a unique naphthoquinone with broad-spectrum antiprotozoal activity. It has been found to be effective against tachyzoites in vitro and may kill bradyzoites within cysts at a higher concentration. Atovaquone is frequently used in combination with other agents in treating CT. Experimental studies have shown that the efficacy of atovaquone was enhanced when other agents were added, such as pyrimethamine, sulfadiazine, clindamycin, or clarithromycin (Guelar et al, 1994). An intravenous preparation is highly effective in murine models with reactivated toxoplasmosis (Schöler et al, 2001; Dunay et al, 2004). In AIDS patients, the only study to report failure with atovaquone during treatment found that a high temperature may induce inactivation of the product in the absence of food intake (Duran et al, 1995). Atovaquone has consistently been found to be a promising therapeutic for salvage therapy in CT patients who were intolerant to or who failed standard regimens (Guelar et al, 1994; Katlama et al, 1996a; Torres et al, 1997; Chirgwin et al, 2002). However, the role of atovaquone in the treatment and prophylaxis of CT in AIDS patients is not well defined and more studies are required before a firm recommendation can be made (Baggish & Hill, 2002). The treatment of choice is often directed by the available therapy, particularly in resource-poor settings. An important question is whether the incidence of secondary reactivation or relapse cases of CT may begin to rise in the future. This depends on how the efficacy of the current treatment regimens and new novel drugs, especially those that can destroy cyst/bradyzoite forms of the *Toxoplasma* parasite. Another important factor is increasing resistance to antiretroviral drugs in HIV-positive patients and the subsequent decline in CD4 cell counts (Kuritzkes et al, 2000) which has been reported in the recent years.

7.2 Primary and secondary chemoprophylaxis

Toxoplasmosis is one of the leading CNS-OIs, that causes morbidity and mortality in advanced stages of HIV-infected patients. Effective primary and secondary prophylaxis has been formulated to prevent the occurrence of CT (Katlama et al, 1996a; Bucher et al, 1997). Before the era of HAART, co-trimoxazole played an important role as a primary prophylactic agent in preventing the reactivation of toxoplasmosis in HIV-positive patients (van Oosterhout et al, 2005). CT was still reported in HIV-infected patients with or without prophylaxis (Nissapatorn et al, 2004; Nissapatorn et al, 2007). To be consistent with previous reports and present situations in most resource limited settings, a current guideline recommends the use of a daily dose of a double-strength tablet of co-trimoxazole in *Toxoplasma*-seropositive patients who have a CD4 cell count below100 cells/cumm (CDC, 2009). For AIDS patients who survive their first episode of CT, the risk of relapse is between 30% and 50% if lifelong suppressive therapy is not provided (Leport et al, 1988; de Gans et al, 1992). Discontinuation of maintenance therapy (secondary/ suppressive therapy) for established CT patients is not recommended (USPHS/IDSA Prevention of opportunistic infections working group, 1997). In the pre HAART era, relapse rates of CT after discontinuation of maintenance therapy was approximately 50% (Katlama et al, 1996b). There are few regimens that have been used for secondary prophylaxis for CT patients; the combination of pyrimethamine (25-50 mg/day) plus sulfadiazine (500 mg every 6 h) plus leucovorin (10-20 mg/day) is a highly effective treatment. The use of this combined thrice-weekly regimen (Podzamczer et al, 1995) or the same doses of sulfadiazine twice a day (Jordan et al, 2004) is an alternative option among non-compliance patients. The recommendation is for pyrimethamine plus clindamycin (600 mg clinidamycin every 8 h) for patients who are intolerant to sulfa drugs (CDC, 2009). Co-trimoxazole (960 mg twice daily) is another potential drug used in secondary prophylaxis for patients with CT (Duval et al, 2004). This agent (2.5/12.5 mg/kg PO every 12 h) is considered as safe, cheap and effective and can be an alternative choice (Pereira-Chioccola et al, 2009) to increase drug adherence in areas where other maintenance therapies are not available.

7.3 Highly active anti-retroviral therapy (HAART)

For more than two decades now, the use of HAART in HIV-infected patients has resulted in an improved quality of life and an increase in the length of time that patients remain free from opportunistic infections (Mocroft et al, 1998; Palella et al, 1998). A higher CNS Penetration-Effectiveness (CPE) score of antiretroviral drugs is increasing the survival rate of CT patients (Lanoy et al, 2011). In CT cases, there is no recommendation for the timing of HAART when CT is present in antiretroviral-naïve patients. However, HAART should be started at least 2 weeks after an anti-*Toxoplasma* regimen was initiated in these patients (Manzardo et al, 2005; Pereira-Chioccola et al, 2009). In HIV-infected patients receiving HAART, primary prophylaxis for CT can be safely discontinued in patients whose CD4 cell counts increase to >200 cells/mm^3 (CDC, 2009). It is a medical challenge to decide whether secondary prophylaxis should be continued while HIV-infected patients are receiving HAART. If maintenance therapy is stopped, recurrence of toxoplasmosis may allow for permanent damage to cerebral and visual functions which is potentially harmful to an affected person (Stout et al, 2002). While maintenance therapy is still essential, evaluation of *T. gondii*-specific immune responses might be the other important step for improving estimates of the individual risk of CT and CT relapse (Hoffmann et al, 2007). Otherwise, secondary prophylaxis can be safely discontinued in CT patients receiving HAART with CD4 cell count of > 200 cells/cumm after 6 months (Pereira-Chioccola et al, 2009). This same prophylaxis should be reintroduced in patients with CD4 cell count of < 200 cells/cumm (CDC, 2009). While, primary and secondary prophylaxis against CT can also be safely discontinued after the CD4 cell count has increased to ≥ 200 cells/cumm for more than 3 months in HIV-infected patients receiving HAART (Miro et al, 2006). These strategies can help in reducing the toxicity, pill overload, and expense associated with complicated therapeutic regimens. Considering that CT patients have a high chance of early death, HAART should be immediately initiated after CT diagnosis and prophylaxis should be maintained in these patients who fail to respond to antiretroviral therapy.

8. Immune Reconstitution Inflammatory Syndrome (IRIS) - from past to future concerns

Anti-retroviral therapy partially restores the immune function of HIV-infected patients, thereby remarkably reducing morbidity and mortality of opportunistic infections in general and CT in particular. The incidence of opportunistic infections, including CT and ECT has decreased, particularly in areas where antiretroviral therapy, including HAART, is accessible (Kaplan et al, 2000; Subsai et al, 2006; Lian et al, 2007). HAART has reduced relapse in cases of toxoplasmosis and has improved survival in these HIV-infected patients. This may be due to the successful suppression of virus replications followed by an increase in CD4+ lymphocytes, a partial recovery of T-cell specific immune responses and decreased susceptibility to both local and systemic opportunistic pathogens (Silva & Araújo, 2005). HIV-associated IRIS is the clinical worsening of opportunistic infections that result from enhancement of pathogen-specific immune responses among patients responding to antiretroviral treatment (Lawn & Wilkinson, 2006). IRIS has been widely recognized in CT patients following initiation of HAART and development of a paradoxical clinical deterioration despite an increased CD4 cell count and decreased HIV viral load which leads to the rapid restoration of the immune system (Gray et al, 2005). So far, more than 20 cases of IRIS-associated CT have been reported in the literature (Table 2). A low CD4 cell count has been identified as a significant risk factor in AIDS patients with CT (Tsambiras et al, 2001; de Boer et al, 2003; Sendi et al, 2006; Chen et al, 2009; Caby et al, 2010; Kung et al, 2011) due to impaired proliferative response to *Toxoplasma* antigen (Belanger et al, 1999), a decreased production of interferon γ (Ullum et al, 1997), and it is found to be more common that IRIS develops in HIV-infected patients (Jevtović et al, 2005). Therefore, monitoring of CD4/CD8 T cells in patients on HAART might serve as a better marker for the restoration of *T. gondii*-specific immune responses than the total number of CD4 cells count (Furco et al, 2008). Immune reconstitution under HAART has been associated with a restoration of immune responses against *T. gondii* (Fournier et al, 2001). In the case where IRIS is suspected in CT patient, close observation for 7-15 days, a higher steroid dose to control IRIS (Venkataramana et al, 2006), uninterrupted HAART, and continued treatment for toxoplasmosis can resolve this problem without biopsy (Tremont-Lukats et al, 2009). Based on reported cases of CT-associated IRIS from different studies, this could verify its association that it can develop in a substantial numbers of HIV-infected patients receiving HAART. No case of IRIS-related toxoplasmosis has ever been reported among AIDS patients in Malaysia even though CT was one of the most common systemic opportunistic infections in AIDS patients (Nissapatorn et al, 2004; Lian et al, 2007). Toxoplasmosis is a common neurological opportunistic infection in industrialized countries for which HAART is often initiated fairly early compared to developing or resource-limited settings. As for the increasing use of HAART worldwide, the care for patients receiving HAART will need to incorporate monitoring for and treating complications of IRIS (Agmon-Levin et al, 2008), including impaired CD4-cell immune reconstitution upon HIV therapy in patients with CT

Reference	Country	No. of cases	Clinical presentation	Baseline CD4 cell count/µL
Rodríguez-Rosado et al, 1998	Spain	3	Cerebral toxoplasmosis	-
González-Castillo et al, 2001	Spain	1	Cerebral toxoplasmosis	456
Tsambiras et al, 2001	USA	1	Cerebral toxoplasmosis	83
de Boer et al, 2003	The Netherlands	1	Cerebral toxoplasmosis	43
Jevtović et al, 2005	Serbia & Montenegro	1	Cerebral toxoplasmosis	<100
Sendi et al, 2006	Switzerland	1	Immune recovery vitritis with isolated toxoplasmic retinochoroiditis	11
Subsai et al, 2006	Thailand	2	Cerebral toxoplasmosis	-
Huruy et al, 2008	Ethiopia	2	Cerebral toxoplasmosis	-
Chen et al, 2009	USA	1	Cerebral toxoplasmosis	29
Klotz et al, 2009	Ethiopia	7	Cerebral toxoplasmosis	50-100
McCombe et al, 2009	Canada	1	Cerebral toxoplasmosis	2
Tremont-Lukats et al, 2009	USA	1	Cerebral toxoplasmosis	14
Cabral et al, 2010	Brazil	1	Cerebral toxoplasmosis	276
Caby et al, 2010	France	1	Placental IRIS	7 (pregnancy)
Martin-Blondel et al, 2010	France	3	Cerebral toxoplasmosis	9, 25, 23
Kung et al, 2011	USA	1	Toxoplasmic myelopathy and myopathy	67
Shah, 2011	India	1 (child)	Cerebral toxoplasmosis	-

Table 2. Summary on reported cases of immune reconstitution inflammatory syndrome (IRIS) associated toxoplasmosis in HIV-infected patients.

(Kastenbauer et al, 2009). As the number of AIDS-associated CT cases treated with HAART increases, the complications of IRIS-CT may become more common and easily recognizable, particularly in areas where toxoplasmosis is endemic. Therefore, increased awareness of IRIS is importance to clinicians along with early diagnosis and appropriate treatment in managing AIDS patients.

9. Conclusion

Despite a decline in both morbidity and mortality in HIV-infected patients in developed countries including the United States and Europe, toxoplasmosis remains an important disease and is unlikely to be eradicated. Toxoplasmosis still occurs in those not diagnosed with HIV and not receiving medical care, those not receiving prophylaxis, and those not taking or not responding to HAART. There are very few reports regarding resistance to the drugs used for toxoplasmosis. Resistance in HIV cases and the action of anti-retroviral therapy with or without IRIS may contribute to an increase in the incidence of CT. In developing countries where anti-retroviral therapy is still lacking, HIV-infected patients are at high risk for CT, these regions include China, India, South America, Southeast Asia and most importantly sub-Saharan Africa. A better understanding of the clinico-epidemiology of toxoplasmosis, and improved efforts in prevention, diagnosis and treatment, are needed. The role of infections with this parasite requires further study, including as to whether infections, such as CT have an impact on HIV/AIDS patients.

10. Acknowledgement

I express my sincere thanks to Assoc. Prof. Dr. Nongyao Sawangjaroen, Department of Microbiology, Faculty of Science, Prince of Songkhla University, Hat Yai, Songkhla, Thailand and Dr. Sucheep Phiriyasamith, Master of Public Administration Program, Graduate School, Kasem Bundit University, Bangkok, Thailand for their assistance during preparation of this chapter. Also, I would like to thank the University of Malaya Research Grant (UMRG094/09HTM) for financial support.

11. References

Agmon-Levin, N., Elbirt, D. & Sthoeger, Z.M. (2008). Immune reconstitution inflammatory syndrome in human immunodeficiency (HIV) infected patients. *Harefuah*, Vol.147, No.5, pp. 439-444, 476, 477, ISSN 0017-7768.

Ajzenberg, D., Year, H., Marty, P., Paris, L., Dalle, F., Menotti, J., Aubert, D., Franck, J., Bessières, M.H., Quinio, D., Pelloux, H., Delhaes, L., Desbois, N., Thulliez, P., Robert-Gangneux, F., Kauffmann-Lacroix, C., Pujol, S., Rabodonirina, M., Bougnoux, M.E., Cuisenier, B., Duhamel, C., Duong ,T.H., Filisetti, D., Flori, P., Gay-Andrieu, F., Pratlong, F., Nevez, G., Totet, A., Carme, B., Bonnabau, H., Dardé, M.L. & Villena, I. (2009). Genotype of 88 *Toxoplasma gondii* isolates associated with toxoplasmosis in immunocompromised patients and correlation with clinical findings. *Journal of Infectious Diseases*, Vol.199, No.8, pp. 1155-1167, ISSN 0022-1899.

Akanmu, A.S., Osunkalu, V.O., Ofomah, J.N. & Olowoselu, F.O. (2010). Pattern of demographic risk factors in the seroprevalence of anti-*Toxoplasma gondii* antibodies in HIV infected patients at the Lagos University Teaching Hospital. *Nigerian Quarterly Journal of Hospital Medicine*, Vol.20, No.1, pp.1-4, ISSN 0189 – 2657.

Alpert, L., Miller, M., Alpert, E., Satin, R., Lamoureux, E. & Trudel, L. (1996). Gastric toxoplasmosis in acquired immunodeficiency syndrome: antemortem diagnosis with histopathologic characterization. *Gastroenterology*, Vol.110, No.1, pp. 258-264, ISSN 0016-5085.

Alves, J.M., Magalhães, V. & Matos, M.A. (2010). Toxoplasmic retinochoroiditis in patients with AIDS and neurotoxoplasmosis. *Arquivos Brasileiros de Oftalmologia*, Vol.73, No.2, pp.150-154, ISSN 0004-2749.

Ammassari, A., Cingolani, A., Pezzotti, P., De Luca, D.A., Murri, R., Giancola, M.L., Larocca, L.M. & Antinori, A. (2000). AIDS-related focal brain lesions in the era of highly active antiretroviral therapy. *Neurology*, Vol.55, No.8, pp. 1194-1200, ISSN 0028-3878.

Amogne, W., Teshager, G. & Zenebe, G. (2006). Central nervous system toxoplasmosis in adult Ethiopians. *Ethiopian Medical Journal*, Vol.44, No.2, pp.113-120, ISSN 0014-1755.

Anekthananon, T., Ratanasuwan, W., Techasathit, W., Rongrungruang, Y. & Suwanagool, S. (2004). HIV infection/acquired immunodeficiency syndrome at Siriraj Hospital, 2002: time for secondary prevention. *Journal of the Medical Association of Thailand*, Vol.87, No.2, pp. 173-179, ISSN 0125-2208.

Apfalter, P., Reischl, U. & Hammerschlag, M.R. (2005). In-house nucleic acid amplification assays in research: how much quality control is needed before one can rely upon the results? *Journal of Clinical Microbiology*, Vol.43, No.12, pp. 5835-5841, ISSN 0095-1137.

Arevalo, J.F., Quiceno, J.I., García, R.F., McCutchan, J.A., Munguia, D., Nelson, J.A. & Freeman, W.R. (1997). Retinal findings and characteristics in AIDS patients with systemic *Mycobacterium avium-intracellulare complex* and toxoplasmic encephalitis. *Ophthalmic Surgery & Lasers*, Vol.28, No.1, pp. 50-54, ISSN 1082-3069.

Armbruster, C., Alesch, F., Budka, H. & Kriwanek, S. (1998). Stereotactic brain biopsy in AIDS patients: a necessary patient-oriented and cost-effective diagnostic measure? *Acta Medica Austriaca*, Vol.25, No.3, pp. 91-95, ISSN 0303-8173.

Arshad, S., Skiest, D. & Granowitz, E.V. (2009). Subacute onset of paralysis in a person with AIDS. *The AIDS Reader*, Vol.19, No.1, pp. 32-35, ISSN 1053-0894.

Artigas, J., Grosse, G., Niedobitek, F., Kassner, M., Risch, W. & Heise, W. (1994). Severe toxoplasmic ventriculomeningoencephalomyelitis in two AIDS patients following treatment of cerebral toxoplasmic granuloma. *Clinical Neuropathology*, Vol.13, No.3, pp. 120-126, ISSN 0722-5091.

Azevedo, K.M., Setúbal, S., Lopes, V.G., Camacho, L.A. & Oliveira, S.A. (2010). Congenital toxoplasmosis transmitted by human immunodeficiency-virus infected women. *The Brazilian Journal of Infectious Diseases*, Vol.14, No.2, pp. 186-189, ISSN 1413-8670.

Bachmeyer, C., Mouchnino, G., Thulliez, P. & Blum, L. (2006). Congenital toxoplasmosis from an HIV-infected woman as a result of reactivation. *Journal of Infection*, Vol.52, No.2, pp. e55-e57, ISSN 0163-4453.

Baggish, A.L. & Hill, D.R. (2002). Antiparasitic agent atovaquone. *Antimicrobial Agents and Chemotherapy*, Vol.46, No.5, pp. 1163-1173, ISSN 0066-4804.

Belanger, F., Derouin, F., Grangeot-Keros, L. & Meyer, L. (1999). Incidence and risk factors of toxoplasmosis in a cohort of human immunodeficiency virus-infected patients: 1988-1995. HEMOCO and SEROCO Study Groups. *Clinical Infectious Diseases*, Vol.28, No.3, pp. 575-581, ISSN 1058-4838.

Berger, B.B., Egwuagu, C.E., Freeman, W.R. & Wiley, C.A. (1993). Miliary toxoplasmic retinitis in acquired immunodeficiency syndrome. *Archives of Ophthalmology*, Vol.111, No.3, pp. 373-376, ISSN 0003-9950.

Béraud, G., Pierre-François, S., Foltzer, A., Abel, S., Liautaud, B., Smadja, D. & Cabié, A. (2009). Cotrimoxazole for treatment of cerebral toxoplasmosis: an observational cohort study during 1994-2006. *The American Journal of Tropical Medicine and Hygiene*, Vol.80, No.4, pp. 583-587, ISSN 0002-9637.

Biedermann, K., Flepp, M., Fierz, W., Joller-Jemelka, H. & Kleihues, P. (1995). Pregnancy, immunosuppression and reactivation of latent toxoplasmosis. *Journal of Perinatal Medicine*, Vol.23, No.3, pp. 191-203, ISSN 0300-5577.

Bossi, P., Caumes, E., Astagneau, P., Li, T.S., Paris, L., Mengual, X., Katlama, C. & Bricaire, F. (1998). Epidemiologic characteristics of cerebral toxoplasmosis in 399 HIV-infected patients followed between 1983 and 1994. *La Revue de Medecine Interne*, Vol.19, No.5, pp. 313-317, ISSN 0248-8663.

Brändle, M., Vernazza, P.L., Oesterle, M. & Galeazzi, R.L. (1995). Cerebral toxoplasmosis with central diabetes insipidus and panhypopituitarism in a patient with AIDS. *Schweizerische medizinische Wochenschrift*, Vol.125, No.14, pp. 684-687, ISSN 0036-7672.

Bretagne, S. (2003). Molecular diagnostics in clinical parasitology and mycology: limits of the current polymerase chain reaction (PCR) assays and interest of the real-time PCR assays. *Clinical Microbiology and Infection*, Vol.9, No.6, pp. 505-511, ISSN 1198-743X.

Brindle, R., Holliman, R., Gilks, C. & Waiyaki, P. (1991). *Toxoplasma* antibodies in HIV-positive patients from Nairobi. *Transactions of the Royal Society of Tropical Medicine and Hygiene*, Vol.85, No.6, pp. 750-751, ISSN 0035-9203.

Brion, J.P., Pelloux, H., Le Marc'hadour, F., Stahl, J.P., Vilde, J.L. & Micoud, M. (1992). Acute toxoplasmic hepatitis in a patient with AIDS. *Clinical Infectious Diseases*, Vol.15, No.1, pp. 183-184, ISSN 1058-4838.

Bucher, H.C., Griffith, L., Guyatt, G.H. & Opravil, M. (1997). Meta-analysis of prophylactic treatments against *Pneumocystis carinii* pneumonia and toxoplasma encephalitis in HIV-infected patients. *Journal of Acquired Immune Deficiency Syndromes and Human Retrovirology*, Vol.15, No.2, pp. 104-114, ISSN 1077-9450.

Cabral, R.F., Valle Bahia, P.R., Gasparetto, E.L. & Chimelli, L. (2010). Immune reconstitution inflammatory syndrome and cerebral toxoplasmosis. *American Journal of Neuroradiology*, Vol.31, No.7, pp.E65-E66, ISSN 0195-6108.

Caby, F., Lemercier, D., Coulomb, A., Grigorescu, R., Paris, L., Touafek, F., Carcelain, G., Canestri, A., Pauchard, M., Katlama, C., Dommergues, M. & Tubiana, R. (2010). Fetal death as a result of placental immune reconstitution inflammatory syndrome. *The Journal of Infection*, Vol.61, No.2, pp. 185-188, ISSN 0163-4453.

Canessa, A., Del Bono, V., De Leo, P., Piersantelli, N. & Terragna, A. (1992). Cotrimoxazole therapy of *Toxoplasma gondii* encephalitis in AIDS patients. *European Journal of Clinical Microbiology & Infectious Diseases*, Vol.11, No.2, pp. 125-130, ISSN 0934-9723.

Cantos, G.A., Prando, M.D., Siqueira, M.V. & Teixeira, R.M. (2000). Toxoplasmosis: occurrence of antibodies anti- *Toxoplasma gondii* and diagnosis. *Revista da Associacao Medica Brasileira* (Sao Paulo), Vol.46, No.4, pp. 335-341, ISSN 0104-4230

Carme, B., M'Pele, P., Mbitsi, A., Kissila, A.M., Aya, G.M., Mouanga-Yidika, G., Mboussa, J. & Itoua-Ngaporo, A. (1988). Opportunistic parasitic diseases and mycoses in AIDS. Their frequencies in Brazzaville (Congo). *Bulletin de la Société de Pathologie Exotique et de ses Filiales*, Vol.81, No.3, pp. 311-316, ISSN 0037-9085.

Carrazana, E.J., Rossitch, E., Jr. & Samuels, M.A. (1989). Parkinsonian symptoms in a patient with AIDS and cerebral toxoplasmosis. *Journal of Neurology, Neurosurgery, and Psychiatry*, Vol.52, No.12, pp. 1445-1447, ISSN 0022-3050.

Carruthers, V.B. (2002). Host cell invasion by the opportunistic pathogen *Toxoplasma gondii*. *Acta Tropica*, Vol.81, No.2, pp.111-122, ISSN 0001-706X.

Carruthers, V.B. & Sibley, L.D. (1997). Sequential protein secretion from three distinct organelles of *Toxoplasma gondii* accompanies invasion of human fibroblasts. *European Journal of Cell Biology*, Vol.73, No.2, pp. 114-123, ISSN 0171-9335.

Castro Figueiredo, J.F., de Lourdes Veronese, R.M., Costa Passos, A.D. Saloum Deghaide, N., Romeo, E., Tokunaga, N.C. & Donadi, E.A. (2000). HLA typing in patients with AIDS and neurotoxoplasmosis. Presented at XIII International AIDS Conference, 9-14 July, Durban, South Africa, (Abstract MoPeB2141).

CDC. (2009). Guidelines for prevention and treatment of opportunistic infection in HIV-infected adults and adolescents. Recommendations from CDC, the National Institutes of Health, and the HIV Medicine Association of the Infectious Diseases Society of America. MMWR. Morbidity and Mortality Weekly Report, Vol.58, No.RR-4, pp. 1-207, ISSN 0149-2195.

Cérède, O., Dubremetz, J.F., Soêten, M., Deslée, D., Vial, H., Bout, D. & Lebrun, M. (2005). Synergistic role of micronemal proteins in Toxoplasma gondii virulence. The Journal of Experimental Medicine, Vol.201, No.3, pp. 453-463, ISSN 0022-1007.

Cesbron-Delauw, M.F. & Capron, A. (1993). Excreted/secreted antigens of Toxoplasma gondii--their origin and role in the host-parasite interaction. Research in Immunology, Vol.144, No.1, pp.41-44, ISSN 0923-2494.

Chaddha, D.S., Kalra, S.P., Singh, A.P., Gupta, R.M. & Sanchetee, P.C. (1999). Toxoplasmic encephalitis in acquired immunodeficiency syndrome. The Journal of the Association of Physicians of India, Vol.47, No.7, pp. 680-684, ISSN 0004-5772.

Chakraborty, J. (1999). HIV/AIDS and ocular manifestations. Journal of the Indian Medical Association, Vol.97, No.8, pp. 299-304, ISSN 14743655.

Chen, K.C., Chen, J.Y. & Tung, G.A. (2009). Case 149: Immune reconstitution inflammatory syndrome. Radiology, Vol.252, No.3, pp. 924-928, ISSN 0033-8419.

Chimenti, C., Del Nonno, F., Topino, S., Abbate, I., Licci, S., Paglia, M.G., Capobianchi, M.R., Petrosillo, N. & Frustaci, A. (2007). Fatal myocardial co-infection by Toxoplasma gondii and Parvovirus B19 in an HIV patient. AIDS, Vol.21, No.10, pp. 1386-1388, ISSN 1473-5571.

Chintana, T., Sukthana, Y., Bunyakai, B. & Lekkla, A. (1998). Toxoplasma gondii antibody in pregnant women with and without HIV infection. Southeast Asian Journal of Tropical Medicine and Public Health, Vol.29, No.2, pp. 383-386, ISSN 0125-1562.

Chirgwin, K., Hafner, R., Leport, C. Remington, J., Andersen, J., Bosler, E.M., Roque, C., Rajicic, N., McAuliffe, V., Morlat, P., Jayaweera, D.T., Vilde, J.L. & Luft, B.J. (2002). Randomized phase II trial of atovaquone with pyrimethamine or sulfadiazine for treatment of toxoplasmic encephalitis in patients with acquired immunodeficiency syndrome: ACTG 237/ANRS 039 Study. AIDS Clinical Trials Group 237/Agence Nationale de Recherche sur le SIDA, Essai 039. Clinical Infectious Diseases, Vol.34, No.9, pp. 1243-1250, ISSN 1058-4838.

Ciricillo, S.F. & Rosenblum, M.L. (1990). Use of CT and MR imaging to distinguish intracranial lesions and to define the need for biopsy in AIDS patients. Journal of Neurosurgery, Vol.73, No.5, pp.720-724, ISSN 0022-3085.

Collazos, J. (2003). Opportunistic infections of the CNS in patients with AIDS: diagnosis and management. CNS Drugs, Vol.17, No.12, pp. 869-887, ISSN 1172-7047.

Corti, M., Metta, H., Villafañe, M.F., Yampolsky, C., Schtirbu, R., Sevlever, G. & Garrido, D. (2008). Stereotactic brain biopsy in the diagnosis of focal brain lesions in AIDS. Medicina, Vol.68, No.4, pp. 285-290, ISSN 0025-7680.

Costa-Silva, T.A., Meira, C.S., Ferreira, I.M., Hiramoto, R.M. & Pereira-Chioccola, V.L. (2008). Evaluation of immunization with tachyzoite excreted-secreted proteins in a novel susceptible mouse model (A/Sn) for *Toxoplasma gondii. Experimental Parasitology,* Vol.120, No.3, pp.227-234, ISSN 0014-4894.

Cota, G.F., Assad, E.C., Christo, P.P., Giannetti, A.V., Santos Filho, J.A. & Xavier, M.A. (2008). Ventriculitis: a rare case of primary cerebral toxoplasmosis in AIDS patient and literature review. *The Brazilian Journal of Infectious Diseases,* Vol.12, No.1, pp. 101-104, ISSN 1413-8670.

Cruz, M.L., Cardoso, C.A., Saavedra, M.C., Santos, E.D. & Melino, T. (2007). Congenital toxoplasmosis infection in an infant born to an HIV-1-infected mother. *Brazilian Journal of Infectious Diseases,* Vol.11, No. 6, pp. 610-611, ISSN 1413-8670.

Dal Pan, G.J. & McArthur, J.C. (1996). Neuroepidemiology of HIV infection. *Neurologic Clinics,* Vol.14, No.2, pp. 359-382, ISSN 0733-8619.

Dankner, W.M., Lindsey, J.C., Levin, M.J., Pediatric AIDS Clinical Trials Group Protocol Teams 051, 128, 138, 144, 152, 179, 190, 220, 240, 245, 254, 300 and 327. (2001). Correlates of opportunistic infections in children infected with the human immunodeficiency virus managed before highly active antiretroviral therapy. *The Pediatric Infectious Disease Journal,* Vol.20, No.1, pp. 40-48, ISSN 0891-3668.

Dardé, M.L. (1996). Biodiversity in *Toxoplasma gondii. Current Topics in Microbiology and Immunology,* Vol.219, pp. 27-41, ISSN 0070-217X.

Dardé, M.L., Bouteille, B. & Pestre-Alexandre, M. (1992). Isoenzyme analysis of 35 *Toxoplasma gondii* isolates and the biological and epidemiological implications. *Journal of Parasitology,* Vol.78, No.5, pp. 786-794, ISSN 0022-3395.

de Boer, M.G., Kroon, F.P., Kauffmann, R.H., Vriesendorp, R., Zwinderman, K. & van Dissel, J.T. (2003). Immune restoration disease in HIV-infected individuals receiving highly active antiretroviral therapy: clinical and immunological characteristics. *The Netherlands Journal of Medicine,* Vol.61, No.12, pp. 408-412, ISSN 0300-2977.

Dedicoat, M. & Livesley, N. (2006). Management of toxoplasmic encephalitis in HIV-infected adults (with an emphasis on resource-poor settings). *Cochrane Database of systematic reviews,* Vol.3, pp. CD005420, ISSN 1613-4125

de Gans, J., Portegies, P., Reiss, P., Troost, D., van Gool, T. & Lange, J.M. (1992). Pyrimethamine alone as maintenance therapy for central nervous system toxoplasmosis in 38 patients with AIDS. *Journal of Acquired Immune Deficiency Syndromes,* Vol.5, No.2, pp. 137-142, ISSN 0894-9255.

Denkers, E.Y. (2003) From cells to signaling cascades: manipulation of innate immunity by *Toxoplasma gondii. FEMS Immunology & Medical Microbiology,* Vol.39, No.3, pp.193-203, ISSN: 1574-695X.

Derouin, F., Pelloux, H. & ESCMID Study Group on Clinical Parasitology. (2008). Prevention of toxoplasmosis in transplant patients. *Clinical Microbiology & Infection,* Vol.14, No.12, pp.1089-1101, ISSN 1198-743X.

Dhiver, C., Milandre, C., Poizot-Martin, I., Drogoul, M.P., Gastaut, J.L. & Gastaut, J.A. (1993). 5-Fluoro-uracil-clindamycin for treatment of cerebral toxoplasmosis. *AIDS,* Vol.7, No.1, pp. 143-144, ISSN 1473-5571.

Dubey, J.P. (1998). Advances in the life cycle of *Toxoplasma gondii. International Journal of Parasitology,* Vol.28, No.7, pp.1019-1024, ISSN 0020-7519.

Dubey, J.P., Lindsay, D.S. & Speer, C.A. (1998). Structures of *Toxoplasma gondii* tachyzoites, bradyzoites, and sporozoites and biology and development of tissue cysts. *Clinical Microbiology Review,* Vol.11, No.2, pp.267-299, ISSN 0893-8512.

Dunay, I.R., Heimesaat, M.M., Bushrab, F.N., Müller, R.H., Stocker, H., Arasteh, K., Kurowski, M., Fitzner, R., Borner, K. & Liesenfeld, O. (2004). Atovaquone maintenance therapy prevents reactivation of toxoplasmic encephalitis in a murine model of reactivated toxoplasmosis. *Antimicrobial Agents and Chemotherapy*, Vol.48, No.12, pp. 4848-4854, ISSN 0066-4804.

Dunn, D., Newell, M.L. & Gilbert, R. (1997). Low risk of congenital toxoplasmosis in children born to women infected with human immunodeficiency virus. *The Pediatric Infectious Disease Journal*, Vol.16, No.1, pp. 84, ISSN 0891-3668.

Dupon, M., Cazenave, J., Pellegrin, J.L., Ragnaud, J.M., Cheyrou, A., Fischer, I., Leng, B. & Lacut, J.Y. (1995). Detection of *Toxoplasma gondii* by PCR and tissue culture in cerebrospinal fluid and blood of human immunodeficiency virus-seropositive patients. *Journal of Clinical Microbiology*, Vol.33, No.9, pp. 2421-2426, ISSN 0095-1137.

Dupouy-Camet, J., de Souza, S.L., Maslo, C., Paugam, A., Saimot, A.G., Benarous, R., Tourte-Schaefer, C. & Derouin, F. (1993). Detection of *Toxoplasma gondii* in venous blood from AIDS patients by polymerase chain reaction. *Journal of Clinical Microbiology*, Vol.31, No.7, pp. 1866-1869, ISSN 0095-1137.

Duran, J.M., Cretel, E., Bagneres, D., Guillemot, E., Kaplanski, G. & Soubeyrand, J. (1995). Failure of atovaquone in the treatment of cerebral toxoplasmosis. *AIDS*, Vol.9, No.7, pp. 812-813, ISSN 1473-5571.

Duval, X., Pajot, O., Le Moing, V., Longuet, P., Ecobichon, J.L., Mentre, F., Leport, C. & Vilde, J.L. (2004). Maintenance therapy with cotrimoxazole for toxoplasmic encephalitis in the era of highly active antiretroviral therapy. *AIDS*, Vol.18, No.9, pp. 1342-1344, ISSN 1473-5571.

Emeka, E.U., Ogunrin, A.O. & Olubunmi, A. (2010). Cerebellar toxoplasmosis in HIV/AIDS: a case report. *West African Journal of Medicine*, Vol.29, No.2, pp. 123-126, ISSN 0189-160X.

Eza, D., Cerrillo, G., Moore, D.A. Castro, C., Ticona, E., Morales, D., Cabanillas, J., Barrantes, F., Alfaro, A., Benavides, A., Rafael, A., Valladares, G., Arevalo, F., Evans, C.A. & Gilman, RH. (2006). Postmortem findings and opportunistic infections in HIV-positive patients from a public hospital in Peru. *Pathology Research and Practice*, Vol.202, No.11, pp. 767-775, ISSN 0344-0338.

Falusi O, French AL, Seaberg EC, Tien, P.C., Watts, D.H., Minkoff, H., Piessens ,E., Kovacs, A., Anastos, K. & Cohen, M.H. (2002). Prevalence and predictors of *Toxoplasma* seropositivity in women with and at risk for human immunodeficiency virus infection. *Clinical Infectious Diseases*, Vol.35, No.11, pp. 1414-1417, ISSN 1058-4838.

Fernandes, R.C., Vasconcellos, V.P., Araújo, L.C. & Medina-Acosta, E. (2009). Vertical transmission of HIV and *Toxoplasma* by reactivation in a chronically infected woman. *The Brazilian Journal of Infectious Diseases*, Vol.13, No.1, pp. 70-71, ISSN 1413-8670.

Fernandez-Martin, J., Leport, C., Morlat, P., Meyohas, M.C., Chauvin, J.P. & Vilde, J.L. (1991). Pyrimethamine-clarithromycin combination for therapy of acute *Toxoplasma* encephalitis in patients with AIDS. *Antimicrobial Agents and Chemotherapy*, Vol.35, No.10, pp. 2049-2052, ISSN 0066-4804.

Ferreira, I.M., Vidal, J.E., Costa-Silva, T.A., Meira, C.S., Hiramoto, R.M., Penalva de Oliveira, A.C. & Pereira-Chioccola, V.L. (2008). *Toxoplasma gondii*: genotyping of strains from Brazilian AIDS patients with cerebral toxoplasmosis by multilocus PCR-RFLP markers. *Experimental Parasitology*, Vol.118, No. 2, pp.221-227, ISSN 0014-4894.

Fournier, S., Rabian, C., Alberti, C., Carmagnat, M.V., Garin, J.F., Charron, D., Derouin, F. & Molina, J.M. (2001). Immune recovery under highly active antiretroviral therapy is associated with restoration of lymphocyte proliferation and interferon-gamma production in the presence of *Toxoplasma gondii* antigens. *The Journal of Infectious Diseases*, Vol.183, No.11, pp. 1586-1591, ISSN 0022-1899.

Frenkel, J.K. (1973). *Toxoplasma* in and around us. *Journal of Biological Sciences*, Vol.23, pp.343-352, ISSN 1727-3048.

Fuentes, I., Rubio, J.M., Ramírez, C. & Alvar, J. (2001). Genotypic characterization of *Toxoplasma gondii* strains associated with human toxoplasmosis in Spain: direct analysis from clinical samples. *Journal of Clinical Microbiology*, Vol.39, No.4, pp. 1566-1570, ISSN 0095-1137.

Furco, A., Carmagnat, M., Chevret, S., Garin, Y.J., Pavie, J., De Castro, N., Charron, D., Derouin, F., Rabian, C. & Molina, J.M. (2008). Restoration of *Toxoplasma gondii*-specific immune responses in patients with AIDS starting HAART. *AIDS*, Vol.22, No.16, pp. 2087-2096, ISSN 1473-5571.

Gagliuso, D.J., Teich, S.A., Friedman, A.H. & Orellana, J. (1990). Ocular toxoplasmosis in AIDS patients. *Transactions of the American Ophthalmological Society*, Vol.90, pp. 63-86, discussion 86-88, ISSN 0065-9533.

Gallo, B.V., Shulman, L.M., Weiner, W.J., Petito, C.K. & Berger, J.R. (1996). HIV encephalitis presenting with severe generalized chorea. *Neurology*, Vol.46, No.4, pp. 1163-1165, ISSN 0028-3878.

Galván Ramírez, M.L., Valdez Alvarado, V., Vargas Gutierrez, G., Jiménez González, O., García Cosio, C. & Vielma Sandoval, M. (1997). Prevalence of IgG and IgM anti-*Toxoplasma* antibodies in patients with HIV and acquired immunodeficiency syndrome (AIDS). *Revista da Sociedade Brasileira de Medicina Tropical*, Vol.30, No.6, pp. 465-467, ISSN 0037-8682.

Genot, S., Franck, J., Forel, J.M., Rebaudet, S., Ajzenberg, D., de Paula, A.M., Dardé, M.L., Stein, A. & Ranque, S. (2007). Severe *Toxoplasma gondii* I/III recombinant-genotype encephalitis in a human immunodeficiency virus patient. *Journal of Clinical Microbiology*, Vol.45, No.9, pp. 3138-3140, ISSN 0095-1137.

Gill, P.S., Graham, R.A., Boswell, W., Meyer, P., Krailo, M. & Levine, A.M. (1986). A comparison of imaging, clinical, and pathologic aspects of space-occupying lesions within the brain in patients with acquired immune deficiency syndrome. *American Journal of Physiologic Imaging*, Vol.1, No.3, pp. 134-141, ISSN 0885-8276.

González-Castillo, J., Blanco, F., Soriano, V., Barreiro, P., Concepción Bravo, M., Jiménez-Nácher, I. & González-Lahoz, J. (2001). Opportunistic episodes in patients infected with the human immunodeficiency virus during the first 6 months of HAART. *Medicina Clinica*, Vol.17, No.3, pp. 81-84, ISSN 0025-7753.

Grant, I.H., Gold, J.W., Rosenblum, M., Niedzwiecki, D. & Armstrong, D. (1990). *Toxoplasma gondii* serology in HIV-infected patients: the development of central nervous system toxoplasmosis in AIDS. *AIDS*, Vol.4, No.6, pp. 519-521, ISSN 0269-9370.

Gray, F., Bazille, C., Adle-Biassette, H., Mikol, J., Moulignier, A. & Scaravilli, F. (2005). Central nervous system immune reconstitution disease in acquired immunodeficiency syndrome patients receiving highly active antiretroviral treatment. *Journal of Neurovirology*, Vol.11, No.Suppl 3, pp. 16-22, ISSN 1355-0284.

Gross, U., Kempf, M.C., Seeber, F., Lüder, C.G., Lugert, R. & Bohne, W. (1997). Reactivation of chronic toxoplasmosis: is there a link to strain-specific differences in the parasite? *Behring Institute Mitteilungen*, Vol.99, pp. 97-106, ISSN 0955-8810.

Guelar, A., Miró, J.M., Mallolas, J., Zamora, L., Cardenal, C., Gatell, J.M. & Soriano, E. (1994). Therapeutic alternatives for cases of cerebral toxoplasmosis in patients with AIDS: clarithromycin and atovaquone. *Enfermedades Infecciosas y Microbiologia Clinica*, Vol.12, No.3, pp. 137-140, ISSN 0213-005X.

Guerot, E., Aissa, F., Kayal, S., Leselbaum, A., Grenier, O., Guerot, C. & Labrousse, J. (1995). *Toxoplasma* pericarditis in acquired immunodeficiency syndrome. *Intensive Care Medicine*, Vol.21, No.3, pp.229-230, ISSN 0342-4642.

Guex, A.C., Radziwill, A.J. & Bucher, H.C. (2000). Discontinuation of secondary prophylaxis for toxoplasmic encephalitis in human immunodeficiency virus infection after immune restoration with highly active antiretroviral therapy. *Clinical Infectious Diseases*, Vol.30, No.3, pp. 602-603, ISSN 1058-4838.

Gupta, S., Shah, D.M. & Shah, I. (2009). Neurological disorders in HIV-infected children in India. *Annals of Tropical Paediatrics*, Vol.29, No.3, pp. 177-181, ISSN 0272-4936.

Gyori, E. & Hyma, B.A. (1998). Fatal automobile crash caused by cerebral toxoplasmosis. *The American Journal of Forensic Medicine and Pathology*, Vol.19, No.2, pp. 178-180, ISSN 0195-7910.

Habegger de Sorrentino, A., López, R., Motta, P., Marinic, K., Sorrentino, A., Iliovich, E., Rubio, A.E., Quarleri, J. & Salomón, H. (2005). HLA class II involvement in HIV-associated toxoplasmic encephalitis development. *Clinical Immunology*, Vol.115, No.2, pp.133-137, ISSN 1521-6616.

Hari, K.R., Modi, M.R., Mochan, A.H. & Modi, G. (2007). Reduced risk of *Toxoplasma* encephalitis in HIV-infected patients--a prospective study from Gauteng, South Africa. *International Journal of STD & AIDS*, Vol.18, No.8, pp. 555-558, ISSN 0956-4624.

Harris, T.M., Smith, R.R., Bognanno, J.R. & Edwards, M.K. (1990). Toxoplasmic myelitis in AIDS: gadolinium-enhanced MR. *Journal of Computer Assisted Tomography*, Vol. 14, No.5, pp. 809-811, ISSN 0363-8715.

Hedriana, H.L., Mitchell, J.L., Brown, G.M. & Williams, S.B. (1993). Normal fetal outcome in a pregnancy with central nervous system with toxoplasmosis and human immunodeficiency virus infection. A case report. *The Journal of Reproductive Medicine*, Vol.38, No.9, pp.747-750, ISSN 0024-7758.

Hierl, T., Reischl, U., Lang, P., Hebart, H., Stark, M., Kyme, P. & Autenrieth, I.B. (2004). Preliminary evaluation of one conventional nested and two real-time PCR assays for the detection of *Toxoplasma gondii* in immunocompromised patients. *Journal of Medical Microbiology*, Vol.53, No.7, pp. 629-632, ISSN 0022-2615.

Hirose, G. (2000). Parkinsonism in a patient with AIDS. *Internal Medicine*, Vol.39, No.12, pp. 1006-1007, ISSN 0918-2918.

Hoffmann, C., Ernst, M., Meyer, P., Wolf, E., Rosenkranz, T., Plettenberg, A., Stoehr, A., Horst, H.A., Marienfeld, K. & Lange, C. (2007). Evolving characteristics of toxoplasmosis in patients infected with human immunodeficiency virus-1: clinical course and *Toxoplasma gondii*-specific immune responses. *Clinical Microbiology and Infection*, Vol.13, No.5, pp. 510-515, ISSN 1198-743X.

Hofman, P., Quintens, H., Michiels, J.F., Taillan, B., Thyss, A., (1993). *Toxoplasma* cystitis associated with acquired immunodeficiency syndrome. *Urology*, Vol.42, No.5, pp.589-592, ISSN 0090-4295.

Holch, A., Opravil, M., Moradpour, D., Siegenthaler, W., Schneider, J. & Lüthy, R. (1993). Disseminated toxoplasmosis in AIDS. *Deutsche Medizinische Wochenschrift*, Vol.118, No.22, pp. 814-819, ISSN 0012-0472.

Holland, G.N., Engstrom, R.E. Jr., Glasgow, B.J., Berger, B.B., Daniels, S.A., Sidikaro, Y., Harmon, J.A., Fischer, D.H., Boyer, D.S. & Rao, N.A. (1988). Ocular toxoplasmosis in patients with the acquired immunodeficiency syndrome. *American Journal of Ophthalmology*, Vol.106, No.6, pp.653-667, ISSN 0002-9394.

Holliman, R.E. (1990). Serological study of the prevalence of toxoplasmosis in asymptomatic patients infected with human immunodeficiency virus. *Epidemiology and Infection*, Vol.105, No.2, pp. 415-418, ISSN 1469-4409.

Honoré, S., Couvelard, A., Garin, Y.J., Bedel, C., Hénin, D., Dardé, M.L. & Derouin, F. (2000). Genotyping of *Toxoplasma gondii* strains from immunocompromised patients. *Pathologie Biologie*, Vol.48, No.6, pp. 541-547, ISSN 0369-8114.

Howe, D.K., Honoré, S., Derouin, F. & Sibley, L.D. (1997). Determination of genotypes of *Toxoplasma gondii* strains isolated from patients with toxoplasmosis. *Journal of Clinical Microbiology*, Vol.35, No.6, pp.1411-1414, ISSN 0095-1137.

Howe, D.K. & Sibley, L.D. (1995). *Toxoplasma gondii* comprises three clonal lineages: correlation of parasite genotype with human disease. *Journal of Infectious Diseases*, Vol.172, No.6, pp.1561-1566, ISSN 0022-1899.

Ho-Yen, D.O. (1992). Immunocompromised patients, In: *Human Toxoplasmosis*, D.O. Ho-Yen, & A.W.L. Joss, (Eds.), 184-213, Oxford University Press, ISBN 0198547501, New York, USA.

Huber, W., Bautz, W., Classen, M. & Schepp, W. (1995). Pyrimethamine-sulfadiazine resistant cerebral toxoplasmosis in AIDS. *Deutsche Medizinische Wochenschrift*, Vol.120, No.3, pp. 60-64, ISSN 0012-0472.

Hung, C.C., Chen, M.Y., Hsieh, S.M., Hsiao, C.F., Sheng, W.H. & Chang, S.C. (2005). Prevalence of *Toxoplasma gondii* infection and incidence of *Toxoplasma* encephalitis in non-haemophiliac HIV-1-infected adults in Taiwan. *International Journal of STD & AIDS*, Vol.16, No.4, pp. 302-6, ISSN 0956-4624.

Huruy, K., Mulu, A., Mengistu, G., Shewa-Amare, A., Akalu, A., Kassu, A., Andargie, G., Elias, D. & Torben, W. (2008). Immune reconstitution inflammatory syndrome among HIV/AIDS patients during highly active antiretroviral therapy in Addis Ababa, Ethiopia. *Japanese Journal of Infectious Diseases*, Vol.61, No.3, pp. 205-209, ISSN 1344-6304.

Ilniczky, S., Debreczeni, R., Kovács, T., Várkonyi, V., Barsi, P. & Szirmai, I. (2006). [Aids-related *Toxoplasma*-encephalitis presenting with acute psychotic episode]. *Ideggyógyászati Szemle*, Vol.59, No.7-8, pp. 289-293, ISSN 0019-1442.

Israelski, D.M., Chmiel, J.S., Poggensee, L., Phair, J.P. & Remington, J.S. (1993). Prevalence of *Toxoplasma* infection in a cohort of homosexual men at risk of AIDS and toxoplasmic encephalitis. *Journal of Acquired Immune Deficiency Syndrome*, Vol.6, No.4, pp. 414-418, ISSN 0894-9255.

Israelski, D.M. & Remington, J.S. (1992). AIDS-associated toxoplasmosis. In: *The medical management of AIDS*, M.A. Sande, & P.A. Volberding (Eds.), 319-345, WB Saunders, ISBN 0721637310, Philadelphia, USA.

Jacobson, J.M., Hafner, R., Remington, J. Farthing, C., Holden-Wiltse, J., Bosler, E. M., Harris, C., Jayaweera, D.T., Roque, C., Luft, B.J. & Members of the ACTG 156 Study Team.

(2001). Dose-escalation, phase I/II study of azithromycin and pyrimethamine for the treatment of toxoplasmic encephalitis in AIDS. *AIDS*, Vol.15, No.5, pp. 583-589, ISSN 1473-5571.

Jevtović, D.J., Salemović, D., Ranin, J., Pesić, I., Zerjav, S. & Djurković-Djaković, O. (2005). The prevalence and risk of immune restoration disease in HIV-infected patients treated with highly active antiretroviral therapy. *HIV Medicine*, Vol.6, No.2, pp. 140-143, ISSN 1464 -2662.

Jordan, M.K., Burstein, A.H., Rock-Kress, D., Alfaro, R.M., Pau, A.K., Kovacs, J.A. & Piscitelli, S.C. (2004). Plasma pharmacokinetics of sulfadiazine administered twice daily versus four times daily are similar in human immunodeficiency virus-infected patients. *Antimicrobial Agents and Chemotherapy*, Vol.48, No.2, pp. 635-637, ISSN 0066-4804.

Jubault, V., Pacanowski, J., Rabian, C. & Viard, J.P. (2002). Interruption of prophylaxis for major opportunistic infections in HIV-infected patients receiving triple combination antiretroviral therapy. *Annales de Médecine Interne*, Vol.151, No.3, pp. 163-168, ISSN 0003-410X.

Kaplan, J.E., Hanson, D., Dworkin, M.S., Frederick, T., Bertolli, J., Lindegren, M.L., Holmberg, S. & Jones, J.L. (2000). Epidemiology of human immunodeficiency virus-associated opportunistic infections in the United States in the era of highly active antiretroviral therapy. *Clinical Infectious Diseases*, Vol.30, No.Suppl 1, pp. S5-S14, ISSN 1058-4838.

Kastenbauer, U., Wolf, E., Kollan, C., Hamouda, O., Bogner, J.R. & ClinSurv Study Group. (2009). Impaired CD4-cell immune reconstitution upon HIV therapy in patients with toxoplasmic encephalitis compared to patients with pneumocystis pneumonia as AIDS indicating disease. *European Journal of Medical Research*, Vol.14, No.6, pp. 244-249, ISSN 0949-2321.

Katlama, C., De Wit, S., O'Doherty, E., Van Glabeke, M. & Clumeck, N. (1996a). Pyrimethamine-clindamycin vs. pyrimethamine-sulfadiazine as acute and long-term therapy for toxoplasmic encephalitis in patients with AIDS. *Clinical Infectious Diseases*, Vol.22, No.2, pp. 268-275, ISSN 1058-4838.

Katlama, C., Mouthon, B., Gourdon, D., Lapierre, D. & Rousseau, F. (1996b). Atovaquone as long-term suppressive therapy for toxoplasmic encephalitis in patients with AIDS and multiple drug intolerance. Atovaquone Expanded Access Group. *AIDS*, Vol.10, No.10, pp. 1107-1112, ISSN 1473-5571.

Khan, A., Su, C., German, M., Storch, G.A., Clifford, D.B. & Sibley, L.D. (2005). Genotyping of *Toxoplasma gondii* strains from immunocompromised patients reveals high prevalence of type I strains. *Journal of Clinical Microbiology*, Vol.43, No.12, pp. 5881-5887, ISSN 0095-1137.

Klotz, S.A., Aziz Mohammed, A., Girmai Woldemichael, M., Worku Mitku, M., Handrich, M. (2009). Immune reconstitution inflammatory syndrome in a resource-poor setting. *Journal of the International association of Physicians in AIDS Care*, Vol.8, No.2, pp. 122-127, ISSN 1545-1097.

Kong, J.T., Grigg, M.E., Uyetake, L., Parmley, S. & Boothroyd, J.C. (2003). Serotyping of *Toxoplasma gondii* infections in humans using synthetic peptides. *The Journal of Infectious Diseases*, Vol.187, No.9, pp. 1484-1495, ISSN 0022-1899.

Kongsaengdao, S. (2009). Neurologic immune reconstitution inflammatory syndrome in HIV/AIDS: outcome and epidemiology. *Neurology*, Vol.73, No.23, pp. 2046-2047, ISSN 0028-3878.

Koppel, B.S. & Daws, M. (1990). Rubral tremor due to midbrain toxoplasmosis abscess. *Movement Disorders*, Vol.5, No.3, pp. 254-256, ISSN 0885-3185.

Kovari, H., Ebnöther, C., Schweiger, A., Berther, N., Kuster, H. & Günthard, H.F. (2010). Pulmonary toxoplasmosis, a rare but severe manifestation of a common opportunistic infection in late HIV presenters: report of two cases. *Infection*, Vol.38, No.2, pp.141-144, ISSN 0300-8126.

Kumarasamy, N., Venkatesh, K.K., Devaleenol, B., Poongulali, S., Yephthomi, T., Pradeep, A., Saghayam, S., Flanigan, T., Mayer, K.H. & Solomon, S. (2010). Factors associated with mortality among HIV-infected patients in the era of highly active antiretroviral therapy in southern India. *Internal Journal of Infectious Diseases*, Vol.4, No.2, pp. e127-e131, ISSN 1201-9712.

Kung, D.H., Hubenthal, E.A., Kwan, J.Y., Shelburne, S.A., Goodman, J.C. & Kass, J.S. (2011). Toxoplasmosis myelopathy and myopathy in an AIDS patient: a case of immune reconstitution inflammatory syndrome? *The Neurologist*, Vol.17, No.1, pp. 49-51, ISSN 1074-7931.

Kuritzkes, D.R., Shugarts, D., Bakhtiari, M., Poticha, D., Johnson, J., Rubin, M., Gingeras, T.R., Kennedy, M., & Eron, J.J. (2000). Emergence of dual resistance to zidovudine and lamivudine in HIV-1-infected patients treated with zidovudine plus lamivudine as initial therapy. *Journal of Acquired Immune Deficiency Syndromes*, Vol.23, No.1, pp. 26-34, ISSN 0894-9255.

Lafeuillade, A., Pellegrino, P., Poggi, C., Profizi, N., Quilichini, R., Chouette, I. & Navarreté, M.S. (1993). Efficacy of atovaquone in resistant toxoplasmosis in AIDS. *Presse médicale*, Vol.22, No.33, pp.1708, ISSN 0755-4982.

Lago, E.G., Conrado, G.S., Piccoli, C.S., Carvalho, R.L. & Bender, A.L. (2009). *Toxoplasma gondii* antibody profile in HIV-infected pregnant women and the risk of congenital toxoplasmosis. *European Journal of Clinical Microbiology & Infectious Diseases*, Vol.28, No.4, pp. 345-351, ISSN 0934-9723.

Lamichhane, G., Shah, D.N., Sharma, S. & Chaudhary, M. (2010). Ocular manifestations in HIV/AIDS cases in Nepal. *Nepalese Journal of Ophthalmology*, Vol.2, No.1, pp. 45-50, ISSN 2072-6805.

Langford, T.D., Letendre, S.L., Larrea, G.J. & Masliah, E. (2003). Changing patterns in the neuropathogenesis of HIV during the HAART era. *Brain Pathology*, Vol.13, No.2, pp. 195-210, ISSN 1015-6305.

Lanjewar, D.N., Jain, P.P. & Shetty, C.R. (1998a). Profile of central nervous system pathology in patients with AIDS: an autopsy study from India. *AIDS*, Vol.12, No.3, pp. 309-313, ISSN 1473-5571.

Lanjewar, D.N., Surve, K.V., Maheshwari, M.B., Shenoy, B.P. & Hira, S.K. (1998b). Toxoplasmosis of the central nervous system in the acquired immunodeficiency syndrome. *Indian Journal of Pathology & Microbiology*, Vol.41, No.2, pp.147-151, ISSN 0377-4929.

Lanoy, E., Guiguet, M., Bentata, M., Rouveix, E., Dhiver, C., Poizot-Martin, I., Costagliola, D., Gasnault, J. & FHDH-ANRS CO4. (2011). Survival after neuroAIDS: Association with antiretroviral CNS Penetration-Effectiveness score. *Neurology*, Vol.76, No.7, pp. 644-651, ISSN 0028-3878.

Lawn, S.D. & Wilkinson, R.J. (2006). Immune reconstitution disease associated with parasitic infections following antiretroviral treatment. *Parasite Immunology*, Vol.28, No.11, pp. 625-633, ISSN 0141-9838.

Leport, C., Bastuji-Garin, S., Perronne, C., Salmon, D., Marche, C., Briçaire, F. & Vilde, J.L. (1989). An open study of the pyrimethamine-clindamycin combination in AIDS patients with brain toxoplasmosis. *Journal of Infectious Diseases*, Vol.160, No.3, pp.557-558, ISSN 0022-1899.

Leport, C., Raffi, F., Matheron, S., Katlama, C., Regnier, B., Saimot, A.G., Marche, C., Vedrenne, C. & Vilde, J.L. (1988). Treatment of central nervous system toxoplasmosis with pyrimethamine/sulfadiazine combination in 35 patients with the acquired immunodeficiency syndrome. Efficacy of long-term continuous therapy. *The American Journal of Medicine*, Vol.84, No.1, pp. 94-100, ISSN 0002-9343.

Letillois, M.F., Laigle, V., Santoro, F., Micoud, M. & Chumpitazi, B.F. (1995). *Toxoplasma gondii* surface antigen-1 in sera of HIV-infected patients as an indicator of reactivated toxoplasmosis. *European Journal of Clinical Microbiology & Infectious Diseases*, Vol.14, No.10, pp. 899-903, ISSN 0934-9723.

Lian, Y.L., Heng, B.S., Nissapatorn, V. & Lee, C. (2007). AIDS-defining illnesses: a comparison between before and after commencement of highly active antiretroviral therapy (HAART). *Current HIV Research*, Vol.5, No.5, pp. 484-489, ISSN 1570-162X.

Lin, D.S. & Bowman, D.D. (1992). *Toxoplasma gondii*: an AIDS enhancing cofactor. *Medical Hypotheses*, Vol.39, No.2, pp. 140-142, ISSN 0306-9877.

Lindström, I., Kaddu-Mulindwa, D.H., Kironde, F. & Lindh, J. (2006). Prevalence of latent and reactivated *Toxoplasma gondii* parasites in HIV-patients from Uganda. *Acta Tropica*, Vol.100, No.3, pp. 218-222, ISSN 0001-706X.

Lucas, S.B., Hounnou, A., Peacock, C., Beaumel, A., Djomand, G., N'Gbichi, J.M., Yeboue, K., Hondé, M., Diomande, M., Giordano, C., Doorly, R., Brattegaard, K., Kestens, L., Smithwick, R., Kadio, A., Ezani, N., Yapi, A. & De Cock, K.M. (1993). The mortality and pathology of HIV infection in a West Africa city. *AIDS*, Vol.7, No.12, pp.1569-1579, ISSN 1473-5571.

Luft, B.J. & Remington, J.S. (1985). Toxoplasmosis of the central nervous system. In: *Current clinical topics in infectious diseases*, J.S. Remington, M.N. Swartz, (Eds.), 315-358, McGraw-Hill, ISBN 0070518556, New York. USA.

Luft, B.J. & RemIngton, J.S. (1988). AIDS Commentary. Toxoplasmic encephalitis. *Journal of Infectious Diseases*, Vol. 157, No.1, pp.1-6. ISSN 0022-1899.

Luft, B.J. & Remington, J.S. (1992). Toxoplasmic encephalitis in AIDS. *Clinical Infectious Diseases*, Vol.15, No.2, pp. 211-222, ISSN 1058-4838.

Machala, L., Malý, M., Hrdá, S., Rozsypal, H., Stanková, M. & Kodym, P. (2009). Antibody response of HIV-infected patients to latent, cerebral and recently acquired toxoplasmosis. *European Journal of Clinical Microbiology & Infectious Diseases*, Vol.28, No.2, pp. 179-182, ISSN 0934-9723.

Maggi, P., de Mari, M., De Blasi, R., Armenise, S., Romanelli, C., Andreula, C., Zimatore, G. & Angarano, G. (1996). Choreoathetosis in acquired immune deficiency syndrome patients with cerebral toxoplasmosis. *Movement Disorders*, Vol.11, No.4, pp. 434-436, ISSN 0885-3185.

Maher, J., Choudhri, S., Halliday, W., Power, C. & Nath, A. (1997). AIDS dementia complex with generalized myoclonus. *Movement Disorders*, Vol.12, No.4, pp. 593-597, ISSN 0885-3185.

Maïga, I., Kiemtoré, P. & Tounkara, A. (2001). Prevalence of antitoxoplasma antibodies in patients with Acquired immunodeficiency syndrome and blood donors in Bamako. *Bulletin de la Société de pathologie exotique*, Vol.94, No.3, pp. 268-270, ISSN 0002-9637.

Mansour, A.M. (1990). Neuro-ophthalmic findings in acquired immunodeficiency syndrome. *Journal of Clinical Neuro-Ophthalmology*, Vol.10, No.3, pp. 167-174, ISSN 0272-846X.

Manzardo, C., Del Mar Ortega, M., Sued, O., García, F., Moreno, A. & Miró, J.M. (2005). Central nervous system opportunistic infections in developed countries in the highly active antiretroviral therapy era. *Journal of Neurovirology*, Vol.11, No.Suppl 3, pp. 72-82, ISSN 1355-0284.

Martin-Blondel, G., Alvarez, M., Delobel, P., Uro-Coste, E., Cuzin, L., Cuvinciuc, V., Fillaux J., Massip, P. & Marchou, B. (2010). Toxoplasmic encephalitis IRIS in HIV-infected patients: a case series and review of the literature. *Journal of Neurology, Neurosurgery, and Psychiatry*, 10.1136/JNNP.2009.199919, ISSN 0022-3050.

Masliah, E., DeTeresa, R.M., Mallory, M.E. & Hansen, L.A. (2000). Changes in pathological findings at autopsy in AIDS cases for the last 15 years. *AIDS*, Vol.14, No.1, pp. 69-74, ISSN 1473-5571.

Mastroianni, A., Coronado, O., Scarani, P., Manfredi, R. & Chiodo, F. (1996). Liver toxoplasmosis and acquired immunodeficiency syndrome. *Recenti Progressi in Medicina*, Vol.87, No.7-8, pp.353-355, ISSN 0034-1193.

McCombe, J.A., Auer, R.N., Maingat, F.G., Houston, S., Gill, M.J. & Power, C. (2009). Neurologic immune reconstitution inflammatory syndrome in HIV/AIDS: outcome and epidemiology. *Neurology*, Vol.72, No.9, pp. 835-841, ISSN 0028-3878.

McFadden, D.C., Camps, M. & Boothroyd, J.C. (2001). Resistance as a tool in the study of old and new drug targets in *Toxoplasma*. *Drug Resistance Updates*, Vol.4, No.2, pp. 79-84, ISSN 1368-7646.

Meira, C.S., Costa-Silva, T.A., Vidal, J.E., Ferreira, I.M., Hiramoto, R.M. & Pereira-Chioccola, V.L. (2008). Use of the serum reactivity against *Toxoplasma gondii* excreted-secreted antigens in cerebral toxoplasmosis diagnosis in human immunodeficiency virus-infected patients. *Journal of Medical Microbiology*, Vol.57, No.Pt 7, pp. 845-850, ISSN 0022-2615.

Meisheri, Y.V., Mehta, S. & Patel, U. (1997). A prospective study of seroprevalence of Toxoplasmosis in general population, and in HIV/AIDS patients in Bombay, India. *Journal of Postgraduate Medicine*, Vol.43, No.4, pp. 93-97, ISSN 0022-3859.

Merzianu, M., Gorelick, S.M., Paje, V., Kotler, D.P. & Sian, C. (2005). Gastric toxoplasmosis as the presentation of acquired immunodeficiency syndrome. *Archives of Pathology & Laboratory Medicine*, Vol.129, No.4, pp.e87-e90, ISSN 0003-9985.

Millogo, A., Ki-Zerbo, G.A., Traoré, W., Sawadogo, A.B., Ouédraogo, I. & Péghini, M. (2000). *Toxoplasma* serology in HIV infected patients and suspected cerebral toxoplasmosis at the Central Hospital of Bobo-Dioulasso (Burkina Faso). *Bulletin de la Société de pathologie exotique*, Vol.93, No.1, pp. 17-19, ISSN 0002-9637.

Minkoff, H., Remington, J.S., Holman, S., Ramirez, R., Goodwin, S. & Landesman, S. (1997). Vertical transmission of toxoplasma by human immunodeficiency virus-infected women. *American Journal of Obstetrics and Gynecology*, Vol.176, No.3, pp. 555-559, ISSN 0002-9378.

Miro, J.M., Lopez, J.C., Podzamczer, D., Peña, J.M., Alberdi, J.C., Martínez, E., Domingo, P., Cosin, J., Claramonte, X., Arribas, J.R., Santín, M., Ribera, E. & GESIDA 04/98 Study Group. (2006). Discontinuation of primary and secondary *Toxoplasma gondii* prophylaxis is safe in HIV-infected patients after immunological restoration with highly active antiretroviral therapy: results of an open, randomized, multicenter clinical trial. *Clinical Infectious Diseases*, Vol.43, No.1, pp. 79-89, ISSN 1058-4838.

Mitchell, C.D., Erlich, S.S., Mastrucci, M.T., Hutto, S.C., Parks, W.P. & Scott, G.B., (1990). Congenital toxoplasmosis occurring in infants perinatally infected with human immunodeficiency virus 1. *The Pediatric Infectious Disease Journal*, Vol.9, No.7, pp. 512-518, ISSN 0891-3668.

Mocroft, A., Vella, S., Benfield, T.L., Chiesi, A., Miller, V., Gargalianos, P., d'Arminio, Monforte, A., Yust, I., Bruun, J.N., Phillips, A.N. & Lundgren, J.D., (1998). Changing patterns of mortality across Europe in patients infected with HIV-1. EuroSIDA Study Group. *The Lancet*, Vol.352, No.9142, pp. 1725-1730, ISSN 0140-6736.

Montoya, J.G. & Liesenfeld, O. (2004). Toxoplasmosis. *The Lancet*, Vol.363, No.9425, pp.1965-1976, ISSN 0140-6736.

Moorthy, R.S., Smith, R.E. & Rao, N.A. (1993). Progressive ocular toxoplasmosis in patients with acquired immunodeficiency syndrome. *American Journal of Ophthalmollogy*, Vol.115, No.6, pp. 742-747, ISSN 1549-4713.

Morisset, S., Peyron, F., Lobry, J.R., Garweg, J., Ferrandiz, J., Musset, K., Gomez-Marin, J.E., de la Torre, A., Demar, M., Carme, B., Mercier, C., Garin, J.F. & Cesbron-Delauw, M.F. (2008). Serotyping of *Toxoplasma gondii*: striking homogeneous pattern between symptomatic and asymptomatic infections within Europe and South America. *Microbes and Infections*, Vol.10, No.7, pp. 742-747, ISSN 1286-4579.

Murakami, T., Nakajima, M., Nakamura, T., Hara, A., Uyama, E., Mita, S., Matsushita, S., Uchino, M.. (2000). Parkinsonian symptoms as an initial manifestation in a Japanese patient with acquired immunodeficiency syndrome and *Toxoplasma* infection. *Internal Medicine*, Vol.39, No.12, pp. 1111-1114, ISSN 0918-2918.

Mwanza, J.C., Nyamabo, L.K., Tylleskär, T. & Plant, G.T. (2004). Neuro-ophthalmological disorders in HIV infected subjects with neurological manifestations. *The British Journal of Ophthalmology*, Vol.88, No.11, pp. 1455-1459, ISSN 0007-1161.

Mzileni, M.O., Longo-Mbenza, B. & Chephe, T.J. (2008). Mortality and causes of death in HIV-positive patients receiving antiretroviral therapy at Tshepang Clinic in Doctor George Mukhari Hospital. *Polskie Archiwum Medycyny Wewnętrznej*, Vol.118, No.10, pp. 548-554, ISSN 0032-3772.

Naito, T., Inui, A., Kudo, N., Matsumoto, N., Fukuda, H., Isonuma, H., Sekigawa, I., Dambara, T. & Hayashida, Y. (2007). Seroprevalence of IgG anti-*Toxoplasma* antibodies in asymptomatic patients infected with human immunodeficiency virus in Japan. *Internal Medicine*, Vol.46, No. 14, pp. 1149-1150.

Nascimento, L.V., Stollar, F., Tavares, L.B., Cavasini, C.E., Maia, I.L., Cordeiro, J.A. & Ferreira, M.U. (2001). Risk factors for toxoplasmic encephalitis in HIV-infected patients: a case-control study in Brazil. *Annals of Tropical Medicine and Parasitology*, Vol.95, No.6, pp. 587-593, ISSN 0003-4983.

Nath, A., Hobson, D.E. & Russell, A. (1993). Movement disorders with cerebral toxoplasmosis and AIDS. *Movement Disorders*, Vol.8, No.1, pp. 107-112, ISSN 0885-3185.

Navia, B.A., Petito, C.K., Gold, J.W., Cho, E.S., Jordan, B.D. & Price, R.W. (1986). Cerebral toxoplasmosis complicating the acquired immune deficiency syndrome: clinical and neuropathological findings in 27 patients. *Annals of Neurology*, Vol.19, No.3, pp. 224-238, ISSN 0364-5134.

Neuen-Jacob, E., Figge, C., Arendt, G., Wendtland, B., Jacob, B. & Wechsler, W. (1993). Neuropathological studies in the brains of AIDS patients with opportunistic diseases. *International Journal of Legal Medicine*, Vol.105, No.6, pp. 339-350, ISSN 0937-9827.

Nissapatorn, V., Wattanagoon, Y., Pungpak, S., Supanaranond, W., Bowonwatnuwong, C., Sukthana, Y., Desakorn, V., Khamboonruang, C., Thang, D.Q. & Kumar, S.M. (2001). Seroprevalence of toxoplasmosis in HIV infected patients in Chonburi regional hospital, Chonburi, Thailand. *Tropical Biomedicine*, Vol.18, No.2, pp. 123-129, ISSN 0127-5720.

Nissapatorn, V., Kamarulzaman, A., Init, I., Tan, L.H., Rohela, M., Norliza, A., Chan, L.L., Latt, H.M., Anuar, A.K. & Quek, K.F. (2002). Seroepidemiology of toxoplasmosis among HIV-infected patients and healthy blood donors. *Medical Journal of Malaysia*, Vol.57, No.3, pp. 304-310, ISSN 0300-5283.

Nissapatorn, V., Lee, C.K. & Khairul, A.A. (2003). Seroprevalence of toxoplasmosis among AIDS patients in Hospital Kuala Lumpur, 2001. *Singapore Medical Journal*, Vol.44, No.4, pp. 194-196, ISSN 0037 - 5675.

Nissapatorn V, Lee C, Quek KF, Leong CL, Mahmud R, Abdullah KA. (2004). Toxoplasmosis in HIV/AIDS patients: a current situation. *Japanese Journal of Infectious Diseases*, Vol.57, No.4, pp. 160-165, ISSN 1344-6304.

Nissapatorn, V., Lim, Y.A., Jamaiah, I., Agnes, L.S., Amyliana, K., Wen, C.C., Nurul, H., Nizam, S., Quake, C.T., Valartmathi, C., Woei, C.Y. & Anuar, A.K. (2005). Parasitic infections in Malaysia: changing and challenges. *Southeast Asian Journal of Tropical Medicine and Public Health*, Vol.36, No.suppl4, pp. 50-59, ISSN 01251562.

Nissapatorn, V., Lee, C.K.C., Lim, Y.A.L., Tan, K.S., Jamaiah, I., Rohela, M., Sim, B.L.H., Ahmad, A., Hadita, S., Lott, P.W., Ng, K.T., Poh, M.E., Zuliana, J. & Khairul Anuar, A. (2007). Toxoplasmosis: a silent opportunistic disease in HIV/AIDS patients. *Research Journal of Parasitology* Vol.2, No.1, pp. 23-31, ISSN 1816-4943.

Nissapatorn, V., Sawangjaroen, N., Hortiwakul, T., Jareonmark, B., Andiappan, H. & Siripaitoon P. Prevalence of latent and reactivated *Toxoplasma gondii* infection in HIV-infected patients from Southern Thailand. (In press).

Nobre, V., Braga, E., Rayes, A., Serufo, J.C., Godoy, P., Nunes, N., Antunes, C.M. & Lambertucci, J.R. (2003). Opportunistic infections in patients with AIDS admitted to an university hospital of the Southeast of Brazil. *Revista do Instituto de Medicina Tropical de São Paulo*, Vol.45, No.2, pp. 69-74, ISSN 0036-4665.

Noël, S., Guillaume, M.P., Telerman-Toppet, N. & Cogan, E. (1992). Movement disorders due to cerebral *Toxoplasma gondii* infection in patients with the acquired immunodeficiency syndrome (AIDS). *Acta neurologica Belgica*, Vol.92, No.3, pp. 148-156, ISSN 0300-9009.

Nogueira, S.A., Guedes, A.L., Machado, E.S., Matos, J.A., Costa, T.P., Cortes, E.M. & Lambert, J.S. (2002). Toxoplasmic encephalitis in an HIV infected pregnant woman: successful outcome for both mother and child. *The Brazilian Journal of Infectious Diseases*, Vol.6, No.4, pp. 201-205, ISSN 1413-8670.

Nolla-Salas, J., Ricart, C., D'Olhaberriague, L., Galí, F. & Lamarca, J. (1987). Hydrocephalus: an unusual CT presentation of cerebral toxoplasmosis in a patient with acquired immunodeficiency syndrome. *European Neurology*, Vol.27, No.2, pp. 130-132, ISSN 0014-3022.

Novati, R., Castagna, A., Morsica, G., Vago, L., Tambussi, G., Ghezzi, S., Gervasoni, C., Bisson, C., d'Arminio Monforte, A. & Lazzarin, A. (1994). Polymerase chain reaction for *Toxoplasma gondii* DNA in the cerebrospinal fluid of AIDS patients with focal brain lesions. *AIDS*, Vol.8, No.12, pp. 1691-1694, ISSN 1473-5571.

Oh, M.D., Park, S.W., Kim, H.B., Kim, U.S., Kim, N.J., Choi, H.J., Shin, D.H., Lee, J.S. & Choe, K.(1999). Spectrum of opportunistic infections and malignancies in patients with human immunodeficiency virus infection in South Korea. *Clinical Infectious Diseases* 1999; Vol.29, No.6, pp. 1524-1528, ISSN 1058-4838.

Oksenhendler, E., Charreau, I., Tournerie, C., Azihary, M., Carbon, C. & Aboulker, J.P. (1994). *Toxoplasma gondii* infection in advanced HIV infection. *AIDS*, Vol. 8, No.4, pp. 483-487, ISSN 0269-9370.

O'Riordan, S.E. & Farkas, A.G. (1998). Maternal death due to cerebral toxoplasmosis. *British Journal of Obstetrics and Gynaecology*, Vol.105, No.5, pp. 565-566, ISSN 0306-5456.

Oshinaike, O.O., Okubadejo, N.U., Ojini, F.I. & Danesi, M.A. (2010). A preliminary study of the frequency of focal neurological deficits in HIV/AIDS patients seropositive for *Toxoplasma gondii* IgG in Lagos, Nigeria. *Nigerian Quarterly Journal of Hospital Medicine*, Vol.20, No.3, pp.104-107, ISSN 0189-2657.

Ouermi, D., Simpore, J., Belem, A.M., Sanou, D.S., Karou, D.S., Ilboudo, D., Bisseye, C., Onadja, S.M., Pietra, V., Pignatelli, S., Gnoula, C., Nikiema, J.B. & Kabre, G.B. (2009). Co-infection of *Toxoplasma gondii* with HBV in HIV-infected and uninfected pregnant women in Burkina Faso. *Pakistan Journal of Biological Sciences*, Vol.12, No.17, pp. 1188-1193, ISSN 1028-8880.

Palella, F.J, Jr., Delaney, K.M., Moorman, A.C., Loveless, M.O., Fuhrer, J., Satten, G.A., Aschman, D.J. & Holmberg, S.D. (1998). Declining morbidity and mortality among patients with advanced human immunodeficiency virus infection. HIV Outpatient Study Investigators. *The New England Journal of Medicine*, Vol.338, No.13, pp. 853-860, ISSN 0028-4793.

Pendry, K., Tait, R.C., McLay, A., Yen, D.H., Baird, D. & Burnett, AK. (1990). Toxoplasmosis after BMT for CML. *Bone Marrow Transplantation*, Vol.5, No.1, pp.65-66, ISSN 0268-3369.

Pereira-Chioccola, V.L., Vidal, J.E. & Su, C. (2009). *Toxoplasma gondii* infection and cerebral toxoplasmosis in HIV-infected patients. *Future Microbiology*, Vol.4, No.10, pp. 1363-1379, ISSN 1746-0913.

Pestre, P., Milandre, L., Farnarier, P. & Gallais, H. (1991). Hemichorea in acquired immunodeficiency syndrome. Toxoplasmosis abscess in the striatum. *Revue Neurologique*, Vol.147, No.12, pp. 833-837, ISSN 0035-3787.

Petito, C.K., Cho, E.S., Lemann, W., Navia, B.A. & Price, R.W. (1986). Neuropathology of acquired immunodeficiency syndrome (AIDS): an autopsy review. *Journal of*

Neuropathology and Experimental Neurology, Vol.45, No.6, pp. 635-646, ISSN 0022-3069.

Peyron, F., Lobry, J.R., Musset, K., Ferrandiz, J., Gomez-Marin, J.E., Petersen, E., Meroni, V., Rausher, B., Mercier, C., Picot, S. & Cesbron-Delauw, M.F. (2006). Serotyping of *Toxoplasma gondii* in chronically infected pregnant women: predominance of type II in Europe and types I and III in Colombia (South America). *Microbes and Infections*, Vol.8, No.9-10, pp. 2333-2340, ISSN 1286-4579.

Pfeffer, G., Prout, A., Hooge, J. & Maguire, J. (2009). Biopsy-proven immune reconstitution syndrome in a patient with AIDS and cerebral toxoplasmosis. *Neurology*, Vol.73, No.4, pp. 321-322, ISSN 0028-3878.

Podzamczer, D., Miró, J.M., Bolao, F., Gatell, J.M., Cosin, J., Sirera, G., Domingo, P., Laguna, F., Santamaria, J., Verdejo, J. & The Spanish Toxoplasmosis Study Group. (1995). Twice-weekly maintenance therapy with sulfadiazine-pyrimethamine to prevent recurrent toxoplasmic encephalitis in patients with AIDS. Spanish Toxoplasmosis Study Group. *Annals of Internal Medicine*, Vol.123, No.3, pp. 175-180, ISSN 0003-4819.

Portegies, P., Solod, L., Cinque, P., Chaudhuri, A., Begovac, J., Everall, I., Weber, T., Bojar, M., Martinez-Martin, P. & Kennedy, P.G. (2004). Guidelines for the diagnosis and management of neurological complications of HIV infection. *European Journal of Neurology*, Vol.11, No.5, pp. 297-304, ISSN 1351-5101.

Potasman, I., Resnick, L., Luft, B.J. & Remington, J.S. (1988). Intrathecal production of antibodies against *Toxoplasma gondii* in patients with toxoplasmic encephalitis and the acquired immunodeficiency syndrome (AIDS). *Annnals of Internal Medicine*, Vol.108, No.1, pp. 49-51, ISSN 0003-4819.

Prigione, I., Facchetti, P., Lecordier, L., Deslée, D., Chiesa, S., Cesbron-Delauw, M.F. & Pistoia, V. (2000). T cell clones raised from chronically infected healthy humans by stimulation with *Toxoplasma gondii* excretory-secretory antigens cross-react with live tachyzoites: characterization of the fine antigenic specificity of the clones and implications for vaccine development. *Journal of Immunology*, Vol.164, No.7, pp.3741-3748, ISSN 0022-1767.

Rabaud, C., May, T., Amiel, C., Katlama, C., Leport, C., Ambroise-Thomas, P. & Canton, P. (1994). Extracerebral toxoplasmosis in patients infected with HIV. A French National Survey. *Medicine*, Vol.73, No.6, pp.306-314, ISSN 0025-7974.

Raffi, F., Aboulker, J.P., Michelet, C., Reliquet, V., Pelloux, H., Huart, A., Poizot-Martin, I., Morlat, P., Dupas, B., Mussini, JM. & Leport, C. (1997). A prospective study of criteria for the diagnosis of toxoplasmic encephalitis in 186 AIDS patients. The BIOTOXO Study Group. *AIDS*, Vol.11, No.2, pp. 177-184, ISSN 0269-9370.

Rajagopalan, N., Suchitra, JB., Shet, A., Khan, ZK., Martin-Garcia, J., Nonnemacher, M.R., Jacobson, J.M. & Wigdahl, B. (2009). Mortality among HIV-Infected Patients in Resource Limited Settings: A case controlled analysis of inpatients at a community care center. *American Journal of Infectious Diseases*, Vol.5, No.3, pp. 219-224, ISSN 1553-6203.

Reischl, U., Bretagne, S., Krüger, D., Ernault, P. & Costa, J.M. (2003). Comparison of two DNA targets for the diagnosis of Toxoplasmosis by real-time PCR using fluorescence resonance energy transfer hybridization probes. *BMC Infectious Diseases*, Vol.3, pp. 7, ISSN 1471-2334.

Reiter-Owona, I., Bialek, R., Rockstroh, J.K. & Seitz, H.M. (1998). The probability of acquiring primary *Toxoplasma* infection in HIV-infected patients: results of an 8-year retrospective study. *Infection*, Vol.26, No.1, pp. 20-25, ISSN 0300-8126.

Richards, F.O Jr., Kovacs, J.A. & Luft, B.J. (1995). Preventing toxoplasmic encephalitis in persons infected with human immunodeficiency virus. *Clinical Infectious Diseases*, Vol.21, No.Suppl 1, pp. S49-S56, ISSN 1058-4838.

Rodríguez-Rosado, R., Soriano, V., Dona, C. & González-Lahoz, J. (1998). Opportunistic infections shortly after beginning highly active antiretroviral therapy. *Antiviral Therapy*, Vol.3, No.4, pp. 229-231, ISSN 1359-6535.

Ruf, B., Schürmann, D., Bergmann, F., Schüler-Maué, W., Grünewald, T., Gottschalk, H. J., Witt, H. & Pohle, H.D. (1993). Efficacy of pyrimethamine/sulfadoxine in the prevention of toxoplasmic encephalitis relapses and *Pneumocystis carinii* pneumonia in HIV-infected patients. *European Journal of Clinical Microbiology & Infectious Diseases*, Vol.12, No.5, pp. 325-329, ISSN 0934-9723.

Ruiz, R., Cu-Uvin, S., Fiore, T. & Flanigan, T.P. (1997). Toxoplasmosis in HIV-positive women: seroprevalence and the role of prophylaxis in preventing disease. *AIDS*, Vol.11, No.1, pp. 119-120, ISSN 0269-9370.

Saba, J., Morlat, P., Raffi, F., Hazebroucq, V., Joly, V., Leport, C. & Vildé J. L. (1993). Pyrimethamine plus azithromycin for treatment of acute toxoplasmic encephalitis in patients with AIDS. *European Journal of Clinical Microbiology & Infectious Diseases*, Vol.12, No.11, pp. 853-856, ISSN 0934-9723.

Sadler, M., Brink, N.S. & Gazzard, B.G. (1998). Management of intracerebral lesions in patients with HIV: a retrospective study with discussion of diagnostic problems. *QJM: Monthly Journal of the Association of Physicians*, Vol.91, No.3, pp. 205-217, ISSN 1460-2725.

Schöler, N., Krause, K., Kayser, O., Müller, R.H., Borner, K., Hahn, H. & Liesenfeld, O. (2001). Atovaquone nanosuspensions show excellent therapeutic effect in a new murine model of reactivated toxoplasmosis. *Antimicrobial Agents and Chemotherapy*, Vol.45, No.6, pp. 1771-1779, ISSN 0066-4804.

Schuman, J.S. & Friedman, A.H. (1983). Retinal manifestations of the acquired immune deficiency syndrome (AIDS): cytomegalovirus, *Candida albicans*, cryptococcus, toxoplasmosis and *Pneumocystis carinii*. *Transactions of the Ophthalmological Societies of the United Kingdom*, Vol.103, No.Pt2, pp. 177-190, ISSN 0078-5334.

Sendi, P., Sachers, F., Drechsler, H. & Graber, P. (2006). Immune recovery vitritis in an HIV patient with isolated toxoplasmic retinochoroiditis. *AIDS*, Vol.20, No.17, pp. 2237-2238, ISSN 0269-9370.

Shah, I. (2011). Immune Reconstitution Syndrome in HIV-1 Infected Children-A Study from India. *Indian Journal of Pediatrics*, Vol.78, No.5, pp. 540-543, ISSN 0019-5456.

Shamilah, H., Hakim, L., Noor Azian, S., Malkith, K.M.Y. & Yisri, M.Y. (2001). Seroprevalence of *Toxoplasma gondii* antibodies in HIV positive and negative patients using the immunofluorescence antibody test (IFAT) methods. *Tropical Biomedicine*, Vol.18, No.2, pp. 137-141, ISSN 0127-5720.

Shankar, S.K., Mahadevan, A., Satishchandra, P., Kumar, R.U., Yasha, T.C., Santosh, V., Chandramuki, A., Ravi, V. & Nath, A. (2005). Neuropathology of HIV/AIDS with an overview of the Indian scene. *The Indian Journal of Medical Research*, Vol.121, No.4, pp. 468-488, ISSN 0971-5916.

Sharma, S.K., Kadhiravan, T., Banga, A., Goyal, T., Bhatia, I. & Saha, P.K. (2004). Spectrum of clinical disease in a series of 135 hospitalised HIV-infected patients from north India. *BMC Infectious Diseases*, Vol.22, No.4, pp. 52. ISSN 1471-2334.

Shivaprakash, M.R., Parija, S.C. & Sujatha, S. (2001). Seroprevalence of toxoplasmosis in HIV infected patients in Pondicherry. *Journal of Communicable Diseases*, Vol.33, No.3, pp. 221-223, ISSN 0019-5138.

Silva, M.T. & Araújo, A. (2005). Highly active antiretroviral therapy access and neurological complications of human immunodeficiency virus infection: impact versus resources in Brazil. *Journal of Neurovirology*, Vol.11, No.Suppl 3, pp. 11-15, ISSN 1355-0284.

Sitoe, S.P., Rafael, B., Meireles, L.R., Andrade, H.F. Jr. & Thompson, R. (2010). Preliminary report of HIV and *Toxoplasma gondii* occurrence in pregnant women from Mozambique. *Revista do Instituto de Medicina Tropical de São Paulo*, Vol.52, No.6, pp. 291-295, ISSN 0036-4665.

Sousa, S., Ajzenberg, D., Vilanova, M., Costa, J. & Dardé, M.L. (2008). Use of GRA6-derived synthetic polymorphic peptides in an immunoenzymatic assay to serotype *Toxoplasma gondii* in human serum samples collected from three continents. *Clinical and Vaccine Immunology*, Vol.15, No.9, pp. 1380-1386, ISSN 1556-6811.

Sousa, S., Ajzenberg, D., Marle, M., Aubert, D., Villena, I., da Costa, J.C. & Dardé, M.L. (2009). Selection of polymorphic peptides from GRA6 and GRA7 sequences of *Toxoplasma gondii* strains to be used in serotyping. *Clinical and Vaccine Immunology*, Vol.16, No.8, pp. 1158-1169, ISSN 1556-6811.

Stout, J.E., Lai, J.C., Giner, J. & Hamilton, C.D. (2002). Reactivation of retinal toxoplasmosis despite evidence of immune response to highly active antiretroviral therapy. *Clinical Infectious Diseases*, Vol.35, No.4, pp. e37-e39, ISSN 1058-4838.

Subsai, K., Kanoksri, S., Siwaporn, C. & Helen, L. (2004). Neurological complications in AIDS patients: the 1-year retrospective study in Chiang Mai University, Thailand. *European Journal of Neurology*, Vol.11, No.11, pp. 755-759, ISSN 1351-5101.

Subsai, K., Kanoksri, S., Siwaporn, C., Helen, L., Kanokporn, O. & Wantana, P. (2006). Neurological complications in AIDS patients receiving HAART: a 2-year retrospective study. *European Journal of Neurology*, Vol.13, No.3, pp. 233-239, ISSN 1351-5101.

Sukthana, Y., Chintana, T. & Lekkla, A. (2000). *Toxoplasma gondii* antibody in HIV-infected persons. *Journal of the Medical Association of Thailand*, Vol.83, No.6, pp. 681-684, ISSN 0125-2208.

Suzuki, Y., Conley, F.K. & Remington, J.S. (1989). Importance of endogenous IFN-gamma for prevention of toxoplasmic encephalitis in mice. *Journal of Immunology*, Vol.143, No.6, pp. 2045-2050, ISSN 0022-1767.

Sýkora, J., Zástěra, M. & Stanková, M. (1992). Toxoplasmic antibodies in sera of HIV-infected persons. *Folia Parasitologica*, Vol.39, No.2, pp. 177-180, ISSN 0015-5683.

Tenter, A.M., Heckeroth, A.R. & Weiss, L.M. (2000). *Toxoplasma gondii*: from animals to humans. *International Journal of Parasitology*, Vol.30, No.12-13, pp.1217-1258, ISSN 0020-7519.

Tilley, M., Fichera, M.E., Jerome, M.E., Roos, D.S. & White, M.W. (1997). *Toxoplasma gondii* sporozoites form a transient parasitophorous vacuole that is impermeable and contains only a subset of dense-granule proteins. *Infection and Immunity*, Vol.65, No.11, pp.4598-605, ISSN 1098-5522.

Tolge, C.F. & Factor, S.A. (1991). Focal dystonia secondary to cerebral toxoplasmosis in a
    patient with acquired immune deficiency syndrome. *Movement Disorders*, Vol.6,
    No.1, pp. 69-72, ISSN 0885-3185.

Torre, D., Speranza, F., Martegani, R., Zeroli, C., Banfi, M. & Airoldi, M. (1998). A
    retrospective study of treatment of cerebral toxoplasmosis in AIDS patients with
    trimethoprim-sulphamethoxazole. *The Journal of Infection*, Vol.37, No.1, pp. 15-18,
    ISSN 3163-4453.

Torres, R.A., Weinberg, W., Stansell, J., Leoung, G., Kovacs, J., Rogers, M. & Scott, J. (1997).
    Atovaquone for salvage treatment and suppression of toxoplasmic encephalitis in
    patients with AIDS. Atovaquone/Toxoplasmic Encephalitis Study Group. *Clinical
    Infectious Diseases*, Vol.24, No.3, pp. 422-429, ISSN 1058-4838.

Touboul, J.L., Salmon, D., Lancastre, F., Mayaud, C., Fermand, J.P., Fouret, P. & Akoun, G.
    (1986). *Toxoplasma gondii* pneumopathy in a patient with the acquired
    immunodeficiency syndrome: demonstration of the parasite by bronchioloalveolar
    lavage. *Revue de Pneumologie Clinique*, Vol.42, No.3, pp. 150-152, ISSN 0761-8417.

Tremont-Lukats, I.W., Garciarena, P., Juarbe, R. & El-Abassi, R.N. (2009). The immune
    inflammatory reconstitution syndrome and central nervous system toxoplasmosis.
    Annals of Internal Medicine, Vol.150, No.9, pp. 656-657, ISSN 0003-4819.

Trujillo, J.R., Jaramillo-Rangel, G., Ortega-Martinez, M., Penalva de Oliveira, A.C., Vidal,
    J.E., Bryant, J. & Gallo, R.C. (2005). International NeuroAIDS: prospects of HIV-1
    associated neurological complications. *Cell Research*, Vol.15, No.11-12, pp. 962-969,
    ISSN 1001-0602.

Tsai, H.C., Lee, S.S., Lin, H.H., Lin, W.R., Chen, Y.S., Huang, C.K., Liu, Y.C. & Chen, E.R.
    (2002). Treatment of *Toxoplasma* brain abscess with clindamycin and sulfadiazine in
    an AIDS patient with concurrent atypical *Pneumocystis carinii pneumonia*. *Journal of
    the Formosan Medical Association*, Vol.101, No.9, pp. 646-649, ISSN 0929-6646.

Tsambiras, P.E., Larkin, J.A. & Houston, S.H. (2001). Case report. *Toxoplasma* encephalitis
    after initiation of HAART. *The AIDS Reader®*, Vol.11, No.12, pp. 608-610, 615-616,
    ISSN 1053-0894.

Tse, W., Cersosimo, M.G., Gracies, J.M., Morgello, S., Olanow, C.W. & Koller, W. (2004).
    Movement disorders and AIDS: a review. *Parkinsonism Related Disorders*, Vol.10,
    No.6, pp. 323-334, ISSN 1353-8020.

Ullum, H., Cozzi Lepri, A., Bendtzen, K., Victor, J., Gøtzsche, P.C., Phillips, A.N., Skinhøj, P.
    & Klarlund Pedersen, B. (1997). Low production of interferon gamma is related to
    disease progression in HIV infection: evidence from a cohort of 347 HIV-infected
    individuals. *AIDS Research and Human Retroviruses*, Vol.13, No.12, pp. 1039-1046,
    ISSN 0889-2229.

Uneke, C.J., Duhlinska, D.D., Njoku, M.O. & Ngwu, B.A. (2005). Seroprevalence of acquired
    toxoplasmosis in HIV-infected and apparently healthy individuals in Jos, Nigeria.
    Parassitologia, Vol.47, No.2, pp. 233-236, ISSN 0048-2951.

USPHS/IDSA Prevention of opportunistic infections working group. (1997). USPHS/IDSA
    guidelines for the prevention of opportunistic infections in persons infected with
    human immunodeficiency virus. *MMWR. Morbidity and Mortality Weekly Report*,
    Vol.46, No.RR-12, pp. 1-46, ISSN 0149-2195.

Vallat-Decouvelaere, A.V., Chrétien, F., Lorin, de la Grandmaison, G., Carlier, R., Force, G.
    & Gray, F. (2003). The neuropathology of HIV infection in the era of highly active

antiretroviral therapy. *Annales de Pathologie*, Vol.23, No.5, pp. 408-423, ISSN 0242-6498.

van Oosterhout, J.J., Laufer, M.K., Graham, S.M., Thumba, F., Perez, M.A., Chimbiya, N., Wilson, L., Chagomerana, M., Molyneux, M.E., Zijlstra, E.E., Taylor, T.E. & Plowe, C.V. (2005). A community-based study of the incidence of trimethoprim-sulfamethoxazole-preventable infections in Malawian adults living with HIV. *Journal of Acquired Immune Deficiency Syndromes*, Vol.39, No.5, pp. 626-631, ISSN 0894-9255.

van Vaerenbergh, K., Debaisieux, L., De Cabooter, N., Declercq, C., Desmet, K., Fransen, K., Maes, B., Marissens, D., Miller, K., Muyldermans, G., Sprecher, S., Stuyver, L., Vaira, D., Verhofstede, C., Zissis, G., Van Ranst, M., De Clercq, E., Desmyter, J. & Vandamme, A.M. (2001). Prevalence of genotypic resistance among antiretroviral drug-naive HIV-1-infected patients in Belgium. *Antiviral Therapy*, Vol.6, No.1, pp. 63-70, ISSN 1359-6535.

Venkataramana, A., Pardo, C.A., McArthur, J.C., Kerr, D.A., Irani, D.N., Griffin, J.W., Burger, P., Reich, D.S., Calabresi, P.A. & Nath, A. (2006). Immune reconstitution inflammatory syndrome in the CNS of HIV-infected patients. *Neurology*, Vol.67, No.3, pp. 383-388, ISSN 0028-3878.

Veronese Rodrigues, M., Demarco, A.L.G., Donadi, E.A., Demarco, L.A., Deghaide, N.H.S., Romão, E. & Figueiredo, J.F.C. (2004). HLA class I profile in patients with AIDS and *Toxoplasma gondii* chorioretinitis. *Investigative Ophthalmology & Visual Science*, Vol.45, pp.E-1672, ISSN 0146-0404.

Vidal, J.E., Hernández, A.V., Oliveira, A.C., de Souza, A.L., Madalosso, G., Silva, P.R. & Dauar, R. (2004a). Cerebral tuberculomas in AIDS patients: a forgotten diagnosis? *Arquivos de Neuro-Psiquiatria*, Vol.62, No.3B, pp. 793-796, ISSN 0004-282X.

Vidal, J.E., Colombo, F.A., de Oliveira, A.C., Focaccia, R. & Pereira-Chioccola, V.L. (2004b). PCR assay using cerebrospinal fluid for diagnosis of cerebral toxoplasmosis in Brazilian AIDS patients. *Journal of Clinical Microbiology*, Vol.42, No.10, pp. 4765-4768, ISSN 0095-1137.

Vidal, J.E., Hernandez, A.V., de Oliveira, A.C., Dauar, R.F., Barbosa, S.P.Jr. & Focaccia, R. (2005a). Cerebral toxoplasmosis in HIV-positive patients in Brazil: clinical features and predictors of treatment response in the HAART era. *AIDS Patient Care and STDs*, Vol.19, No.10, pp. 626-634, ISSN 1087-2914.

Vidal, J.E., Penalva, de Oliveira, A.C., Bonasser Filho, F., Schiavon Nogueira, R., Dauar, R.F., Leite, A.G., Lins, D.L. & Coelho, J.F. (2005b). Tuberculous brain abscess in AIDS patients: report of three cases and literature review. *Internal Journal of Infectious Diseases*, Vol.9, No.4, pp. 201-207, ISSN 1201-9712.

Vidal, J.E., Dauar, R.F. & de Oliveira, A.C. (2008). Utility of brain biopsy in patients with acquired immunodeficiency syndrome before and after introduction of highly active antiretroviral therapy. *Neurosurgery*, Vol.63, No.6, pp. E1209, ISSN 0148-396X.

Wadia, R.S., Pujari, S.N., Kothari, S., Udhar, M., Kulkarni, S., Bhagat, S.& Nanivadekar, A. (2001). Neurological manifestations of HIV disease. *The Journal of the Association of Physicians of India*, Vol.49, pp. 343-348, ISSN 0004-5772.

Wainstein, M.V., Wolffenbuttel, L., Lopes, D.K., González, H.E., Golbspan, L., Ferreira, L., Sprinz, E., Kronfeld, M. & Edelweiss, M.I. (1993). The sensitivity and specificity of the clinical, serological and tomographic diagnosis of *Toxoplasma gondii* encephalitis in the acquired immunodeficiency syndrome (AIDS). *Revista da Sociedade Brasileira de Medicina Tropical*, Vol.26, No.2, pp. 71-75, ISSN 0037-8682.

Wallace, M.R., Rossetti, R.J. & Olson, P.E. (1993). Cats and toxoplasmosis risk in HIV-infected adults. *The Journal of the American Medical Association*, Vol.269, No.1, pp. 76-77, ISSN 0098-7484.

Wanachiwanawin, D., Sutthent, R., Chokephaibulkit, K., Mahakittikun, V., Ongrotchanakun, J. & Monkong, N. (2001). *Toxoplasma gondii* antibodies in HIV and non-HIV infected Thai pregnant women. *Asian Pacific Journal of Allergy and Immunology*, Vol.19, No.4, pp. 291-293, ISSN 0125-877X.

Welker, Y., Geissmann, F., Benali, A., Bron, J., Molina, J.M. & Decazes, J.M. (1994). *Toxoplasma*-induced cystitis in a patient with AIDS. *Clinical Infectious Diseases*, Vol.18, No.3, pp.453-454, ISSN 1058-4838.

Woldemichael, T., Fontanet, A.L., Sahlu, T., Gilis, H., Messele, T., Rinke de Wit, T.F., Yeneneh, H., Coutinho, R.A. & Van Gool, T. (1998). Evaluation of the Eiken latex agglutination test for anti-*Toxoplasma* antibodies and seroprevalence of *Toxoplasma* infection among factory workers in Addis Ababa, Ethiopia. *Transactions of the Royal Society of Tropical Medicine and Hygiene*, Vol.92, No.4, pp. 401-403, ISSN 0035-9203.

Wongkamchai, S., Rungpitaransi, B., Wongbunnate, S. & Sittapairochana, C. (1995). *Toxoplasma* infection in healthy persons and in patients with HIV or ocular disease. *Southeast Asian Journal of Tropical Medicine and Public Health*, Vol.26, No.4, pp. 655-658, ISSN 0125-1562.

Yap, G., Pesin, M. & Sher, A. (2000). Cutting edge: IL-12 is required for the maintenance of IFN-gamma production in T cells mediating chronic resistance to the intracellular pathogen, *Toxoplasma gondii*. *Journal of Immunology*, Vol.165, No.2, pp.628-631, ISSN 0022-1767.

Yeo, K.K., Yeo, T.T., Chan, C.Y., Sitoh, Y.Y., Teo, J. & Wong, S.Y. (2000). Stereotactic brain biopsies in AIDS patients--early local experience. *Singapore Medical Journal*, Vol.41, No.4, pp. 161-166, ISSN 0037-5675.

Yoong, K.Y. & Cheong, I. (1997). A study of Malaysian drug addicts with human immunodeficiency virus infection. *International Journal of STD & AIDS*, Vol.8, No.2, pp. 118-123, ISSN 0956-4624.

Zajdenweber, M., Muccioli, C. & Belfort, R. Jr. (2005). Ocular involvement in AIDS patients with central nervous system toxoplasmosis: before and after HAART. *Arquivos Brasileiros de Oftalmologia*, Vol.68, No.6, pp. 773-775, ISSN 0004-2749.

Zhou, X.W., Kafsack, B.F., Cole, R.N., Beckett, P., Shen, R.F. & Carruthers, V.B. (2005). The opportunistic pathogen *Toxoplasma gondii* deploys a diverse legion of invasion and survival proteins. *The Journal of Biological Chemistry*, Vol.280, No.40, pp. 34233-44, ISSN 0021-9258.

Zufferey, J., Sugar, A., Rudaz, P., Bille, J., Glauser, M.P. & Chave, J.P. (1993). Prevalence of latent toxoplasmosis and serological diagnosis of active infection in HIV-positive patients. *European Journal of Clinical Microbiology & Infectious Diseases*, Vol.12, No.8, pp. 591-595, ISSN 0934-9723.

Zumla, A., Savva, D., Wheeler, R.B., Hira, S.K., Luo, N.P., Kaleebu, P., Sempala, S.K., Johnson, J.D. & Holliman, R. (1991). *Toxoplasma* serology in Zambian and Ugandan patients infected with the human immunodeficiency virus. *Transactions of the Royal Society of Tropical Medicine and Hygiene*, Vol.85, No.2, pp. 227-229, ISSN 0035-9203.

5

Bacterial and Parasitic Agents of Infectious Diarrhea in the Era of HIV and AIDS - The Case of a Semi Rural Community in South Africa

Samie A.[1], Bessong P.O.[1], Obi C.L.[2], Dillingham R.[3] and Guerrant R.L.[3]
[1]*AIDS Virus Research Laboratory, Department of Microbiology,*
University of Venda, Thohoyandou,
[2]*Academic and Research Directorate, Walter Sisulu University,*
Nelson Mandela Drive Eastern Cape,
[3]*Centre for Global Health, University of Virginia, Charlottesville,*
[1,2]*South Africa*
[3]*USA*

1. Introduction

Infection by the human immunodeficiency virus (HIV) is a worldwide public health concern. In the Southern African region, the HIV and AIDS pandemic has grown faster than in any other parts of the world, from infection rate, in pregnant women, of 0.8% in 1990 to 30.2% in 2005 in South Africa and 29.4% in 2009 (DOH, 2000; DOH, 2006; DOH 2010). Due to its destructive effect on the immune system, HIV infection further exposes the individual to multiple opportunistic infections. From the beginning of the HIV pandemics in the 1980s, gastrointestinal diseases have been demonstrated to be a major problem in patients with HIV and AIDS, and diarrhea is reported in up to 60% of patients with AIDS in developed countries and up to 90% in developing countries (Siddiqui et al., 2007; Silva et al., 2010). Recent studies by Bradshaw *et al.,* (2005) have indicated that HIV/AIDS is the leading cause of premature mortality for all provinces in South Africa and mortality due to pre-transitional causes, such as diarrhea, is more pronounced in the poorer and more rural provinces. In Limpopo Province as well as other poorer provinces in South Africa, diarrheal diseases are the first cause of mortality after HIV/AIDS (Bradshaw *et al.,* 2005). However, data on specific etiologies is sparse (Obi and Bessong, 2002) and such information will be crucial in the specific management of HIV and AIDS.

Although diarrheagenic organisms have been studied in different parts of the African continent, most research activities targeted specific organisms and their role in the production of diarrhea with little consideration to the presence of other organisms, their role in the production of inflammation which might be a considerable part of the pathogenesis of the organisms (Nel et al., 2010). Elsewhere, the combination of environmental factors, new ways of living and structural changes in the genetic material of most microorganisms have led to the appearance of emerging and re-emerging diseases (Lashley, 2006). Combined to the increasing recognition of a widening array of enteric pathogens associated with illnesses of the gastrointestinal tract, these factors highlight the growing need for the understanding of the epidemiology and transmission of the different organisms involved in infectious diarrhea in specific settings, using the more specific and sensitive molecular tools, for a better management of these diseases and the improvement of the quality of life of the concerned populations.

Gastrointestinal infections are major causes of morbidity and mortality throughout the world and particularly in developing countries where mortality rates due to infectious diarrhea could be as high as 56% (WHO, 2004). Children and young adults are the most affected, particularly in regions with limited resources and where hygienic measures are not strictly followed (Guerrant et al., 2005; Opintan et al., 2010). In Africa, diarrhea has been estimated to be responsible for 25 to 75% of all childhood illnesses (Kirkwood, 1991), and episodes of diarrhea lead to about 14% of outpatient visits, 16% of hospital admissions, and account for an average of 35 days of illness per year in children less than five years old (Greenwood et al., 1987). Causes of diarrhea in endemic areas include a wide variety of bacteria, viruses and parasites. Intestinal parasites are associated with serious clinical disease and mortality, and are known to cause malnutrition, growth, learning and physical development impairment in children. It is thus necessary to have a fairly accurate picture of the situation in order to target intervention strategies in affected areas.

It has been suggested that intestinal parasites occur at unacceptably high levels throughout South Africa. However, accurate prevalence data for the whole country are not currently available. With the exception of mapping being undertaken in KwaZulu-Natal, the medical geography of intestinal parasitic infections is stale, very fragmented and almost useless for planning, implementing and monitoring effective interventions (Fincham et al., 1997). In Cape Town, surveys at primary schools in urban and rural communities have revealed soil transmitted helminthiasis prevalence range between 7% and 83% (Kirkwood, 1991). However, there is scanty information, if any, on the prevalence of intestinal parasitic infections in the Limpopo Province.

Bacterial organisms such as *Campylobacter spp*, *Salmonella spp*, *Shigella spp* and different groups of enteropathogenic *E. coli* are well known as causes of gastrointestinal diseases all over the world. These organisms have been demonstrated in water and stools from the Vhembe district (Obi et al., 2004; Larsen et al., 2011). Infections by most of these organisms can be asymptomatic, or can be treated with rehydration solutions particularly in case of viruses and some bacteria. The use of antibiotics might shorten the duration of diarrhea and limit the shedding of the organisms which otherwise might continue to pollute the environment and pose further risk of infections. Antibiotics such as erythromycin and gentamicin have been proven to be effective in some communities. However, antibiotic resistance is an overgrowing problem and there is a need to monitor the susceptibility of common bacterial isolates to drugs used in the community in order to provide guidelines for the empirical treatment of bacterial infections.

Diarrhea is a common final expression of infection with a myriad of pathogens. Appropriate management requires knowledge of the setting in which the patient became ill, the underlying disease state, presence and extent of dehydration and other clinical symptoms, travel history, known outbreaks, and pathogenic mechanism (invasive or toxigenic) and the physical findings and laboratory results at the time the patient presented with the condition (de Truchis and de Truchis, 2007; Beatty, 2010). Optimal evaluation and treatment of each of these infections (as well as of cases caused by noninfectious organisms) can limit the duration of illness, the morbidity rate, the cost of work-up, and the spread of secondary infection (Goodman and Segreti, 1999). Although the differential diagnosis of infectious diarrhea is broad, the clinical history can help guide the clinician toward the appropriate evaluation for each patient. For those patients with diarrhea of 2-3 days' duration, work-up is rarely necessary unless fever, bloody diarrhea, or severe abdominal pain is present. A detailed history of recent travel (within 6 months), recent antibiotic use (within 6-8 weeks), and contact with individuals who are ill and specific dietary ingestions during foodborne outbreaks can suggest an infectious etiology (DuPont, 1997). Infection with HIV is also a common cause of diarrhea. Therefore, medical history should include looking for risk factors for HIV and other comorbid illness that may result in immunosuppression (eg, diabetes, liver disease, organ transplantation) (Quinn et al., 1983).

Clinical signs of dehydration, including dry mucous membranes, low urine output, or tachycardia, suggest severe infection. Other symptoms of severe infection include fever, severe abdominal pain, distension of the abdomen, and decreased bowel sounds. Although these findings are less helpful in determining the etiology of the diarrhea, they are helpful in deciding if the patient requires any immediate treatment or hospitalization.

Most cases of acute infectious diarrhea do not need medical evaluation or intervention because they will resolve spontaneously and rapidly (Herickstad et al., 2002). However, if patients have any of the following clinical signs or presentations, they should undergo medical evaluation: (1) dehydration secondary to profuse watery diarrhea or inability to tolerate oral fluids; (2) fever (temperature >= 38.5 °C or 101.3 °F); (3) stools containing blood and mucus; (4) passage of 6 or more stools in a 24-hour period or duration of illness 48 hours or longer; (5) diarrhea with severe abdominal pain in patients 50 years of age or older; or (6) diarrhea in individuals 70 years of age or older or in those with known immunosuppression (eg, AIDS, transplant patients, patients who have recently received chemotherapy) (Guerrant et al., 2001).

The distinction between inflammatory and non-inflammatory diarrhea has long been useful in the diagnosis of diarrhea and in the creation of treatment algorithms for managing diarrhea (Guerrant et al., 2001; Thielman and Guerrant, 2004). The highly inflammatory diarrheas (or overt dysenteries) are caused by cultivable and potentially treatable pathogens, such as Shigella species, Campylobacter jejuni, E. histolytica, C. difficile and more recently Enteroaggregative E. coli and sometimes, Salmonella species (Huang et al., 2003; Jiang et al., 2010; Hou et al., 2010). The currently available tests, microscopy for fecal leukocytes and an immunoassay for fecal lactoferrin (a simpler, quicker and more sensitive marker for the presence of fecal leukocytes), provide supporting evidence of inflammatory diarrhea and may be useful when such clinical features are equivocal (Victora et al., 2000; Mercado et al, 2011). Recent studies have indicated that infections with Cryptosporidium parvum or Giardia species may result in mild intestinal inflammation that leads to detectable levels of fecal lactoferrin (Alcantara et al., 2003). In equivocal cases, the negative predictive value of fecal lactoferrin testing may help to determine the need for routine bacteriologic culture for organisms such as Campylobacter spp, Salmonella spp, and Shigella spp (Thielman and Guerrant, 2004).

Stool cultures are considered to be the gold standard for the diagnosis of bacterial causes of gastroenteritis. However, their clinical use is limited to organisms that are routinely cultured (Choi et al., 1996). The choice of the organisms to be cultured for depends on epidemiological data available for the region as well as outbreak and travel history. For example, most laboratories only attempt to culture for Salmonella spp, Shigella spp, and Campylobacter spp. Culture has also been used for diagnosis purposes in cases of Entamoeba histolytica suspicion. However this method is cumbersome and lack both sensitivity and specificity for the detection and identification of *E. histolytica* (Abd-Alla *et al.*, 1998). Considerable savings may be achieved if cultures for bacterial enteric pathogens are restricted to samples from patients hospitalized for ≤ 3 days (Valenstein *et al.*, 1996). Common organisms that can cause diarrhea, such as enteroinvasive *E. coli* and enterotoxigenic *E. coli* are not routinely looked for since these organisms can only be identified by molecular methods which are mostly restricted to research laboratories or few laboratories in developed countries. Unusual organisms such as *Yersinia* species and *Vibrio* species, which may be important in certain locations, are not routinely tested for.

Microscopy is the traditional method commonly used in developing countries for the detection of ova and trophozoites of parasites and some times can be helpful in the detection of bacterial organisms such as *Campylobacter* spp. In developed countries such as the USA, stool examination for ova and parasites is generally performed particularly if a patient is potentially immunosuppressed or returning from a developing country. However, in Africa microscopy is the mostly used method for diagnosis of parasitic infections and can be used in direct stools examination, or after staining by different methods such as the simplified Ritchie technique and Ziehl Neelsen modified coloration (Kassi *et al.*, 2004). The method used also depends on the suspected microorganism. In some cases such as in cryptosporidiosis where shedding of oocysts can be intermittent, up to 3 stool specimens may be needed for diagnosis (Goodgame *et al.*, 1993; Chappell *et al.*, 1996). By use of a modified acid-fast stain (Kinyoun), oocysts appear as red spheres of 4 - 6μm in diameter; no other organisms should be easily confused with *Cryptosporidium* species on the basis of size and appearance. Unfortunately, acid-fast staining is relatively insensitive, requiring 10,000 oocysts/g of watery stool and 500,000 oocysts/g of formed stool to make the diagnosis. Microscopy remains the best available test for acid-fast *Cyclospora cayetanensis* infections.

Traditionally, infections by *Giardia* as well as other organisms such as *E. histolytica*, *Dientamoeba fragilis*, *Balantidium coli* and other helminthes have been diagnosed by means of ova and parasite examination of fecal or small bowel specimens (including small bowel specimens obtained using the "string" test) (Stark *et al.*, 2006; Kurniawan et al., 2009). The physical characteristics of the cysts or ova may prove helpful in the differentiation of the organisms involved. For example, *Giardia* cysts are ovoid or ellipsoid and measure 11–15 μm in diameter while trophozoites are approximately the same size, with 2 anteriorly placed nuclei and 8 flagella best visualized by staining with trichrome or with the iron hematoxylin method (Shetty *et al.*, 1988; El-Naggar *et al.*, 2006). Although microscopy might be useful in a rural setting, its use is limited by its insensitivity and lack of specificity which might lead to over diagnosis of some infections such as those of *E. histolytica* (Kebede *et al.*, 2003; Nesbitt *et al.*, 2004). More sensitive methods have thus been introduced which are easier and have higher sensitivities and specificities.

The development of molecular methods has tremendously improved the detection and identification of infecting agents. A variety of PCRs have been described for the detection of different bacteria such as *Shigella, Salmonella, Campylobacter* spp, diarrheagenic *E. coli, Aeromonas* spp and *Plesiomonas* spp as well as parasitic organisms such as *Cryptosporidium, E. histolytica*, Micrsoporidia, *Cyclospora, Isospora* and *Giardia* species (Marshall *et al.*, 1999; Sturbaum *et al.*, 2001, Larsen et al., 2011) . The sensitivity of detection by PCR is greater than that by microscopy, making it of great use for detection of low numbers of parasites in stool samples (Bialek et al., 2002). PCR for the detection of Cryptosporidium species, for example, has a sensitivity of 93% and a specificity of 95%, compared with 67% and 99%, respectively, for the Direct immunofluorescence assay (DFA) assay and 68% and 58%, respectively, for

Enzyme Immuno Assay (EIA) (Bushen et al., 2004; Kar et al., 2011). In addition to identifying protozoa, the use of real-time PCR—restriction fragment—length polymorphism (RFLP) analysis can detect as few as 5 *Cryptosporidium* oocysts and can differentiate between 5 genotypes and, more recently, subtypes (Limor *et al.*, 2002). PCR-RFLP analysis is more sensitive, as it may detect 50–500 oocysts/mL of liquid stool or <1 pg of DNA and <10 oocysts from environmental samples (Sturbaum *et al.*, 2001). Detection of diarrheagenic *E. coli* such as EAEC has required a specific test for one of the characteristic virulence traits of this group of organisms. Because an entire cassette of potential virulence traits is regulated by the transcriptional activator AggR, some have proposed that genetic probes for this trait may be the single best test for EAEC at the present time, and such genetic probes have been incorporated into a multiplex PCR test (Cerna *et al.*, 2003). With the introduction of easier, more-sensitive methods that reduce labor, time, and reagent costs, the possibility of combining assays for the detection of different targets into one assay has become a possibility. A multiplex real-time PCR and an oligonucleotide microarray may be new methods for the detection of *Campylobacter* spp, *Salmonella* spp, *Shigella* spp, *E. histolytica, Giardia lamblia,* and *C. parvum,* with excellent, perhaps unprecedented, sensitivity and specificity in either fecal or water samples (Wang *et al.*, 2004; Verweij *et al.*, 2004). Work on these and potential new methods to detect fecal contamination in water may help to identify and ameliorate inadequate sanitation and contaminated water that perpetuates the devastating illness burdens associated with enteric infections around the world (Dillingham and Guerrant, 2004).

The causes of infectious diarrhea include a wide array of viruses, bacteria, and parasites, many of which have been recognized only in the last decade or two (Steiner *et al.*, 2006). The occurrence of the different pathogens depends on region. While enterotoxigenic *Escherichia coli* and rotaviruses predominate in developing areas, Norwalk-like viruses, *Campylobacter jejuni,* and cytotoxigenic *Clostridium difficile* are seen with increasing frequency in developed areas; and *Shigella, Salmonella, Cryptosporidium* species, and *Giardia lamblia* are found throughout the world (Taylor, 1993). Bacterial gastroenteritis generally produces more severe symptoms than viral infection, including more frequent and bloody stools and severe cramping. The importance of each pathogen depends on the region. In a study in Mozambique for example, diarrheagenic *Escherichia coli* (22%) were the most frequently isolated pathogens, followed by *Ascaris lumbricoides* (9.3%). Others detected pathogens included *Salmonella* spp. and *Giardia lamblia* (2.5% each) and *Campylobacter* spp. (1.7%). *A. lumbricoides* and *Strongyloides stercolaris* (100% versus 0%; P=0.008) were most frequently isolated in children older than 12 months of age (Mandomando *et al.*, 2007).

The prevalence of *Cryptosporidium* varies widely from country to country and from one region to another. In Korea, for example, Lee *et al.* (2005) reported a prevalence of 1% (among HIV patients) while in Tanzania, Houpt *et al.* (2005) described a prevalence of 17.3% amongst HIV patients. In Guinea Bissau, *Cryptosporidium parvum* had a prevalence of 7.7% and was the second most common parasite with a marked seasonal variation, with peak prevalence found consistently at the beginning of or just before the rainy seasons, May through July. In South Africa, studies by Kfir *et al.* (1995) indicated that *Giardia* cysts and *Cryptosporidium* oocysts were found in all types of water tested including surface water, sewage or treated effluents. Studies by Moodley *et al.* (1991) in Durban, South Africa showed that *Cryptosporidium* was the second most common enteric pathogen isolated from children admitted to hospital with gastroenteritis with infection rates varying between 1.2 and 20.9% according to season with the highest prevalence in the summer months, and 10%

of the children infected with *Cryptosporidium* died. However the prevalence of *Cryptosporidium* infections is not known in Limpopo Province, and particularly in the Vhembe district.

With the advent of HIV and AIDS, it has become more important to determine the distribution of parasitic infections such as *E. histolytica* and *E. dispar* amongst HIV infected individuals. In Mexico, *E. histolytica* prevalence of 25.3% in the HIV/AIDS group and 18.5% in the HIV negative group was described using PCR (Moran *et al.*, 2005). Likewise in Taiwan, persons infected with HIV were at increased risk for invasive amoebiasis and exhibited a relatively high frequency of elevated antibody titers and intestinal colonization with *E. histolytica* (Hung *et al.*, 2005). Previous studies in South Africa have been based in the Durban area in the eastern coast of the country where a prevalence of 10% using the PCR has been described (Zaki *et al.*, 2003). However no study to our knowledge has been conducted in the Limpopo Province and particularly in the Vhembe district. The first case of human microsporidial infection was described in 1959 and as early as 2 years after the identification of HIV as the causative agent of AIDS, the microsporidial species *Enterocytozoon bieneusi* was discovered in HIV-infected patients with chronic diarrhea (Desportes *et al.*, 1985). Although infections in immunocompetent patients are usually self-limiting, infections in immune compromised host can be life threatening, especially in patients with AIDS (Desportes *et al.*, 1985). Studies in Cape Town have indicated prevalence up to 22% of all *Campylobacter* spp when the filter method is used for isolation (Lastovica and Roux, 2000). In Venda, the infection level by *Campylobacter spp* was found to be around the same level (20%) amongst HIV infected individuals (Obi and Bessong, 2002). However, the isolates were not ascertained by the use of molecular methods and very few studies have determined the genetic variability of *Campylobacter* spp in Africa. Enteroaggregative *Escherichia coli* (EAEC) is an emerging diarrheagenic pathogen associated with diarrheal illnesses among patients in developed and developing countries. Recent studies have implicated EAEC in persistent diarrhea in patients infected with human immunodeficiency virus (HIV) (Wanke *et al.*, 1998; Nataro *et al.*, 2006).

Clostridium difficile is a spore-forming, anaerobic Gram positive bacillus that produces exotoxins that are pathogenic to humans. Infection can lead to asymptomatic carriage or clinical disease, ranging from mild diarrhea to life threatening pseudomembranous colitis (Cleary, 1998). *Clostridium difficile* associated disease (CDAD) is an important clinical problem that is believed to occur predominantly following hospitalisation and administration of antibiotics and especially affects the elderly (Wilcox, 1996). Community-acquired disease has been reported but the incidence is felt to be low and the rate of disease resulting in hospitalization is reported as negligible. For example a Swedish study of 5 133 cases of *C. difficile* diarrhea defined 28% as being community acquired (Karlström *et al.*, 1998). Recent events in the USA, Canada and Europe have indicated the changing epidemiology of *Clostridium difficile* associated diarrhea (CDAD) with the occurrence of serious CDAD in otherwise healthy patients with minimal or no exposure to a health-care setting (Kuijper *et al.*, 2006; Reichardt *et al.*, 2007). However, the occurrence of *C. difficile* in developing regions such as the Vhembe district has not been reported. In the present study, molecular biology methods were used for the detection of different emerging bacterial and parasitic organisms including *Campylobacter* spp, *Arcobacter* spp, Enteroaggregative *E. coli*, *Clostridium difficile*, *Cryptosporidium* spp, *Entamoeba histolytica* and microsporidia, in relation to their pathogenicity among HIV positive and HIV negative individuals visiting different hospitals in the Vhembe district of South Africa.

2. Material and methods

2.1 Ethical Issues

Ethical approval of this research was granted by the Health, safety and Research Ethics Committee of the University of Venda. Authorization was also sought and obtained from the Department of Health and Welfare Limpopo Province, South Africa. The different hospitals and schools were then approached and the research objectives thoroughly explained to the study participants in the local language (TshiVenda) for their consent. Informed consent was obtained from all participants either directly or through their legal and competent guardians. Only consenting individuals were accepted in the study.

2.2 Study sites and sample collection

The study was conducted in the Vhembe district, of the Vhembe district, Limpopo Province, South Africa. Thohoyandou, meaning "head of the elephant" in tshiVenda, is the former capital of the independent homeland and the proud heart of the VhaVenda people. Thohoyandou is home to the University of Venda and is also the headquarters of the Vhembe district and is the tenth most populated town in the country with 584,469 people while the population of the region is approximately 1.2 million. The Vhembe district is semi urban and agriculture is the main activity practiced by the population. Main hospitals in the region include Elim, Tshilidzini, Vhufhuli (Donald Frazer) and Siloam hospitals. These hospitals deliver care directly to the population and are referral centers for smaller clinics in the region. The Vhembe district is bounded on the north by the Limpopo River, on the west by Sand River, on the south and east by the Levubu River and the remainder of the southern boundary by the farms adjoining the south of the Sinthumule location. The bulk of the people are today concentrated in locations and crown lands approximately from longitude 29*40'E-30*50'E and latitude 22*20'S-23*10'S. In normal seasons the rain starts in October/November and from that time onwards the weather becomes moist and hot, the shade temperature ranging from 80-90 degrees and north of the mountains being 110 degrees or more.

For sample collection two groups of population were considered for the study including patients attending four main public hospitals in the region namely Elim, Vhufuli, Siloam and Tshilidzini hospitals, and pupils from two public primary schools both situated in Wuwani, locality situated at about 6km from the Tshilidzini hospital. At the primary schools, the objectives of the study were explained to the parents in a meeting with the authority of the schools who then distributed the collection bottles to the pupils whose parents had agreed to the study and signed a consent form. The pupils then brought the collection bottles home and with the help of their parents collected the stool in the bottles. The samples were collected the following morning from the schools and transported without any further delay to the Laboratory of Microbiology, University of Venda. Samples that were not analysed the same day were stored at -20oC. A total of 322 stool samples were collected. 255 samples were from patients attending the three public hospitals with abdominal complaints or diarrhea while 67 were from apparently healthy pupils attending two public primary schools.

2.3 Lactoferrin latex agglutination assay

Stool supernatants were tested according to the manufacturer's specifications including appropriate kit controls (LEUKO-TEST; Tech Lab, Blacksburg, VA). Stool sample dilution was conducted as described by the manufacturer in the following way: one drop (50 µl) of stool was added to 375 µl of diluent yielding a 1:25 dilution. Using the pipette provided with the Kit, one drop of the diluted sample was mixed with one drop of sensitized latex (lactoferrin antibody-coated latex beads) or negative latex beads for 3min and the agglutination was observed for positive samples. Each test was run in parallel with a negative control as indicated by the manufacturer. Positive controls provided with the test kits were also performed. Agglutination reaction was graded with the unaided eye from 0 (no agglutination) to 4+ (large agglutination with a clear background).

2.4 Lactoferrin quantitative assay
The lactoferrin content in the lactoferrin positive stools samples was quantified using the ELISA method with the IBD scan kit from Techlab (Blacksburg, Virginia) following the instructions of the manufacturer.

2.5 Test for occult blood
The presence of occult blood in the stool samples was tested by the Hemoccult test kit (Beckman Coulter, Inc Harbor Blvd, Fullerton, CA, USA) following the instructions of the manufacturer.

2.6 Detection of pathogenic organisms
2.6.1 DNA purification
Four different methods were used and compared for the purification of total genomic DNA from stool samples. This would then allow for the detection of most parasites from the same sample and avoid conducting several DNA extractions from the same samples for the molecular detection of different pathogens. The first method involved the treatment of 200µg of stool sample by a freeze-thaw procedure using liquid nitrogen and boiling water followed by the use of the QIAamp DNA Stool Mini Kit from Qiagen (Valencia, CA, USA) according to the manufacturer's recommendations. The second method involved the use of the QIAamp DNA Stool Mini Kit, with higher temperature (95oC) for the first incubation. The third method involved the used of alkaline treatment following a modified version of the method described by Haque *et al.*, (1998). Briefly, fifty microliters of 1M KOH and 18 µl of 1M dithiothreitol were added to 250mg or 250 µl of stool. The samples were mixed thoroughly by stirring with a pipette tip, followed by brief shaking. After incubation at 65°C for 15 min, the samples were neutralized with 8 µl of 25% HCl and buffered with 80 µl of 2M Tris–HCl (pH 8.3) and the suspension was mixed by briefly vortexing. The genomic DNA was then purified from the suspension using the QIAamp DNA Stool Mini Kit from Qiagen (Valencia, CA, USA) following the manufacturer's instructions. The last method was the use of glass beads in order to physically dreak open the cells, cysts, oocysts and spore that could be in the stool samples. Following the bead beating the QIA amp DNA Stool Mini Kit from Qiagen for final DNA purification.

The comparison of all the pretreatment methods showed that a combination of two pretreatment methods including one which is either the bead beating or the alkaline treatment or freeze and thaw with a surplus stool portion added untreated and the whole used in the Qiagen with an increased temperature at 95oC for 15 min gave bettwe detectionof all pathogens including bacterial and parasites. The purified DNA was stored at -20oC until further used in the different PCR and Real time PCR procedures.

2.6.2 Detection and genotyping of *Cryptosporidium*

Cryptosporidium species detection and genotyping was conducted as previously described using a real time PCR for the screening and PCR –RFLP for genotyping (Samie et al., 2006a).

2.6.3 Detection and genetic characterisation of *Entamoeba histolytica*

Entamoeba histolytica was detected from the samples using the Techlab (TechLab, Inc. Blacksburg, VA, USA) *E. histolytica* II antigen detection kit . The identification of the different species of *Entamoeba* mainly *E. histolytica* and *E. dispar* was conducted as previously described (Samie et al., 2006b). Genotyping of *E. histolytica* was conducted as previously described through the polymorphism of the serine-rich *E. histolytica* protein (SREHP) followed by enzymatic digestion (Samie et al., 2008).

2.6.4 PCR amplification for the detection of microsporidia

The PCR method described by Fedorko *et al* (1995) and further developed by Samie et al., (2007) was used with minor modification as indicated followed by restriction analysis.

2.6.5 Detection of *Campylobacters*

2.6.5.1 Culture and maintenance of reference strains

Reference strains used in this study included *Campylobacter jejuni* subsp. jejuni (ATCC 33291), *Campylobacter coli* (ATCC 33559) , *Campylobacter concisus* (ATCC 33237), *Campylobacter fetus* subsp. *fetus* (ATCC 27374), *Campylobacter hyointestinalis* (ATCC 35217), *Campylobacter upsaliensis* (ATCC 43954), *Helicobacter pylori* (ATCC 43504), *Arcobacter butzleri* (ATCC 49616), *Campylobacter jejuni* (ATCC 33560), *Campylobacter jejuni* (ATCC 81116), *Campylobacter jejuni* (ATCC 11168), *Campylobacter coli* (ATCC 33559) and *Campylobacter lari* (ATCC 35221). The cultures were sub-cultured in blood agar supplemented with 10% tryptose and 0.1% yeast extract and were preserved in Bolton broth and 25% sterile glycerol. Prior to DNA isolation, 500 µl of the preserved culture was added to 10ml of brain Heart infusion or Bolton broth and incubated in a Microaerophilic environment for 24hours and inoculated to blood agar or mCCDA. The culture method using a charcoal based media (mCCDA) was used to detect *Campylobacter* spp from 37 diarrheal stool samples collected from Donald Frazer hospital as indicated in the Cape Town protocol (Lastovica and Le Roux, 2000) and suspected colonies were confirmed using a *Campylobacter* haemagglutination kit "Campy Dry Spot" (Oxoid, England) as recommended by the manufacturer.

2.6.5.2 PCR detection of Campylobacteria

The genomic DNA purified as described above was used for the detection of *Campylobacter* spp, *Arcobacter* spp and *Helicobacter* spp by the PCR- RFLP as described by Marshall et al (1999) and Samie et al., (2007a).

Restriction profiles were generated with   *DdeI, TaqI*, or *BsrI* (New England Biolabs, Inc., Beverly, Mass.) in a 20-µl reaction mixture including 10 µl of the PCR amplicon with 10 U of the restriction endonuclease following conditions recommended by the manufacturer. Ten microliters of each digest was analyzed electrophoretically at 5 V/cm for 2 h with a 3% agarose gel in 1× TAE buffer. The gels were stained in ethidium bromide and photographs were taken for the analysis of the profiles. **Further specific detection and confirmation of** *Campylobacter jejuni* **and** *coli* was conducted as previously described (Linton et al., 1997; Samie al., 2007a)

Campylobacter concisus was detected from the samples using the method described by conventional and real time PCR protocols based on the methods previously described by Matsheka et al (2001).

A real time PCR for the rapid detection of *Campylobacter concisus* was developed based on the method described by Matsheka *et al.* (2001) and Samie et al (2008) using the primers pcisus1 and pcisus6 and the iQTM SYBR® Green Supermix (Bio-Rad, CA),

2.6.5.3 Specific detection of *Helicobacter Pylori*

The specific detection of H. pylori was conducted as previously described (Samie et al., 2007b) using the primers consisting of two specific 16S rRNA oligonucleotides, designated HPF and HPR, which generates a 138-bp product.

2.6.5.4 Use of a multiplex PCR assay for the simultaneous detection and identification of *Arcobacter butzleri*, *Arcobacter cryaerophilus* and *Arcobacter skirrowii*

A multiplex PCR reaction described by Houf et al (2000) and modified by Samie et al was used to identify the three main *Arcobacter* species.

2.6.6 Detection of Enteroaggregative *E. coli* from stool samples

A quantitative real time PCR using SYBR-Green -490 (Bio-Rad, CA) based on the protocol described by Samie et al., (2007c) used to confirm the presence of the *AggR* gene of EAEC in the stool samples. Standard cultures with known numbers of EAEC cells were used as reference and positive controls, while water and *E. coli* K-12 were used as negative controls in each reaction. The level of positivity of the samples was indicated by the Ct values.

2.6.6.1 Multiplex PCR detection of EAEC virulence genes from stool samples

A multiplex PCR protocol previously described was used with modifications in order to determine the presence of three EAEC genes in the stool samples (Cerna *et al.*, 2003; Samie et al., 2007c). Only the presence of the correctly sized gene PCR product(s) was interpreted as a positive test.

2.6.7 Detection of *Clostridium difficile* from stool samples

A PCR protocol targeting a species-specific internal fragment of the triose phosphate isomerase (*tpi*) housekeeping gene was used as described by Lemee *et al.*, (2004) for the detection of C. *difficile* in the stool samples (Samie et al., 2008c). The presence of the binary toxin was ascertained by two different reactions using two different primer pairs for the enzymatic and the binding components of the *cdt* gene using the conditions previously described by Stubbs *et al.*, (2000). The negative regulator gene was detected by using two different primer pairs as previously described by Spigaglia and Mastrantonio (2002). The first primer pair (C1 and C2) detects a fragment of the *tcdC* gene while the second primer pair (Tim 1 and Struppi 2) amplifies and internal fragment of the first PCR product. The PCR products were observed in 2% agarose gel except for the products of the second PCR for the *tcd* gene that was run in 3% agarose gel. This helped to observe any size difference that could exist in the amplification products.

2.7 Statistical analysis

All data was analysed using the statistical package for social sciences (SPSS) program (Version 13.1). The potential relationship between the presence of the different pathogens and the pathogenesis variables such as diarrhea, intestinal inflammation (through the measurement of the intestinal lactoferrin in the stool samples) and the presence of occult blood was determined by cross tabulation and the chi squarre test, risk evaluation and the Mantel-Haenszel Common Odds Ratio Estimate was used for statistical analysis. The difference was considered significant if the p value was less than 0.05. The Pathogenicity index (PI) as well as the Inflammatory index (II) were calculated. These were the ratios of the number of samples that were diarrheal (for PI) or were positive for Lactoferrin (for II) and positive for the pathogen in consideration over the number of samples that were positive for the pathogen but not positive for lactoferrin or diarrhea. This indicates the strength of the involvement of the organisms in the specific pathogenicity (diarrhea or intestinal inflammation).

3. Results

3.1 Population demographics and characteristics of stool specimens

From a total of 322 samples from 322 individuals of whom 44 were HIV positive patients while 211 were HIV negative patients and 67 were apparently healthy school children. The age of the hospital patients varied between 2 weeks and 88 years with most patients aged between 10 and 39 years old while the school children were aged between 3 and 15 years. At the hospital 148 (58%) were females while at the schools 34 (51%) were females. Diarrhea was common among hospital patients (65%) as well as intestinal inflammation indicated by elevated lactoferrin level in the stool samples (56%), and the presence of occult blood in the stools (43%). Diarrhea was common in the age groups 0 – 2 and 2 – 5 yeas old, and also in the age groups 40 – 49 and > 60. Diarrhea was more common amongst the HIV positive group compared to the HIV negative (x^2= 12.452, p = 0.002 < 0.05). Of the 44 samples collected from HIV positive individuals, 11 (25%) were non diarrheal, 32 (72.7%) were diarrheal and 1 (2.3%) had bloody diarrhea. Of the 44 HIV positive patients 27 (61.4%) were females. HIV positive individuals were found at all age groups but the highest percentage was among those older than 20 years.

3.2 Gender distribution of diarrheagenic organisms in the study population

There was no significant difference in the distribution of the different pathogens tested in the present study according to gender, except for *Campylobacter coli* and *H. pylori* both of which were more common in males compared to females (Table 1a). *C. parvum* was more common among females while *C. hominis* was more common among males, however, the difference was not significant (Table 1b). For *E. histolytica*, 16% of the females had *E. histolytica* DNA with about 4% *E. histolytica* single infection and 13% mixed infections with *E. dispar*, while 12.2% had *E. dispar* DNA alone. Of the 109 stool samples from males, 16 (14.7%) had *E. histolytica* with 2 (1.8%) *E. histolytica* alone and 14 (12.8%) mixed infections. Seven (6.4%) had *E. dispar* DNA alone. *Campylobacter concisus* was more common among females (although the difference was not statistically significant) unlike *C. coli* that was more common in males. Similarly, *Cryptosporidium parvum* was more common among males while *C. hominis* was more common among females. *Enterocytozoon bieneusi* and *Entamoeba histolytica* were all more common in females compared to males, but with no significant difference.

	C. jejuni	C. coli	C. concisus	H. pylori	A. butzleri	A. skirrowii	A cryaerophilus
Females	19 (10.4%)	7 (3.8%)	7 (3.8%)	76 (41.8%)	10 (5.5%)	4 (2.2%)	7 (3.8%)
Males	14 (10.0%)	14 (10%)	3 (2.1%)	75 (53.6%)	10 (7.1%)	2 (1.4%)	2 (1.4%)
Sub-total	33 (10.2%)	21 (6.5%)	10 (3.1%)	151 (46.9%)	20 (6.3%)	6 (1.9%)	9 (2.8%)
χ^2,	0.017	4.915	0.763	4.434	0.369	0.256	1.702
p value	0.897	0.027	0.382	0.035	0.544	0.613	0.192

Table 1a. Distribution of diarrheagenic pathogens by gender.

	C. parvum	C. hominis	E. bieneusi	E. histolytica	C. difficile	EAEC
Females	6 (4.4%)	18 (13.3%)	23 (12.6%)	22 (16.3%)	27 (14.8%)	29 (15.9%)
Males	2 (1.8%)	18 (16.5%)	13 (9.3%)	16 (14.7%)	18 (12.8%)	23 (16.4%)
Sub-total	8 (3.3%)	36 (14.8%)	36 (%11.2)	38 (15.6%)	45 (14%)	52 (16.1%)
χ^2,	1.295	0.485	0.895	0.120	0.258	0014
p value	0.255	0.486	0.344	0.729	0.612	0.905

Table 1b.

3.3 Age distribution of different pathogens in Vhembe according to sample origin
In the population studied, all age groups were affected by infections. However, patients in the age group between 3 and 5 years were the most infected particularly with organisms like *C. jejuni*, *H. pylori*, *A. butzleri* and Enteroaggregative *E. coli* for the bacterial organisms as well as *C. hominis* and *E. histolytica* among the parasites (Table 2a and 2b). Other species of *Arcobacter* did not occur among patients less than 5 years of age. *Cryptosporidium parvum* did not occur among patients aged less than 10 years (Table 2b). For *Cryptosporidium*, the age group the most affected were 2–5 years old (28.6%) 30–39 years old (23.5%), and 40–49, and 4 (27.7%). None of the samples from individuals aged >60 was positive for *Cryptosporidium*. For *E. histolytica*, the age groups most infected were 0 – 2 (33%) followed by the age group 20 – 29 (27%). *E. bieneusi* was also common among the patients aged between 3 and 5 years old. The prevalence of *A. butzleri* was lower in the older population compared to the younger populations.

3.4 Diarrhea related pathogens in the studied population
Of all the samples analyzed, 31% of diarrheal samples did not have any pathogen while 66% of the non diarrheal samples had no pathogens detected. *Helicobacter pylori* was the most commonly detected organisms using polymerase chain reaction from both diarrheal and non- diarrheal samples, However, the difference was not significant. Of the 10 bacterial organisms tested, *C. jejuni*, toxigenic *C. difficile*, Enteroaggregative *E. coli* and *C. coli* were the most commonly detected and associated with diarrhea among the patients in the total population. These organisms also had the highest pathogenic indexes indicating their potential involvement in diarrheal cases. Of the 4 parasitic organisms tested, *E. histolytica* and *Cryptosporidium hominis* were more common and statistically associated with diarrhea with pathogenic indexes of 8 for *E. histolytica* and 2.1 for *C. hominis*. The prevalence of the different organisms in both diarrheal and non diarrheal samples is shown in Table 3 below as well as the pathogenic indexes of the organisms. Briefly, *C. jejuni* was the most pathogenic bacterial organisms (in relation to diarrhea) while *E. histolytica* was the most diarrheagenic parasitic organism in this population.

Origin	Age group	Total	C. jejuni	C. coli	C. concisus	H. pylori	A butzleri	A. skirrowii	A cryaerophilus
Hospitals	0 – 2	18	2 (11.1%)	0	1 (5.5%)	9 (50%)	2(11.1%)	0	0
	3 – 5	16	3 (18.7%)	1 (6.2%)	0	9 (56.2%)	1 (6.2%)	0	0
	6 – 9	16	2 (12.5%)	0	0	8 (50%)	1 (6.2%)	0	0
	10 – 19	65	4 (6.2%)	3 (4.6%)	4 (6.1%)	29 (44.6%)	6 (9.2%)	1 (1.5%)	1 (1.5%)
	20 – 29	62	9 (14.5%)	7 (11.3%)	1 (1.6%)	26 (41.9%)	4 (6.5%)	2 (3.2%)	2 (3.2%)
	30 – 39	42	6 (14.3%)	1 (2.3%)	0	29 (69%)	4 (9.5%)	2 (4.8%)	4 (9.5%)
	40 – 49	18	4 (22.2%)	2 (11.1%)	1 (5.5%)	8 (44.4)	0	0	1 (5.5%)
	50 – 59	10	1 (10%)	2 (20%)	0	4 (40%)	0	0	0
	≥ 60	8	1 (12.5%)	2 (25%)	0	4 (50%)	1(12.5%)	0	1 (12.5%)
	Subtotal	255	32 (12.5%)	18 (7%)	7 (2.7%)	126(49.4%)	19(7.5%)	5 (2%)	9 (3.5%)
Schools	3 – 5	5	0	0	1 (20%)	4 (80%)	0	0	0
	6 – 9	4	0	0	0	1 (25%)	0	0	0
	10 – 15	58	1 (1.7%)	3 (5.2%)	2 (3.4%)	32 (55.2%)	1 (1.7%)	1 (1.7%)	0
	Subtotal	67	1 (1.5%)	3 (4.4%)	3 (4.5%)	37 (55.2%)	1 (1.5%)	1 (1.5%)	0
Total		322	33 (10.2%)	21 (6.5%)	10 (3.1%)	163 (50.6%)	20 (6.2%)	6 (1.9%)	9 (2.8%)
χ²			7.052	0.580	0.871	0.717	4.853	0.064	2.433
P value			0.008	0.446	0.351	0.397	0.028	0.801	0.119

Table 2a

Origin	Age group	Total	C. parvum	C. hominis	E. bieneusi	E. histolytica	C. diff	EAEC
Hospitals	0 – 2	18		1 (9.1%)		3 (27.3%)	3 (16.7%)	1 (5.6%)
	3 – 5	16		4 (28.6%)	4 (25.0%)	4 (28.6%)	2 (12.5%)	5 (31.3%)
	6 – 9	16		2 (15.4%)		2 (15.4%)	1 (6.3%)	2 (12.5%)
	10 – 19	65	2 (4.3%)	5 (10.6%)	6 (9.2%)	6 (12.8%)	10 (15.4%)	11 (16.9%)
	20 – 29	62	1 (2.1%)	7 (14.6%)	11 (17.7%)	13 (27.1%)	11 (17.7%)	12 (19.4%)
	30 – 39	42	5 (14.7%)	3 (8.8%)	9 (21.4%)	5 (14.7%)	12 (28.6%)	11 (26.2%)
	40 – 49	18		2 (13.3%)	2 (11.1%)	3 (20.0%)	1 (5.6%)	5 (27.8%)
	50 – 59	10		4 (50.0%)			2 (20.0%)	3 (30.0%)
	≥ 60	8			1 (12.5%)	1 (14.3%)	1 (12.5%)	
	Subtotal	255	8 (4.1%)	28 (14.2%)	33 (12.9%)	37 (18.8%)	43 (17%)	50 (19.6%)
Schools	3 – 5	5		2 (50.0%)				2 (40.0%)
	6 – 9	4						
	10 – 15	58		6 (14.6%)	3 (5.2%)	1 (2.4%)	2 (3.4%)	
	Subtotal	67		8 (17.0%)	3 (4.5%)	1 (2.1%)	2 (3.0%)	2 (3.0%)
Total		322			36 (11.2%)	38 (15.6%)	45 (13.9%)	52 (16.1%)
χ²								
P value								

Table 2b.

Table 2. Distribution of bacterial and parasitic agents of diarrhea in the study population according to age group.

3.5 Diarrheagenic organisms and intestinal inflammation

Intestinal inflammation was measured by the amount of lactoferrin produced in the stool samples. Previous studies have correlated the occurrence of lactoferrin in the stool samples with leukocytes which is a marker of intestinal inflammation and even better because fecal leukocytes are generally difficult to count since they die faster once out of the body. Therefore, fecal lactoferrin is the best marker of intestinal inflammation. The inflammatory index was calculated in the same manner as the pathogenic index by dividing the prevalence of the organisms in lactoferrin positive samples by that of the organisms in lactoferrin negative samples. Of all the bacterial organisms tested *Campylobacter jejuni* was the most significantly associated with intestinal inflammation. Enteroaggregative *E. coli* was the next most inflammatory bacterial organism followed by *C. coli* and *C. concisus* (Table 4). Of all the parasitic organisms tested in the present study, *E. histolytica* was significantly associated with intestinal inflammation.

Characteristics	Diarrheal stools	Non-diarrheal stools	Total	χ^2, p value	PI
No Infection	53 (31.2%)	101 (66.4%)	154 (47.8%)		
All infections					
C. jejuni	29 (17.1%)	4 (2.6%)	33 (10.2%)	**18.159 (0.000)**	**6.6**
C. coli	16 (9.4%)	5 (3.3%)	21 (6.5%)	**4.934 (0.026)**	**2.8**
C. concisus	8 (4.5%)	2 (1.4%)	10 (3.1%)	1.226(0.268)	3.2
A. butzleri	14 (8.2%)	6 (3.9%)	20 (6.2%)	2.533 (0.112)	2.1
A. skirrowii	3 (1.8%)	3 (2.0%)	6 (1.9%)	0.019 (0.890)	0.9
A. cryaerophilus	4 (2.4%)	5 (3.3%)	9 (2.8%)	0.259 (0.611)	0.7
H. pylori	91 (51.7%)	60 (41.1%)	151 (46.9%)	2.652(0.103)	1.2
C. diff	34 (19.3%)	11 (7.5%)	45 (13.9%)	**9.21 (0.002)**	2.6
Toxigenic C. diff	20 (11.4%)	3 (2.1%)	23 (7.1%)	**10.48 (0.001)**	5.4
Non Toxigenic C. diff	14 (8%)	8 (5.5%)	22 (6.8%)	0.768 (0.381)	1.4
EAEC	36 (21.2%)	16 (10.5%)	52 (16.1%)	**6.722 (0.010)**	2.01
Parasitic organisms					
E. histolytica	34 (27%)	4 (3.4%)	38 (15.6%)	**25.544 (0.000)**	**8**
C. parvum	4 (3.2%)	4 (3.4%)	8 (3.3%)	0.009 (0.925)	1
C. hominis	25 (19.8%)	11 (9.3%)	36 (14.8%)	**5.361 (0.021)**	**2.1**
E. bieneusi	23 (13.1%)	13 (8.9%)	36 (11.2%)	1.393 (0.238)	1.5

Table 3. Prevalence of different diarrheagenic pathogens in diarrheal and non diarrheal stool samples in the general population in the Vhembe district of South Africa as detected by different Polymerase Chain Reaction methods. The pathogenic indexes show the potential association of the organisms with diarrhea.

3.6 Occurrence of organisms and occult blood in the stool samples

Occult blood was tested in the samples and correlated with the presence of the different organisms. Of all the organisms tested, 4 bacterial species were significantly associated with occult blood and these included in order of statistical importance Enteroaggregative *E. coli*, *Campylobacter jejuni*, *C. difficile* and *Campylobacter coli*. Of all the parasitic organisms tested, only *Entamoeba histolytica* showed a statistically significant correlation with occult blood. The pathogenicity index in terms of occult blood occurrence in the stool samples in association

Characteristics	Lactoferrin positive stools	Lactoferrin negative stools	Total	χ^2, p value	OR (95%CI)	II
All infections						
C. jejuni	26 (17.4%)	7 (4.0%)	33 (10.2%)	**16.586 (0.000)**	5.231 (2.2 – 12.4)	4.4
C. coli	14 (9.6%)	7 (4.0%)	21 (6.5%)	**4.122 (0.042)**	2.561 (1 – 6.5)	2.4
C. concisus	8 (5.5%)	2 (1.1%)	10 (3.1%)	**5.002 (0.025)**	5.043 (1 – 24.1)	5
A. butzleri	11 (7.5%)	9 (5.1%)	20 (6.2%)	0.803 (0.370)	1.5 (0.6 – 3.7)	1.5
A. skirrowii	2 (1.4%)	4 (2.3%)	6 (1.9%)	0.356 (0.551)	0.597 (0.1 – 3.3)	0.6
A. cryaerophilus	3 (2.1%)	6 (3.4%)	9 (2.8%)	0.539 (0.463)	0.594 (0.1 – 2.4)	0.6
H. pylori	69 (47.3%)	82 (46.6%)	151 (46.9%)	0.014 (0.905)	1.027 (0.6 - 15)	1.01
C. diff	25 (17.1%)	23 (13.1%)	48 (14.9%)			
EAEC	32 (21.9%)	20 (11.4%)	52 (16.1%)	**6.565 (0.010)**	2.189 (1.2 – 4)	1.9
E. histolytica	27 (26%)	11 (7.9%)	38 (15.6%)	**14.875 (0.000)**	4.112 (1.9 – 8.7)	3.3
C. parvum	3 (2.9%)	5 (3.6%)	8 (3.3%)	0.089 (0.766)	0.802 (0.2 – 3.4)	0.8
C. hominis	18 (17.3%)	18 (12.9%)	36 (14.8%)	0.940 (0.332)	1.419 (0.6 – 2.8)	1.3
E. bieneusi	16 (11%)	20 (11.4%)	36 (11.2%)	0.013 (0.909)	0.960 (0.4 – 1.9)	1

Table 4. Diarrheagenic organisms and intestinal inflammation as indicated by the detection of lactoferrin in the stool samples.

with the organisms was calculated using the same formula described above for lactoferrin and diarrhea. EAEC had the highest index followed by *Campylobacter jejuni*, *Campylobacter coli* and *Clostridium difficile* for the bacteria and *E. histolytica* among the parasites. The summary of these results is shown in table 4. EAEC infections were significantly associated with intestinal inflammation (χ^2=6.565, P=0.010) and 61.5% of stools that were positive for EAEC genes had elevated lactoferrin compared to 42.2% for samples negative for EAEC genes. Stool samples positive for EAEC genes were more likely to have occult blood (Odd ratio=5.069; 95%CI: 2.665 – 9.644) even when the number of cells carrying the *AggR* gene was lower in the stool. Of the samples positive for at least one EAEC gene, 69.2% had occult blood compared to only 30.7% for samples negative for EAEC genes (χ^2=27.725, P<0.00001). The occult blood pathogenicity index was higher for samples containing *AggR* compared to the other two genes. In general, most bacterial and parasitic organisms tested were more common in samples with occult blood. However, the difference was not significant (P>0.05) (Table 5).

3.7 Occurrence of infections in HIV positive and HIV negative patients with or without diarrhea

In the present study, the presence of bacterial and parasitic organisms was determined according to HIV status of the patients. In order to have a better indication on how important could a pathogen be to the HIV positive group, we calculated the HIV relatedness index (HI) by dividing the prevalence of these infections in HIV positive by the prevalence of the same organism among HIV negative patients. A higher HI indicates that the organism was more common among HIV positive patients. Generally a HI higher than 2 was a good

Characteristics	Occult blood positive stools (n=119)	Occult blood negative stools (n=203)	Total	χ^2, p value	OR (95%CI)	PI
All infections						
C. jejuni	21 (17.6%)	12 (5.9%)	33 (10.2%)	**11.233 (0.001)**	3.411 (1.6 – 7.2)	2.9
C. coli	2 (10.1%)	9 (4.4%)	21 (6.5%)	**3.929 (0.047)**	2.417 (0.9 – 5.9)	2.3
C. concisus	6 (5.0%)	4 (2.0%)	10 (3.1%)	2.35 (0.125)	2.642 (0.7 – 9.5)	2.5
A. butzleri	10 (8.4%)	10 (4.9%)	20 (6.2%)	1.557 (0.212)	1.771 (0.7 – 4.3)	1.7
A. skirrowii	2 (1.7%)	4 (2.0%)	6 (1.9%)	0.034 (0.853)	0.850 (0.1 – 4.7)	0.85
A. cryaerophilus	5 (4.2%)	4 (2.0%)	9 (2.8%)	1.275 (0.241)	2.182 (0.5 – 8.2)	2.1
H. pylori	58 (48.7%)	93 (45.8%)	151 46.9(%)	0.258 (0.611)	1.125 (0.7 – 1.7)	1.06
C. diff	26 (21.8%)	22 (10.8%)	48 (14.9%)	**7.171 (0.007)**	2.300 (1.2 – 4.2)	2.01
EAEC	36 (30.3%)	16 (7.9%)	52 (16.1%)	**27.725 (0.000)**	5.069 (2.7 – 9.6)	3.8
E. histolytica	21 (23.3%)	17 (11%)	38 (15.6%)	**6.530 (0.011)**	2.453 (1.2 – 4.9)	2.1
C. parvum	4 (4.4%)	4 (2.6%)	8 (3.3%)	0.611 (0.434)	1.7 (0.7 – 4.1)	1.7
C. hominis	17 (18.9%)	19 (12.3%)	36 (14.8%)	1.938 (0.164)	1.655 (0.8 – 3.4)	1.5
E. bieneusi	18 (15.1%)	18 (8.9%)	36 (11.2%)	2.960 (0.085)	1.832 (0.9 – 3.6)	1.7

Table 5. Diarrheagenic organisms and occult blood in the stool samples.

indication that the specific pathogen was correlated with HIV infections. Of all the organisms tested in the present study, EAEC, C. jejuni and C. coli appeared to be important bacterial pathogens in HIV positive patients while E. bieneusi was the most common parasitic organism among HIV positive patients.

The prevalence of EAEC infection among HIV positive individuals was significantly higher (χ^2=5.360, P=0.021) with 13 (29.5%) infections than the rest of the study population with 39 (14%) infections. Of the HIV positive patients tested, 8 were positive for E. histolytica. Of these individuals 5 were females and three were males. Among the HIV negative individuals, 29 (13.8%) males and 28 (13.3%) females were infected (χ^2=0.754, P= 0.385). Five samples from HIV positive patients were genotyped for E. histolytica. Of these, 3 (60%) belonged to the same profile mostly (3 out of 4 [75%]) found in HIV positive patients with diarrhea (2 out of 3) or without diarrhea (1 out of 3). One other profile was found mostly (7 out of 8) in HIV negative patients while one other profile was unique to a HIV positive individual. In the present study, we found a higher Campylobacter infection rate: 18.2% and 11.4% among HIV positive patients compared to 11.4% and 6.2% in HIV negative individuals for C. jejuni and C. coli respectively. The prevalence of these Campylobacter's infection among HIV positive individuals was significantly higher (χ^2=5.360, P=0.021) with 13 (29.5%) infections than the rest of the study population with 39 (14%) infections. When compared to HIV negative individuals, HIV positive individuals were more likely to have microsporidiosis (χ^2=4.414, p=0.036). In the HIV negative population, males were more infected than females. However, in the HIV positive population, females were significantly more infected than males (p<0.001). In the HIV negative subgroup, E. bieneusi was more common in individuals without diarrhea (15.9%) than individuals with diarrhea (9.0%), but this was not statistically significant. In the HIV positive group, *E. bieneusi* was found only in diarrheal samples indicating the possible involvement of these organisms in the production of diarrhea in immunocompromised hosts. The prevalence of infection by *C. difficile* was generally higher in HIV negative individuals (14.4%) than HIV positive individuals (11.4%), but the difference was not significant (χ^2=0.289, p=0.591). However, all the toxigenic *C. difficile* in HIV positive patients were found in diarrheal samples, with elevated lactoferrin and occult blood while the non-toxigenic strains were found in stool samples negative for the lactoferrin test and for occult blood indicating that even though *C. difficile* infections are not more prevalent among HIV positive patients, they might be more susceptible to these infections.

		C. jejuni	C. coli	C. concisus	H. pylori	A butzleri	A. skirrowii	A cryaerophilus
HIV positive	Diarrheal	8 (21.1%)	5 (13.2%)	2 (5.3%)	19 (50%)	1 (2.6%)	1 (2.6%)	2 (5.3%)
	Non diarrheal	0	0	0	3 (50%)	0	0	0
	Sub-total	8 (18.2%)	5 (11.4%)	2 (4.5%)	22 (50%)	1 (2.3%)	1 (2.3%)	2 (4.5%)
HIV negative	Diarrheal	21 (15.9%)	12 (9.1%)	6 (4.5%)	68 (51.5%)	13 (9.8%)	2 (1.5%)	3 (2.3%)
	Non diarrheal	4 (2.7%)	4 (2.7%)	2 (1.4%)	61 (41.8%)	6 (4.1%)	3 (2.1%)	4 (2.7%)
	Sub-total	25 (9%)	16 (5.8%)	8 (2.9%)	129 (46.4%)	19 (6.8%)	5 (1.8%)	7 (2.5%)
	χ^2, p value	3.487 (0.062)	1.960 (0.162)	0.351 (0.553)	0.197 (0.657)	1.357 (0.244)	0.047 (0.829)	0.575 (0.448)
	PI	2	2	1.5	1.1	0.3	1.3	1.8

Table 6a

		C. parvum	C. hominis	E. bieneusi	E. histolytica	C. difficile	EAEC
HIV positive	Diarrheal	1 (3.8%)	3 (11.5%)	9 (23.7%)	4 (15.4%)	5 (13.2%)	12 (31.6%)
	Non diarrheal	0	0	0	1 (16.7%)	0	1 (16.7%)
	Sub-total	1 (3.1%)	3 (9.4%)	9 (20.5%)	5 (15.6%)	5 (11.4%)	13 (29.5%)
HIV negative	Diarrheal	2 (2.1%)	19 (20.2%)	13 (9.8%)	30 (31.9%)	28 (20.3%)	25 (18.9%)
	Non diarrheal	5 (4.2%)	14 (11.9%)	14 (9.6%)	3 (2.5%)	12 (8.6%)	14 (9.6%)
	Sub-total	7 (3.3%)	33 (15.6%)	27 (9.7%)	33 (15.6%)	40 (14.4%)	39 (14.0%)
	χ^2, p value	0.003 (0.958)	0.847 (0.357)	4.414 (0.036)	0.000 (0.993)	0.504 (0.478)	6.754 (0.009)
	PI	1	0.6	2.1	1	0.8	2.1

Table 6b.

Table 6. Distribution of bacterial and parasitic organisms among HIV positive and HIV negative patients. The statistics compare the values for the HIV positive and the HIV negative patients. The HIV relatedness index (HI) was the ratio of the occurrence of infection among HIV positive patients to the prevalence of that same infection among HIV negative patients.

4. Discussion

Intestinal bacterial and parasitic infections are common in developing countries and responsible for most acute and chronic diarrhea cases amongst HIV/AIDS patients (Silva et al., 2010). The objective of this study was to determine the prevalence and genotype distribution of bacterial and parasitic organisms in the general population including school children and among HIV positive and HIV negative individuals in the Vhembe district of South Africa; a semi urban area situated in Limpopo Province in the northern part of the country. The organisms detected include *Cryptosporidium species, Entamoeba histolytica,* Microsporidia, *Campylobacter* spp, *Arcobacter* spp, *Helicobacter pylori,* Emteroaggregative *E. coli* and *Clostridium difficile.*

According to the South African Department of Health, the HIV prevalence in the general population was 10.8% for all South Africans over the age of 2 years in 2005 (DOH, 2010). Among those between 15 and 49 years old, the estimated HIV prevalence was 16.2% in 2005. Females were more affected (13.3%) than males (8.2%). In the Limpopo Province, the prevalence in the whole population was 8%. In our study, 15.7% of the patients visiting the hospitals were positive for HIV. This is closer to the national prevalence for individuals between 15 and 49 years of age. These rates are still high compared to countries from other parts of the African continent such as Mali (1.9%), but is comparable with the rates in other countries in the Southern African sub-region such as Malawi (14.2%) and Zambia (16.5%) (Banerjee *et al.,* 2004). It is well known that chronic diarrhea is one of the major AIDS-defining illnesses in WHO Classification and occurs in 60-90% of HIV infected patients in Africa and in a Swiss Cohort Study, diarrhea was found to be an independent predictor of poor survival amongst HIV and AIDS patients (Tadesse and Kassu, 2005; Humphreys et al., 2010). In our study, diarrhea was very common and was present in 74.2% of fecal specimens submitted from cases in the HIV population and is thus in agreement with data from previous studies.

Studies in other parts of the world have indicated that *Cryptosporium* spp represented by *C. Parvum* are the most common diarrheagenic parasitic organisms, however, few studies have compared rates among HIV negative and HIV positive patients. The prevalence and species distribution of *Cryptosporidium spp* vary greatly with the regions or country studied and even within specific groups of the population. This creates a complex picture of the epidemiology of infection by these organisms whose understanding will be helpful in shaping the appropriate measures for their control. In Limpopo Province, the HIV prevalence is 16.2% as determined by the report of the Department of Health and Welfare of South Africa (DOH, 2003). Previous studies in Limpopo Province have targeted different bacterial infections in HIV/AIDS patients; however no attempt has been made to isolate parasites (Obi and Bessong, 2002). This study is thus the first to use a molecular approach for the detection, genetic diversity and pathogenicity of the bacterial and parasitic infections in the region.

The real time quantitative PCR (qPCR) is a very sensitive, specific and easy to use method for the identification and quantification of organisms from a variety of sources. The qPCR used in the present study for the detection of *Cryptosporidium* has been tested for specificity and sensitivity using stools spiked with different numbers of oocysts and proved to be highly effective (Houpt *et al.,* 2005; Taniuchi et al 2011). Studies in various tropical countries have demonstrated highest prevalence of cryptosporidiosis in children younger than 2 years. In rural areas children of between 2 – 5 years old are more exposed to infections since this is the period when they begin to be active on their own. In Zimbabwe, Simango and Mutikani (2004) demonstrated that *Cryptosporidium* was common amongst children aged less than 5 years old with infection rate of 11.2%. In India, studies conducted in twin cities of Hyderabad and Secunderabad indicated that children in the age group of six months to one year were the most vulnerable with 14.3% infections compared to 8.2% among children less than five years of age while in Malaysia the prevalence was 7.5% and 33.3% in Egypt (Nagamani et al., 2007; Al-Mekhlafi et al., 2011).

It has been demonstrated in some countries such as Mexico (Javier-Enriquez *et al.*, 1997), Brazil (Newman *et al.*, 1999; de Oliveira-Silva et al 2007), and Indonesia (Katsumata *et al.*, 2000; Moyo et al., 2011) that *Cryptosporidium* transmission in children is usually associated with the rainy season, and waterborne transmission is considered a major route in the epidemiology of cryptosporidiosis in these areas. Although water contamination with *Cryptosporidium* has been demonstrated in other parts of South Africa, such research needs to be completed in the Limpopo Province in order to confirm the source of transmission in the region. Considering the presence of *Cryptosporidium* in the hospitals as well as in the schools, it can be hypothesized that water is a widespread transmission vector in the region. A study in Peruvian children has demonstrated that cryptosporidiosis was more frequent in children from houses without a latrine or toilet (Bern *et al.*, 2002). Previous studies in Venda have also indicated poor level of hygiene in Venda (Potgieter *et al.*, 2005). However, more detailed studies need to be conducted in order to clarify the role of hygienic habits in the transmission of *Cryptosporidium* as well as other parasitic organisms in the Vhembe district.

Cryptosporidium parasitizes the small intestinal epithelium. Infection results in accelerated loss of villous enterocytes, leading to severe villous atrophy and a malabsorptive and secretory diarrhea. The most common symptom of cryptosporidiosis is watery diarrhea. Other symptoms include: dehydration, weight loss, stomach cramps or pain, fever, nausea, and vomiting. Abdel-Messih *et al.* (2005) in Egypt demonstrated that clinical findings associated with *Cryptosporidium* diarrhea included vomiting, persistent diarrhea and the need for hospitalization. Studies by Alcantara *et al.* (2003) indicated that *Cryptosporidium* was associated with inflammation as indicated by the lactoferrin test and the presence of IL8 and TNF-α. In this study, *Cryptosporidium* was also associated with inflammation and more than 59.1% of *Cryptosporidium* infections might lead to inflammation. However more detailed study is required to clarify the real impact of *Cryptosporidium* infections as well as other protozoan parasitic infections in the production of intestinal inflammation in Venda. Another study in Haiti by Kirkpatrick *et al.* (2002) indicated that malnourished children with acute cryptosporidiosis mount inflammatory (with high lactoferrin content), Th-2, and counter regulatory intestinal immune responses. Studies of Peruvian as well as Brazilian children have demonstrated malnutrition, particularly stunting with lack of growth catch-up after even asymptomatic *C. parvum* infection (Checkley *et al.*, 1998; Antonios et al., 2010).

The existence of two *Entamoeba* species morphologically identical but genetically different was suggested as early as 1925 by Brumpt. However, it was not until 1993 that enough biochemical, immunological and genetic data were gathered to re-classify *E. histolytica* into 2 separate species: *E. histolytica* which can invade the gut mucosa, causes diarrhea and extra-intestinal disease, and *E. dispar*, which causes only asymptomatic colonization (Diamond and Clark, 1993). Following the reclassification of *Entamoeba histolytica*, the epidemiology of amoebiasis needed to be redefined by the use of methods that are able to differentiate between *E. histolytica* and *E. dispar*. Thus different PCR methods have been developed with variable efficiencies. A nested PCR previously described has been successfully used to differentiate between E. *histolytica* and E. *dispar* (Haque *et al*, 1998; Ali *et al.*, 2003). Using the same method; we were able to differentiate between E. *histolytica* from E. *dispar* in samples collected from patients visiting public hospitals with gastrointestinal complaints or diarrhea; and pupils attending public primary schools in the Vhembe district. E. *histolytica* was found both in the hospital and in the Schools. However, E. *histolytica* was less common amongst primary School children aged between five and fifteen. These findings underscore the potential role of E. *histolytica* in morbidity in the study area since the association between E. *histolytica* infections and diarrhea was statistically significant ($P < 0.05$). Similar results have been found in other countries around the world such as Thailand (Haghighi *et al.*, 2003).

Infection rates as well as species diversity (ratio between the occurrence of E. *histolytica* and E. *dispar*) varied tremendously from one region to the other. In Italy, more patients were found to be infected with E. *dispar* (8.3%) than E. *histolytica* (5.6%) using PCR assays (Calderaro *et al.*, 2005). In Sweden, amoebiasis is a notifiable disease and 400–500 cases are reported annually to the Swedish Institute for Infectious Disease Control (SMI). The PCR analysis showed that 165 (79.7%) patients were positive for E. *dispar*, whereas only 10 (4.8%) patients were positive for E. *histolytica* (Lebbad and Svard, 2005). In contrast, higher rates of E. *histolytica* infections was found in Mexico as compared to E. *dispar* infections (13.8% versus 9.6%), using PCR (Ramos *et al.*, 2005). Similarly in the Philippines, 74 cases (65.48%) were positive for E. *histolytica* and 6 cases (5.30%) positive for E. *dispar* from a mental institution (Rivera *et al.*, 2006). In the Gaza strip, Palestine, E. *histolytica* was identified by PCR in 64 (69.6%) of the samples and that of E. *dispar* in 21 (22.8%) (Al-Hindi *et al.*, 2005).

In the present study, we found a rate of 15.5% for E. *histolytica* which is higher than the rate found in Durban by Gathiram and Jackson (1985). This can be explained by the fact that our population was potentially ill and thus had a higher risk of been infected which was not the case in the group without diarrhea in whom there were no mixed infections and only one asymptomatic case of E. *histolytica* was found. The antigen detection test from Techlab (Blacksburg, Virginia, USA) has previously been shown to be suitable for the diagnosis of amoebiasis in endemic areas (Abd-Alla and Ravdin, 2002). In the present study, ELISA had a high specificity. It should be noted that samples positive for PCR and negative with the ELISA test were generally mixed infections with E. *histolytica* and E. *dispar*. This might have a hindering effect on the ability of the ELISA test to detect these samples and might also be related to the pathogenicity or virulence of the strains involved. It has been indicated elsewhere that when both organisms are present in an individual, E. *dispar* generally outgrows E. *histolytica*. However, since E. *dispar* is non pathogenic, the result of the infection will probably be asymptomatic. Mixed infections have also been described in Mexico where 13% of individuals were found harboring E. *histolytica* and E. *dispar* at the same time, particularly amongst HIV positive individuals (Moran *et al.*, 2005).

The mechanisms of disease production following an infection by E. *histolytica* are not fully understood. Most E. *histolytica* infections remain asymptomatic. However, other studies have suggested that amebic colitis may be encountered during colonoscopic examination even in subjects who are asymptomatic (Okamoto *et al.*, 2005). E. *histolytica* has also been associated with traveler's diarrhea. In a study in Sweden, when the patients were divided into immigrants and travelers, the percentages with E. *histolytica* were 3.8% and 9.5%, respectively (Barwick *et al.*, 2002). In invasive amoebiasis, white blood cells can be present in the stool, and in severe cases pus can be visible, but faecal leukocyte numbers are generally not as high as in shigellosis (Speelman *et al.*, 1984). Indeed, virulent *E. histolytica* can destroy neutrophils upon contact; hence may induce inflammation but show only pyknotic leukocytes in the stools (Guerrant *et al.*, 1981; Callendar, 1933). Such a process would be expected to cause evidence of inflammation (i.e. lactoferrin) even without morphologically clear PMNs in the stool. Inflammation occurs most often and previous studies have demonstrated that fecal lactoferrin was the best way to indicate the presence of PMN in stool samples. In our study, 85.7% of samples with *E. histolytica* DNA were positive for lactoferrin with 43% of cases presenting with high level of lactoferrin while *E. dispar* positive samples had only 1 (4.3%) case with a high lactoferrin level. This further confirms the pathogenic differences between the two species. When we excluded other detected organisms, the association of *E. histolytica* with diarrhea and with lactoferrin was even stronger. Other studies had indicated low levels of lactoferrin with *E. histolytica* and *S. hematobium* infections compared to shigellosis and other UTI infections (Aly *et al.*, 2005). However, *E. histolytica* infections had not been ascertained by specific test such as PCR.

Whether risk of invasive amebiasis due to *E. histolytica* is higher among human immunodeficiency virus (HIV)-infected persons than uninfected persons remains unclear, although intestinal colonization by *E. histolytica/dispar* has been reported to be higher among HIV positive individuals (Moran *et al.*, 2005). While studies in Thailand have indicated that *E. histolytica* was more common among HIV positive patients (P<0.001), studies in Mexico were not conclusive on this issue (Hung *et al.*, 2005). We had recently described a much higher seroprevalence of *Entamoeba histolytica* among HIV and AIDS patients compared to HIV negative patients (Samie et al., 2010). In a study on the genetic diversity of *E. histolytica*, we found that one profile was more common among HIV positive individuals indicating that the increased susceptibility of HIV positive individual to *E. histolytica* might depend on the genetic profile of the infecting *E. histolytica* strain. In a recent study in Uzbekistan, HIV-infected patients were found to have virtually all parasites, such as *Giardia lamblia*, *Cryptosporidium parvum*, *Chilomastix mesnili*, *Entamoeba coli*, *Iodamoeba butschlii*, *Entamoeba histolytica/dispar*, *Endolimax nana*, *Blastocystis hominis*, *Enlerobius vermicularis*, *Ascaris lumbricoides*, *Hymenolepis nana*, detectable in the population of Tashkent (Nurtaev *et al.*, 2006). Of special interest was the fact that in all the forms (stages) of HIV infection, the infestation with *E. histolytical/dispar* was 10 times greater than that in non HIV infected individuals.

Since their successful isolation from stools in the 1970s *Campylobacter spp* have risen from obscurity to notoriety as important food borne agents of gastroenteritis with present isolation rates superceding those of other enteric pathogens such as *Salmonella* spp. and *Shigella* spp. in most developed countries and higher prevalence among children in the developing world (Crushell *et al.*, 2004; Fernández-Cruz et al., 2010). Although their implication in human infections has been described worldwide, their epidemiology varies in different regions of the world and the knowledge of their prevalence using molecular methods is essential for the designing of efficient control measures adapted to each area. Acute self-limited gastrointestinal illness, characterized by diarrhea, fever and abdominal cramps, is the most common presentation of *C. jejuni/C. coli* infection (Butzler, 2004). In this study we found a significant association of *C. jejuni* and *C. coli* infections with diarrhea and inflammation. *Campylobacter spp* other than *C jejuni/coli* have also been implicated in human and animal diseases (Lastovica and Skirrow, 2000; Moran, 2010). In this study, we detected *C. concisus* in 10 (3.1%) samples with 6 (60%) cases present in diarrheal stools indicating the possibility of the involvement of this *Campylobacter species* in disease production in the Vhembe district. In Cape Town, studies by Lastovica and LeRoux indicated that C. *concisus* was the second most isolated *Campylobacter* after C. *jejuni* and constituted 23.55% of all *Campylobacter* isolates (Lastovica and Le Roux, 2000).

Unlike its close phenotypically related neighbour *Campylobacter, Arcobacter* is not currently a major public health concern, but is considered as an emerging human pathogen, and is of significance in animal health (Snelling *et al.*, 2006; Kalischuk and Buret, 2010). In the present study 70% of A. *butzleri* containing samples was diarrheal and 55% with elevated level of lactoferrin indicating possible involvement in inflammatory processes. However more research needs to be conducted in order to confirm its involvement in human disease. *H. pylori* was found in 163 (50.6%) of all the samples among which 55.9% of H. *pylori* positive samples were diarrheal and that *Helicobacter pylori* was common among school children and hospital patients. These results are similar to previous studies that have indicated that *H. pylori* is a common human pathogen estimated to colonize 50% of the world's population (Van Der Hulst *et al.*, 1996). Epidemiological evidence has suggested that H. *pylori* is spread by fecal-oral and oral-oral routes. Although there are no known environmental reservoirs for H. pylori, H. *pylori* has been cultured from the feces (Thomas *et al.*, 1992) of infected individuals and has been detected by polymerase chain reaction (PCR) in dental plaque (Nguyen *et al.*, 1993). The prevalence found in the present study was lower compared to other recent studies in Pretoria, South Africa, where H. *pylori* was found in 84% of stomach biopsies from Healthy individuals but not in dental samples (Olivier *et al.*, 2006). It has been estimated that the relationship between chronic diarrhea, retarded growth, iron-deficient anaemia, and H. *pylori* infection in children especially from developing countries remains controversial (Raymond *et al.*, 2005). However, more research is needed in order to determine their involvement in gastric ulcers as well as any other pathogenic features in the Vhembe district.

Over the past few years, enteroaggregative E. *coli* have been increasingly characterized in developing countries and recent data have suggested that EAEC are emerging as diarrheal agents in developed nations as well (Nataro *et al.*, 2006; Opintan et al., 2010). However; the true distribution of these organisms as well as their pathogenicity is not well studied in South Africa particularly in the Vhembe district. In the present study, we detected the presence of three EAEC pathogenic genes employing a recently developed multiplex PCR. We evaluated these genes in relation to HIV status, diarrheal symptoms, intestinal inflammation, determined by elevated lactoferrin, and occult blood in a sample population composed of hospital patients with known HIV status and school children in the Vhembe district of South Africa. Different methods have been described for the detection of EAEC and have suggested the existence of two different categories of EAEC including Typical and Atypical EAEC (Jenkins *et al.*, 2006). Typical EAEC carry the pAA plasmid originally detected by the AA probe. Enteroaggregative E. *coli* have also been associated with weakened immune system such as in patients with HIV and AIDS. EAEC have been described as the most common pathogen among HIV positive patients in many countries even though the rates of infection vary from country to country. In this study we found a higher rate of EAEC infection among HIV positive patients (29.5%) compared to Senegal (West Africa) where EAEC was found in 19.6 % of HIV patients and was the most common pathogen amongst these individuals (Gassama *et al.*, 2001). In Switzerland, EAEC genes were detected in 22% of HIV positive patients with diarrhea while in Zambia, EAEC was found in both HIV patients and control even though cytotoxic phenotypes were only isolated from the AIDS patients with no evidence of seasonality in the frequency of isolation, and no evidence of long-term carriage (Kelly *et al.*, 2003; Crump et al., 2011).

Different markers of pathogenesis have been described in EAEC infections including fecal cytokines such as IL-8 and IL-1R, lactoferrin, and occult blood (Steiner *et al.*, 1998, Greenberg *et al.*, 2002). Volunteer challenge studies have demonstrated heterogeneity in the ability of EAEC isolates to cause disease and several studies have been unable to make clear associations with EAEC and diarrhea. In this study, more EAEC positive samples had elevated lactoferrin and diarrhea, and the presence of EAEC in the stools was significantly associated with occult blood (P<0.001). Although EAEC have been associated with bloody stool samples the relationship with occult blood has not been clearly described (Durrer *et al.*, 2000). A study in Central African Republic indicated that EAEC were the most frequently identified agents in HIV positive patients with persistent diarrhea and 42.8% of the patients with EAEC as sole pathogens had bloody diarrhea (Germani *et al.*, 1998). The presence of occult blood in the stools of individuals infected with EAEC was tested in a previous study that did not find a significant association between EAEC infection and the presence of occult blood in the stools since only 4 (31.1%) of EAEC positive stool samples had occult blood, while 27 (60.0%) of EAEC positive stool samples had lactoferrin (Bouckenooghe *et al.*, 2000). Our study is thus the first that found significant association between EAEC infections and occult blood in the stool and might indicate a different pathogenic manifestation of these organisms in this part of the world.

Studies elsewhere have indicated that the best characterized *E. coli* pathotypes require multiple genes to be fully/highly virulent. For example enterotoxigenic *E. coli* (ETEC) with heat-labile toxin (LT), heat-stable toxin (ST) and colonization factor antigens (CFAs) are the most virulent; Enteropathogenic *E. coli* (EPEC) with Bundle Forming Pilus (BFP) and the *eae* gene encoding the adhesin intimin, responsible for the intimate attachment of the bacteria to the epithelial cell are most virulent; Shiga-toxin-producing *E. coli* (STEC) with Shiga-like toxin (Stx) and eaeA, encoding intimin involved in attachment of bacteria to enterocytes and plasmid are most virulent (Qadri *et al.*, 2000 ; Rappelli *et al.*, 2001 ; Scaletsky *et al.*, 2002 ; Karch *et al.*, 2006; Turner *et al.*, 2006; Medina et al., 2010). However, the presence of multiple genes has not been associated with pathogenesis in EAEC. This study has shown that strains with all the three genes were more pathogenic in terms of diarrhea production, intestinal inflammation indicated by the lactoferrin level in the stools and occult blood.

Two species of microsporidia, *Enterocytozoon bieneusi* and *Encephalitozoon* (*Septata*) *instestinalis,* are known to cause intestinal microsporidiosis. Even though *E. bieneusi* is responsible for about 90% of reported infections (Orenstein, 1994), other microsporidial species such as the Vittaforma-like species were recently described in stool samples from both HIV positive and HIV negative individuals in Portugal (Sulaiman *et al.*, 2003). In our study, only *E. bieneusi* was detected in stool samples, even though the PCR method used could detect all of the *Encephalitozoon spp.* in addition to *E. bieneusi*. Other studies have also indicated that *E. bieneusi* was the most common microsporidia infecting HIV negative as well as HIV positive individuals (Sarfati *et al.*, 2006) and that PCR based assays can be used successfully for microsporidian species differentiation from stool specimens, thus obviating the need for invasive biopsy procedures (Liguory *et al.*, 1997).

To date, the pathogenicity of Microsporidia is not clearly defined and the mechanisms by which Microsporidia induce diarrhea in HIV patients have not been determined. A wide range of pathology has been associated with Microsporidia; these include inflammation and cell death, and symptoms such as shortness of breath, sinusitis, and diarrhea with wasting (Orenstein, 2003; Stark et al., 2009). In our study we found that even though HIV positive patients infected by *E. bieneusi* had more diarrhea than those non-infected, they actually had less inflammation as compared to the non-infected HIV positive individuals as demonstrated by the lactoferrin test. This could be explained by the occurrence of multiple infections in these individuals. The high level of lactoferrin could thus be due to infections by other organisms such as *Cryptosporidium* spp, *Entamoeba histolytica*, Enteroaggregative *E. coli*, *Clostridium difficile* and *Campylobacter jejuni / coli* also found in these stool samples. Compared to previous studies we have conducted in the same region, *E. bieneusi* was more common than *Cryptosporidium spp* among HIV patients (Samie et al., 2006a). However, HIV positive patients infected with *Cryptosporidium* had more diarrhea and more lactoferrin than those who were not infected, indicating that the expected outcome would be worse with *Cryptosporidium* than with *E. bieneusi* in this population. This observation is similar to those described by Bern et al. (2005) in Peru, where microsporidiosis did not appear to have a major impact on survival among AIDS patients compared to cryptosporidiosis, even though some genotypes of *E. bieneusi* caused chronic diarrhea in these patients.

E. bieneusi was not associated with intestinal inflammation in our study, as demonstrated by the lactoferrin test in HIV negative and HIV positive individuals even though most HIV positive individuals without microsporidia had elevated lactoferrin, indicating high level of intestinal inflammation. This could be due to the effect of HIV itself as previously demonstrated (Kotler et al., 1993; Maingat et al., 2011). This is in line with some studies where multiple small intestinal biopsies showed atrophy with acute and chronic inflammation in HIV seropositive individuals even without apparent pathogens (Orenstein et al., 1992; Snijders et al., 1995; Idris et al 2010). It thus suggests that microsporidia might be cause of secretory diarrhea in HIV patients while most HIV negative individuals remain asymptomatic in the Vhembe district.

This study also determined the prevalence of community acquired *C. difficile* toxigenic characteristics among hospital outpatients and school children and evaluated the association between different pathologic features and the presence and toxigenic profiles of the isolates. *C. difficile* was less frequent among apparently healthy school children. The two positive samples obtained from the schools were non toxigenic as opposed to the toxigenic strains obtained from the hospital outpatients. We also identified the existence of a mutation on the *tcdC* gene associated with increased virulence of associated *C. difficile* infections and this is in harmony with a previous repport (Cloud et al., 2007). The prevalence of *C. difficile* associated diarrhea among HIV patients have been demonstrated to vary according to different studies (Cappell 1993; Lu 1994). In a study of *C difficile* associated diarrhea among HIV positive patients in Illinois, USA, CDAD was observed in 32% of all study patients with diarrhea especially those with advanced HIV disease (Pulvirenti et al., 2002). Other reports have suggested that clinical manifestations and response to therapy in HIV infected patients with *C. difficile* associated diarrhea (CDAD) were similar to that of patients without HIV (DeLalla 1992; Hutin 1993; Cozart 1993) while others have noted a more severe, refractory presentation in HIV infected patients (Colarian 1988; Beaugerie 1994). In our study *C. difficile* did not appear to be associated with HIV. However like other studies, our HIV population was very little (44 patients) and was not clearly characterized in terms of CD4+ counts or HIV disease state. Thus more studies are needed to confirm the role of *C. difficile* as diarrheal agent among HIV positive patients in the Vhembe district and in South Africa in general.

Toxin-A-negative, toxin-B-positive (A- B+) *Clostridium difficile* isolates were identified in several studies (Wultanska *et al.*, 2005). We found that only 3 (6.7%) of all *C. difficile* positive samples were A-B+ variants which is lower compared to those found in horses by Arroyo *et al.*, (2007) and around the same level as those described by Pituch *et al*, (2003) in Poland were about 7% of the strains isolated from CDAD patients had the variant A-B+ isolates. Recent studies have also reported on the existence of cluster of A- B+ *C. difficile*, universally resistant to the fluoroquinolones tested including ofloxacin, ciprofloxacin, levofloxacin, moxifloxacin and gatifloxacin, with MICs > 32 mg/mL, associated with a novel transversion mutation in gyrB (Drudy *et al.*, 2006). The high prevalence of A-B+ *C. difficile* strains might have a negative impact on the detection of toxigenic *C. difficile* in stool samples when the ELISA test is used. This further underscores the importance of the implementation of molecular methods in the detection and characterization of *C. difficile* in specific settings.

5. Conclusions

The quantitative real time PCR using SYBR green is a simple and fast method for the detection of different infectious organisms including bacteria and parasites. Different pre-treatment methods can be used to improve DNA purification for the detection of bacterial and parasitic organisms in stool samples for molecular epidemiological studies. These include the alkaline treatment of the stool sample, the use of the freeze and thaw and the use of glass beads prior to DNA purification by the traditional phenol chloroform method or the use of different kits such as the Qiagen. This study has demonstrated a high prevalence of microsporidia, *Cryptosporidium* infections in the Vhembe district and its implications in the production of diarrhea and inflammation. *C. hominis* was more common and related to pathogenesis than *C. parvum*. HIV positive patients did not appear to be more likely to be infected by *Cryptosporidium*. However, more studies are needed using larger number of HIV positive samples. The study of antigenic profiles of these organisms will provide insight for the development of effective vaccines.

E histolytica appears to be common in the Vhembe district of South Africa. Mixed infections were especially frequent as opposed to other areas in the world such as Japan (Ali *et al.*, 2003). *E. dispar* was less associated with diarrhea or fecal lactoferrin and occurred more often than *E. histolytica* in the general population. Fecal lactoferrin may provide a useful indicator of acute invasive *E. histolytica* infections and could be used as screening test for inflammatory diarrhea including *E. histolytica* in the Vhembe district considering its simplicity. This study also shows the susceptibility of females infected with HIV to *E. histolytica*, which is also commonly seen in males with or without HIV. The study of genetic and antigenic profiles will shed more light on the pathogenicity of this important protozoal infection and provide insight into improved control measures such as improved water and sanitation, vaccine and drug development.

We successfully used different PCR methods for the detection and identification of Enteroaggregative E. Coli, *Campylobacter*, *Helicobacter* and *Arcobacter* spp from stool samples. Of interest was the development of a fast and efficient real time PCR using SYBR GREEN for the detection of *C. concisus*. EAEC was an important etiological agent of diarrhea in the Vhembe district, South Africa as indicated by its high prevalence among hospital patients and particularly among HIV positive patients. Furthermore, EAEC may be a treatable cause of diarrhea in patients with AIDS (Wanke *et al.*, 1998b). Toxigenic *C. difficile* was associated with pathologic conditions among the patients. Typical preventive measures against infections by these organisms include careful personal hygiene, especially promotion of hand washing through health education programs. Major therapeutic intervention for all individuals with diarrhea consists of fluid and electrolyte therapy. However, when antimicrobial therapy is appropriate, selection of a specific agent should be made based upon susceptibility patterns of the pathogen or information on local susceptibility patterns.

Quantitative real time PCR showed that a certain threshold, related to the number of cells, was needed for the EAEC to cause pathologic symptoms such as diarrhea and inflammation. HIV positive individuals are at a higher risk of infection by EAEC and had higher level of lactoferrin when compared to HIV negative individuals. This is the first study to significantly associate EAEC with the presence of occult blood in the stools which might be due to pathogenic factors such as the plasmid encoded toxin (Pet) which is highly homologous to the EspP protease of EHEC and to EspC of EPEC as well as the protein involved in colonization (Pic) .

The current study has demonstrated that *E. bieneusi* is the most common microsporidian species occurring in the Vhembe district particularly among HIV positive patients and *E. bieneusi* is a cause of secretory diarrhea among HIV positive individuals as opposed to inflammatory diarrhea. This study has demonstrated that the pathogenicity of Enteroaggregative *E. coli* could be directly related to the genetic profile of the infecting strains. This is important in the understanding of the pathogenicity of these organisms with possible effect on the development of control methods including diagnostics, drug target molecules (genes) and vaccination procedures. This study also associated EAEC infections with occult blood which might indicate a possible relation/link between the pathogenicity of this organism and that of Enterohemorrhagic *E. coli* (EHEC) often involved in hemolytic uremic syndrome (HUS) and bloody diarrhea.

The pathogenicity index determines the importance of the infecting agent as a pathogen in a specific community. The pathogenicity index indicated that *E. histolytica, Cryptosporidium hominis, C. jejuni/coli, C. concisus, Clostridium difficile* and Enteroaggregative *E. coli* were the most diarrheagenic organisms in the Vhembe population while *E. histolytica, C. jejuni/coli, C. concisus, Clostridium difficile* were the most inflammatory. Enteroaggregative *E. coli* was the most associated with occult blood followed by *E. histolytica, C. jejuni/coli,* and *Clostridium difficile*. This further indicates the importance of the lactoferrin and occult tests as screening methods for diarrheal organisms in hospitals and will probably reduce the cost of infectious diarrheal diagnosis and improve the quality of service. HIV positive patients are more susceptible to infections, therefore, the implementation of molecular methodologies is recommended for an improved diagnosis of gastrointestinal infections among these patients and the quality of their lives. Diarrheal diseases can be prevented through access to clean, safe drinking water and through proper sanitation measures, including hand washing and safe disposal of human waste. Thus increased health education in schools as well as in the communities is highly recommended and could help prevent the transmission of diarrheal diseases in the population. Proper management and treatment of waste and waste water is recommended through increased investments in water and sanitation systems at least in fast growing areas. Such strategies could alleviate a great deal of unnecessary suffering and loss of productivity; reduce the number of lives lost to these diseases, and result in significant savings in health care costs.

6. Acknowledgements

The present study was supported in part by the Pfizer and Ellison foundations through the Centre for Global Health of the University of Virginia, The National research foundation of South Africa, The International Society for Infectious diseases and the United Nations educational, scientific and cultural organization (UNESCO) and the University of Venda. Samples were collected thanks to the collaboration of primary schools' staff and the Hospitals' staff. Authorization was obtained from the Department of Health in Limpopo, South Africa.

7. References

Abd-Alla MD, and Ravdin JI (2002). Diagnosis of amebic colitis by antigen capture ELISA in patients presenting with acute amebic diarrhea in Cairo Egypt. *Tropical Medicine and International Health*, 7, 365--370.

Abd-Alla MD, Jackson TG and Ravdin JI (1998). Serum IgM antibody response to the galactose-inhibitable adherence lectin of *E. histolytica*. *American Journal of Tropical Medicine and Hygiene*, 59, 431-434.

Abdel-Messih IA, Wierzba TF, Abu-Elyazeed R, Ibrahim AF, Ahmed SF, Kamal K, Sanders J, French R (2005). Diarrhea associated with *Cryptosporidium parvum* among young children of the Nile River Delta in Egypt. *Journal of Tropical Pediatrics* 51, 154–159.

Alcantara CS, Yang CH, Steiner TS, Barret LJ, Lima AA, Chappell CL, Okhuysen PC, White JrAC, Guerrant RL (2003). Interleukin- 8, tumor necrosis factor alpha, and lactoferrin in immunocompetent hosts with experimental and Brazilian children with acquired cryptosporidiosis. *American Journal of Tropical Medicine and Hygiene*, 68, 325–328.

Al-Hindi A, Shubair ME, Marshall I, Ashford RW, Sharif FA, Abed AA, Kamel EG (2005). *Entamoeba histolytica* or *Entamoeba dispar* among children in Gaza, Gaza Strip? *Journal of the Egyptian Society of Parasitology*, 35(1), 59--68.

Ali IK, Hossain MB, Roy S, Ayeh-Kumi PF, Petri WA Jr, Haque R, Clark CG (2003). *Entamoeba moshkovskii* infections in children in Bangladesh. *Emerg Infect Dis* 9:580--584.

Al-Mekhlafi HM, Mahdy MA, 'azlin MY, Fatmah MS, Norhayati M (2011). Childhood *Cryptosporidium* infection among aboriginal communities in Peninsular Malaysia. Annals of Tropical Medicine and Parasitology, 105(2):135-43.

Aly SM, El-Zawawy LA, Said DE, Fathy FM, Mohamed On (2005). The utility of lactoferrin in differentiating parasitic from bacterial infections. *Journal of the Egyptian Society of Parasitology*, 35(3 Suppl):1149--1162.

Antonios SN, Tolba OA, Othman AA, Saad MA (2010). A preliminary study on the prevalence of parasitic infections in immunocompromised children. *Journal of the Egyptian Society of Parasitology*, 40(3), 617-30.

Arroyo LG, Staempfli H, Weese JS (2007). Molecular analysis of *Clostridium difficile* isolates recovered from horses with diarrhea. *Veterinary Microbiology*, 120, 179-83.

Banerjee B, Hazra S and Bandyopadhyay D (2004). Diarrhea Management Among Under Fives. *Indian Pediatrics* 41: 255 --260.

Barwick RS, Uzicanin A, Lareau S, Malakmadze N, Imnadze P, Iosava M, Ninashvili N, Wilson M, Hightower AW, Johnston S, Bishop H, Petri WA Jr, Juranek DD (2002). Outbreak of amebiasis in Tbilisi, Republic of Georgia, 1998. *American Journal of Tropical Medicine and Hygiene* , 67(6), 623--631.

Beatty GW (2010). Diarrhea in patients infected with HIV presenting to the emergency department. Emergency Medicine Clinics of North America, 28(2), 299-310.

Beaugerie L, Ngo Y, Goujard F, Gharakhanian S, Carbonnel F, Luboinski J, Malafosse M, Rozenbaum W, Le Quintrec Y (1994). Etiology and management of toxic megacolon in patients with human immuno deficiency virus infection. *Gastroenterology*, 107, 858-63.

Bern C, Kawai V, Vargas D, Rabke-Verani J, Williamson J, Chavez-Valdez R, Xiao L, Sulaiman I, Vivar A, Ticona E, Navincopa M, Cama V, Moura H, Secor WE, Visvesvara G, Gilman RH (2005). The epidemiology of intestinal microsporidiosis in patients with HIV/AIDS in Lima, Peru. *Journal of Infectious Diseases*, 191, 1658-64.

Bern C, Ortega Y, Checkley W, Roberts JM, Lescano AG, Cabrera L, Verastegui M, Black RE, Sterling C, Gilman RH (2002). Epidemiologic differences between cyclosporiasis and cryptosporidiosis in Peruvian children. *Emerging Infectious Diseases*, 8, 581–585.

Bialek R, Binder N, Dietz K, Joachim A, Knobloch J, Zelck UE (2002). Comparison of fluorescence, antigen and PCR assays to detect *Cryptosporidium parvum* in fecal specimens. Diagnostic Microbiology and Infectious Diseases, 43(4), 283-8.

Bouckenooghe AR, DuPont HL, Jiang ZD, Adachi J, Mathewson JJ, Verenkar MP, Rodrigues S, Steffen R (2000). Markers of enteric inflammation in enteroaggregative *Escherichia coli* diarrhea in travellers. *American Journal of Tropical Medicine and Hygiene*, 62, 711–713.

Bradshaw D, Nannan N, Groenewald P, Joubert J, Laubscher R, Nojilana B, Norman R, Pieterse D and Schneider M (2005). Provincial mortality in South Africa, 2000: priority-setting for now and a benchmark for the future. *South African Medical Journal*, 95 (7), 496-503.

Bushen OY, Davenport JA, Lima AB, Piscitelli SC, Uzgiris AJ, Silva TM, Leite R, Kosek M, Dillingham RA, Girao A, Lima AA, Guerrant RL (2004). Diarrhea and reduced levels of antiretroviral drugs: improvement with glutamine or alanyl-glutamine in a randomized controlled trial in northeast Brazil. *Clinical Infectious Diseases*, 38(12), 1764-70.

Butzler JP (2004). *Campylobacter*, from obscurity to celebrity. *Clin Microbiol Infect* 2004; 10:868-76.

Calderaro A, Gorrini C, Bommezzadri S, Piccolo G, Dettori G, and Chezzi C (2005). *Entamoeba histolytica* and *Entamoeba dispar*: comparison of two PCR assays for diagnosis in a non-endemic setting. *Transactions of the Royal Society of Tropical Medicine and Hygiene*, 100(5), 450--457.

Callendar GR (1933). The differential pathology of dysentery. *American Journal of Tropical Medicine and Hygiene* , 14, 207 - 233.

Cappell MS, Philogene C (1993). *Clostridium difficile* infection is a treatable cause of diarrhea in patients with advanced human immunodeficiency virus infection: a study of seven consecutive patients admitted from 1986 to 1992 to a university teaching hospital. *American Journal of Gastroenterology*, 88, 891-7.

Cerna JF, Nataro JP, Estrada-Garcia T (2003). Multiplex PCR for detection of three plasmid-borne genes of enteroaggregative *Escherichia coli* strains. *Journal of Clinical Microbiology*, 41, 2138-2140.

Chappell CL, Okhuysen PC, Sterling CR, DuPont HL (1996). *Cryptosporidium parvum*: intensity of infection and oocyst excretion patterns in healthy volunteers. *Journal of Infectious Diseases*, 173(1), 232-6.

Checkley W, Epstein LD, Gilman RH, Black RE, Cabrera L, Sterling CR (1998). Effects of *Cryptosporidium parvum* infection in Peruvian children: growth faltering and subsequent catch-up growth. *American Journal of Epidemiology*, 148, 497-506.

Choi SW, Park CH, Silva TM, Zaenker EI, Guerrant RL (1996). To culture or not to culture: fecal lactoferrin screening for inflammatory bacterial diarrhea. *Journal of Clinical Microbiology*, 34(4), 928-32.

Cleary RK (1998). *Clostridium difficile*-associated diarrhea and colitis: Clinical manifestations, diagnosis, and treatment. Diseases of the Colon & Rectum, 41, 1435-49.

Cloud J, Kelly CP (2007). Update on *Clostridium difficile* associated disease. *Curr Opin Gastroenterol* 23:4-9.

Colarian J (1988). *Clostridium difficile* colitis following antiviral therapy in the acquired immunodeficiency syndrome. *Am J Med* 84: 1081.

Cozart JC, Kalangi SS, Clench MH, Taylor DR, Borucki MJ, Pollard RB, Soloway RD (1994). *Clostridium difficile* diarrhea in patients with AIDS versus non-AIDS controls. Methods of treatment and clinical response to treatment. *J Clin Gastroenterol* 16:192-4.

Crump JA, Ramadhani HO, Morrissey AB, Msuya LJ, Yang LY, Chow SC, Morpeth SC, Reyburn H, Njau BN, Shaw AV, Diefenthal HC, Bartlett JA, Shao JF, Schimana W, Cunningham CK, Kinabo GD. Invasive bacterial and fungal infections among hospitalized HIV-infected and HIV-uninfected children and infants in northern Tanzania. Trop Med Int Health. 2011 Apr 7. doi: 10.1111/j.1365-3156.2011.02774.x.

Crushell E, Harty S, Sharif F, Bourke B (2004). Enteric *Campylobacter*: Purging Its Secrets? *Pediatr Res* 55: 3-12.

de Lalla F, Nicolin R, Rinaldi E, Scarpellini P, Rigoli R, Manfrin V, Tramarin A (1992). Prospective study of oral teicoplanin versus oral vancomycin for therapy of pseudomembranous colitis and *Clostridium difficile*-associated diarrhea. Antimicrobial Agents and Chemotherapy, 36, 2192-6.

de Oliveira-Silva MB, de Oliveira LR, Resende JC, Peghini BC, Ramirez LE, Lages-Silva E, Correia D (2007). Seasonal profile and level of CD4+ lymphocytes in the occurrence of cryptosporidiosis and cysto-isosporidiosis in HIV/AIDS patients in the Triângulo Mineiro region, Brazil. *Revista da Sociedade Brasileira de Medicina Tropical*. 40(5):512-5.

de Truchis P, de Truchis A (2007). Acute infectious diarrhea]. *Presse Medicale*, 36(4 Pt 2), 695-705.

Department of Health (DOH) (2006). National HIV and syphilis antenatal seroprevalence survey in South Africa: 2005.

Department of Health, "National HIV and Syphilis Antenatal Sero-prevalence Survey in South Africa 2000.

Department of Health, 2010. National Antenatal Sentinel HIV and Syphilis. Prevalence Survey in South Africa, 2009.

Desportes I, Le Charpentier Y, Galian A, Bernard F, Cochand-Priollet B, Lavergne A, Ravisse P, Modigliani R (1985). Occurrence of a new microsporidan: Enterocytozoon bieneusi n.g., n. sp., in the enterocytes of a human patient with AIDS. *Journal of Protozoology*, 32(2), 250-4.

Diamond LS and Clark CG (1993). A redescription of *Entamoeba histolytica* Schaudinn, 1903 (emended Walker, 1911) separating it from *Entamoeba dispar* Brumpt, 1925, Journal of Eukaryotic Microbiology, 40, 340-344.

Dillingham R, Guerrant RL (2004). Childhood stunting: measuring and stemming the staggering costs of inadequate water and sanitation. *Lancet,* 363(9403), 94-5.

Drudy D, Quinn T, O'Mahony R, Kyne L, O'Gaora P, Fanning S (2006). High-level resistance to moxifloxacin and gatifloxacin associated with a novel mutation in gyrB in toxin-A-negative, toxin-B-positive *Clostridium difficile*. *Journal of Antimicrobial Chemotherapy,* 58, 1264-7.

DuPont HL (1997). Guidelines on acute infectious diarrhea in adults. The Practice Parameters Committee of the American College of Gastroenterology. *American Journal of Gastroenterology*, 92(11), 1962-75.

Durrer P, Zbinden R, Fleisch F, Altwegg M, Ledergerber B, Karch H, Weber R (2000). Intestinal infection due to enteroaggregative *Escherichia coli* among human immunodeficiency virus-infected persons. *J Infect Dis* 182:1540-1544.

el-Naggar SM, el-Bahy MM, Abd Elaziz J, el-Dardiry MA (2006). Detection of protozoal parasites in the stools of diarrhoeic patients using different techniques. *Journal of the Egyptian Society of Parasitology*, 36(2), 487-516.

Fedorko DP, Nelson NA, Cartwright CP (1995). Identification of microsporidia in stool specimens by using PCR and restriction endonucleases. *Journal of Clinical Microbiology*, 33, 1739–1741.

Fernández-Cruz A, Muñoz P, Mohedano R, Valerio M, Marín M, Alcalá L, Rodriguez-Créixems M, Cercenado E, Bouza E. *Campylobacter* bacteremia: clinical characteristics, incidence, and outcome over 23 years. *Medicine (Baltimore).* 2010, 89(5):319-30.

Fincham JE, Jackson TFHG, Schoeman S, Evans AC, Markus MB, Mwamba JC. Intestinal parasites in children: the need for community-based interventions. Tygerberg: Medical Research Council, 1997:1-2. (MRC policy brief no. 3).

Gassama A, Thiaw B, Dia NM, Fall F, Camara P, Hovette P, Perret JL, Gueye – Ndiaye A, Mboup S, Sow PS, Aidara-Kane A, (2001). [Infective etiology of diarrhea in adults with HIV infection in Dakar: a case-control study on 594 patients]. *Dakar Medical* 46:46-50.

Gathiram V, Jackson TF (1985). Frequency distribution of *Entamoeba histolytica* zymodemes in a rural South African population. *Lancet* 30 (8431):719--721. 35.

Germani Y, Minssart P, Vohito M, Yassibanda S, Glaziou P, Hocquet D, Berthelemy P, Morvan J, (1998). Etiologies of acute, persistent, and dysenteric diarrheas in adults in Bangui, Central African Republic, in relation to human immunodeficiency virus serostatus. *Am J Trop Med Hyg* 59:1008-1014.

Goodgame RW, Genta RM, White AC, Chappell CL (1993). Intensity of infection in AIDS-associated cryptosporidiosis. Journal of Infectious Diseases, 167(3), 704-9.

Goodman L, Segreti J (1999). Infectious diarrhea. Dis Mon. 1999 Jul; 45(7):268-99.

Greenberg DE, Jiang ZD, Steffen R, Verenker MP, DuPont HL, (2002). Markers of inflammation in bacterial diarrhea among travelers, with a focus on enteroaggregative *Escherichia coli* pathogenicity. *Journal of Infectious Diseases, 185,* 944–949.

Greenwood BM. Greenwood AM. Bradley AK. Tulloch S. Hayes R. Oldfield FS. Deaths in infancy and early childhood in a well-vaccinated, rural, West African population. *Ann Trop Paediatr.* 1987;7:91–9.

Guerrant RL, Brush J, Ravdin JI, Sullivan JA, Mandell GL (1981). Interaction between *Entamoeba histolytica* and human polymorphonuclear neutrophils. *J Infect Dis* 143(1):83--93.

Guerrant RL, Oria R, Bushen OY, Patrick PD, Houpt E, Lima AA (2005). Global impact of diarrheal diseases that are sampled by travelers: the rest of the hippopotamus. *Clin Infect Dis* 1; 41 Suppl 8:S524-30.

Guerrant RL, Van Gilder T, Steiner TS, Thielman NM, Slutsker L, Tauxe RV, Hennessy T, Griffin PM, DuPont H, Sack RB, Tarr P, Neill M, Nachamkin I, Reller LB, Osterholm MT, Bennish ML, Pickering LK; Infectious Diseases Society of America (2001). Practice guidelines for the management of infectious diarrhea. *Clinical Infectious Diseases,* 32(3), 331-51.

Haghighi A, Kobayashi S, Takeuchi T, Thammapalerd N, Nozaki T (2003). Geographic diversity among genotypes of *Entamoeba histolytica* field isolates. *Journal of Clinical Microbiology,* 41, 3748-56.

Haque R, Ali IKM, Akther S, Petri JrWA (1998). Comparison of PCR, isoenzyme analysis, and antigen detection for diagnosis of *Entamoeba histolytica* infection. *Journal of Clinical Microbiology,* 36, 449–452.

Herikstad H, Yang S, Van Gilder TJ, Vugia D, Hadler J, Blake P, Deneen V, Shiferaw B, Angulo FJ (2002). A population-based estimate of the burden of diarrhoeal illness in the United States: FoodNet, 1996-7. Epidemiology and Infection, 129(1), 9-17.

Hou Y, Mortimer L, Chadee K (2010). Entamoeba histolytica cysteine proteinase 5 binds integrin on colonic cells and stimulates NFkappaB-mediated pro-inflammatory responses. *Journal of Biological Chemistry,* 285(46), 35497-504.

Houf K, Tutenel A, De Zutter L, Van Hoof J, Vandamme P (2000). Development of a multiplex PCR assay for the simultaneous detection and identification of *Arcobacter butzleri, Arcobacter cryaerophilus* and *Arcobacter skirrowii. FEMS Microbiol Lett* 193:89-94.

Houpt E, Bushen OY, Sa NE, Kohli A, Asgharpour A, Ng CT, Calfee DP, Guerrant RL, Maro V, Ole-Nguvaine S, Shao JF (2005). Short report: asymptomatic *Cryptosporidium hominis* infection among human immunodeficiency virus-infected patients in Tanzania. *American Journal of Tropical Medicine and Hygiene,* 73, 520–522.

Huang DB, Jiang ZD, Dupont HL (2003). Association of virulence factor-positive and -negative enteroaggregative Escherichia coli and occurrence of clinical illness in travelers from the United States to Mexico. *American Journal of Tropical Medicine and Hygiene,* 69(5), 506-8.

Humphreys EH, Smith NA, Azman H, McLeod D, Rutherford GW. Prevention of diarrhoea in children with HIV infection or exposure to maternal HIV infection. *Cochrane Database of Systematic Reviews*, 16(6), CD008563.

Hung CC, Deng HY, Hsiao WH, Hsieh SM, Hsiao CF, Chen MY, Chang SC, Su KE (2005). Invasive amebiasis as an emerging parasitic disease in patients with human immunodeficiency virus type 1 infection in Taiwan. *Archives of Internal Medicine*, 165, 409-15.

Hutin Y, Molina JM, Casin I, Daix V, Sednaoui P, Welker Y, Lagrange P, Decazes JM, Modai J (1993). Risk factors for *Clostridium difficile*-associated Diarrhea in HIV-infected patients. *AIDS* 7, 1441-7.

Idris NS, Dwipoerwantoro PG, Kurniawan A, Said M. Intestinal parasitic infection of immunocompromised children with diarrhoea: clinical profile and therapeutic response. *The Journal of Infection in Developing Countries*, 4(5), 309-17.

Javier-Enriquez F, Avila CR, Ignacio-Santos J, Tanaka-Kido J, Vallejo O, Sterling CR (1997). *Cryptosporidium* infections in Mexican children: clinical, nutritional, enteropathogenic, and diagnostic evaluations. *American Journal of Tropical Medicine and Hygiene*, 56, 254–257.

Jenkins C, Chart H, Willshaw GA, Cheasty T, Smith HR, (2006). Genotyping of enteroaggregative *Escherichia coli* and identification of target genes for the detection of both typical and atypical strains. *Diagnostic Microbiology and Infectious Disease*, 55(1), 13-19.

Jiang ZD, DuPont HL, La Rocco M, Garey KW (2010). In vitro susceptibility of *Clostridium difficile* to rifaximin and rifampin in 359 consecutive isolates at a university hospital in Houston, Texas. *Journal of Clinical Pathology*, 63(4), 355-8.

Kalischuk LD, Buret AG. A role for *Campylobacter jejuni*-induced enteritis in inflammatory bowel disease? *The American Journal of Physiology: Gastrointestinal and Liver Physiology*, 298(1), G1-9.

Kar S, Gawlowska S, Daugschies A, Bangoura B (2011). Quantitative comparison of different purification and detection methods for *Cryptosporidium parvum* oocysts. *Veterinary Parasitology*, 177(3-4), 366-70.

Karch H, Friedrich AW, Gerber A, Zimmerhackl LB, Schmidt MA, Bielaszewska M, (2006). New aspects in the pathogenesis of enteropathic hemolytic uremic syndrome. *Seminars in Thrombosis and Hemostasis*, 32, 105-12.

Karlström O, Fryklund B, Tullus K, Burman LG (1998). A prospective nationwide study of *Clostridium difficile*-associated diarrhea in Sweden. The Swedish *C. difficile* Study Group. *Clinical Infectious Diseases*, 26,141-5.

Kassi RR, Kouassi RA, Yavo W, Barro-Kiki CP, Bamba A, Menan HI, Kone M (2004). Cryptosporidiosis and isosporiasis in children suffering from diarrhoea in Abidjan]. Bull Soc Pathol Exot. 97(4):280-2.

Katsumata T, Hosea D, Ranuh IG, Uga S, Yanagi T, Kohno S (2000). Short report: possible *Cryptosporidium muris* infection in humans. *American Journal of Tropical Medicine and Hygiene*, 62, 70–72.

Kebede A, Verweij JJ, Endeshaw T, Messele T, Tasew G, Petros B, Polderman AM (2004). The use of real-time PCR to identify *Entamoeba histolytica* and *E. dispar* infections in prisoners and primary-school children in Ethiopia. *Annals of Tropical Medicine and Parasitology*, 98(1), 43--48.

Kelly P, Hicks S, Oloya J, Mwansa J, Sikakwa L, Zulu I, Phillips A (2003). Escherichia coli enterovirulent phenotypes in Zambians with AIDS-related diarrhoea. *Transactions of the Royal Society of Tropical Medicine and Hygiene*, 97(5), 573-6.

Kelly P, Hicks S, Oloya J, Mwansa J, Sikakwa L, Zulu I, Phillips A, (2003). *Escherichia coli* enterovirulent phenotypes in Zambians with AIDS-related Diarrhea. *Transactions of the Royal Society of Tropical Medicine and Hygiene*, 97, 573-6.

Kfir R, Hilner C, du Preez M, Bateman B (1995). Studies on the prevalence of giardia cysts and *Cryptosporidium* oocysts in South African water. *Water Science and Technology*, 31, 435–438.

Kirkpatrick BD, Daniels MM, Jean SS, Pape JW, Karp C, Littenberg B, Fitzgerald DW, Lederman HM, Nataro JP, Sears CL (2002). Cryptosporidiosis stimulates an inflammatory intestinal response in malnourished Haitian children. *J Infect Dis* 186, 94–101.

Kirkwood BR. *In: Feachem RG, Jamison DT, editors. Disease and mortality in sub-Saharan Africa*. New York, NY: Oxford University Press; 1991. Diarrhoea; pp. 134–57.

Kotler DP, Reka S, Chow K, Orenstein JM (1993). Effects of enteric parasitoses and HIV infection upon small intestinal structure and function in patients with AIDS. *Journal of Clinical Gastroenterology*, 16, 10-5.

Kuijper EJ, Coignard B, Tull P; the ESCMID Study Group for *Clostridium difficile* (ESGCD)* (2006). EU Member States and the European Centre for Disease Prevention and Control (ECDC) Emergence of *Clostridium difficile*-associated disease in North America and Europe. *Clinical Microbiology and Infections*, 6, 2-18.

Kurniawan A, Karyadi T, Dwintasari SW, Sari IP, Yunihastuti E, Djauzi S, Smith HV (2009) Intestinal parasitic infections in HIV/AIDS patients presenting with diarrhoea in Jakarta, Indonesia. *Transactions of the Royal Society of Tropical Medicine and Hygiene*, doi: 10.1016/j.trstmh.2009.02.017.

Larsen IK, Gradel KO, Helms M, Hornstrup MK, Jürgens G, Mens H, Rosager CL, Clausen TH, Kronborg G, Nielsen H (2011). Non-typhoidal *Salmonella* and *Campylobacter* infections among HIV-positive patients in Denmark. Scand J Infect Dis. 43(1):3-7.

Lashley FR (2006). Emerging infectious diseases at the beginning of the 21st century. Online J Issues Nurs. 31;11(1):2.

Lastovica AJ, Le Roux E (2000). Efficient isolation of campylobacteria from stools. *Journal of Clinical Microbiology*, 38, 2798–9.

Lastovica AJ, Skirrow MB (2000). Clinical significance of *Campylobacter* and related species other than *C. jejuni* and *C. coli*, p 89-120. *In* I. Nachamkin and M. J. Blaser (ed.), *Campylobacter*, 2nd ed. American Society for Microbiology, Washington, D.C. 2000.

Lebbad M, Svard SG (2005). PCR differentiation of *Entamoeba histolytica* and *Entamoeba dispar* from patients with amoeba infection initially diagnosed by microscopy. *Scandinavian Journal of Infectious Diseases*, 37(9), 680-685.

Lee JK, Song HJ, Yu JR (2005). Prevalence of diarrhea caused by *Cryptosporidium parvum* in non-HIV patients in Jeollanam-do, Korea. *Korean Journal of Parasitology*, 43, 111–114.

Lemee L, Dhalluin A, Testelin S, Mattrat MA, Maillard K, Lemeland JF, Pons JL (2004). Multiplex PCR targeting tpi (triose phosphate isomerase), tcdA (Toxin A), and tcdB (Toxin B) genes for toxigenic culture of *Clostridium difficile*. *Journal of Clinical Microbiology*, 42, 5710-4.

Liguory O, David F, Sarfati C, Schuitema AR, Hartskeerl RA, Derouin F, Modai J, Molina JM (1997). Diagnosis of infections caused by *Enterocytozoon bieneusi* and *Encephalitozoon intestinalis* using polymerase chain reaction in stool specimens. *AIDS*. 11, 723-726.

Limor JR, Lal AA, Xiao L (2002). Detection and differentiation of *Cryptosporidium* parasites that are pathogenic for humans by real-time PCR. *Journal of Clinical Microbiology*, 40(7), 2335-8.

Linton D, Lawson AJ, Owen RJ, Stanley J (1997). PCR detection, identification to species level, and fingerprinting of *Campylobacter jejuni* and *Campylobacter coli* direct from diarrheic samples. *Journal of Clinical Microbiology*, 35, 2568-2572.

Lu SS, Schwartz JM, Simon DM, Brandt LJ (1994). *Clostridium difficile*-associated diarrhea in patients with HIV positivity and AIDS: a prospective controlled study. *Americal Journal of Gastroenterology*, 89, 1226-9.

Maingat F, Halloran B, Acharjee S, van Marle G, Church D, Gill MJ, Uwiera RR, Cohen EA, Meddings J, Madsen K, Power C. Inflammation and epithelial cell injury in AIDS enteropathy: involvement of endoplasmic reticulum stress. FASEB Journal, 2011 Mar 22.

Mandomando IM, Macete EV, Ruiz J, Sanz S, Abacassamo F, Vallès X, Sacarlal J, Navia MM, Vila J, Alonso PL, Gascon J (2007). Etiology of diarrhea in children younger than 5 years of age admitted in a rural hospital of southern Mozambique. *American Journal of Tropical Medicine and Hygiene*, 76(3), 522-7.

Marshall SM, Melito PL, Woodward DL, Johnson WM, Rodgers FG, Mulvey MR (1999). Rapid identification of *Campylobacter*, *Arcobacter*, and *Helicobacter* isolates by PCR-restriction fragment length polymorphism analysis of the 16S rRNA gene. *J Clin Microbiol* 37:4158-60.

Matsheka MI, Lastovica AJ, Elisha BG (2001). Molecular identification of *Campylobacter concisus*. *Journal of Clinical Microbiology*, 39, 3684-9.

Medina AM, Rivera FP, Romero LM, Kolevic LA, Castillo ME, Verne E, Hernandez R, Mayor YE, Barletta F, Mercado E, Ochoa TJ. Diarrheagenic Escherichia coli in human immunodeficiency virus (HIV) pediatric patients in Lima, Peru. *American Journal of Tropical Medicine and Hygiene*, 83(1), 158-63.

Mercado EH, Ochoa TJ, Ecker L, Cabello M, Durand D, Barletta F, Molina M, Gil AI, Huicho L, Lanata CF, Cleary TG (2011). Fecal Leukocytes in Children Infected with Diarrheagenic Escherichia coli. *Journal of Clinical Microbiology*, 49(4), 1376-81.

Moodley D, Jackson TFHG, Gathiram V, van den Ende J (1991). *Cryptosporidium* infections in children in Durban. *South African Medical Journal*, 79, 295-297.

Moran AP (2010). The role of endotoxin in infection: Helicobacter pylori and *Campylobacter jejuni*. *Subcellular Biochemistry*, 53, 209-40.

Moran P, Ramos F, Ramiro M, Curiel O, Gonzalez E, Valadez A, Gomez A, Garcia G, Melendro EI, Ximenez C (2005). *Entamoeba histolytica* and/or *Entamoeba dispar*: infection frequency in HIV+/AIDS patients in Mexico city. *Experimental Parasitology*, 110, 331-4.

Moyo SJ, Gro N, Matee MI, Kitundu J, Myrmel H, Mylvaganam H, Maselle SY, Langeland N (2011). Age specific aetiological agents of diarrhoea in hospitalized children aged less than five years in Dar es Salaam, Tanzania. BMC Pediatrics, 23; 11:19.

Nagamani K, Pavuluri PR, Gyaneshwari M, Prasanthi K, Rao MI, Saxena NK (2007). Molecular characterisation of Cryptosporidium: an emerging parasite. Indian Journal of Medical Microbiology, 25(2),133-6.

Nataro JP, Mai V, Johnson J, Blackwelder WC, Heimer R, Tirrell S, Edberg SC, Braden CR, Glenn Morris J Jr, Hirshon JM, (2006). Diarrheagenic Escherichia coli infection in Baltimore, Maryland, and New Haven, Connecticut. Clinical Infectious Diseases, 43, 402-407.

Nel ED, Rabie H, Goodway J, Cotton MF. A Retrospecive Study of Cryptosporidial Diarrhea in a Region with High HIV Prevalence. Journal of Tropical Pediatrics, 2010 Oct 14.

Nesbitt RA, Mosha FW, Katki HA, Ashraf M, Assenga C, Lee CM (2004). Amebiasis and comparison of microscopy to ELISA technique in detection of Entamoeba histolytica and Entamoeba dispar. Journal of the National Medical Association, 96(5), 671--677.

Newman RD, Sears CL, Moore SR, Nataro JP, Wuhib T, Agnew DA, Guerrant RL, Lima AAM (1999). Longitudinal study of Cryptosporidium infection in children in Northeastern Brazil. Journal of Infectious Diseases, 18 (1), 167–175.

Nguyen AM, Engstrand L, Genta RM, Graham DY, El-Zaatari FA (1993). Detection of Helicobacter pylori in dental plaque by reverse transcription polymerase chain reaction. Journal of Clinical Microbiology, 3 1, 783-787.

Nurtaev KhS, Badalova NS, Zalialieva MV, Osipova SO (2005). [Intestinal parasitic diseases in HIV-infected patients in Uzbekistan]. Med parazitol parazit bol 3, 45-9.

Obi CL, Bessong PO (2002). Diarrheagenic bacterial pathogens in HIV-positive patients with Diarrhea in rural communities of Limpopo province, South Africa. Journal of Health Population and Nutrition, 20, 230–234.

Obi CL, Green E, Bessong PO, de Villiers B, Hoosen AA, Igumbor EO and Potgieter N, (2004). Gene encoding virulence markers among Escherichia coli isolates from diarrhoeic stool samples and river sources in rural Venda communities of South Africa. Water SA 30: 515-519.

Obi CL, Momba MNB, Samie A, Igumbor JO, Green E and Musie E (2007). Microbiological, physico-chemical and management parameters impinging on the efficiency of small water treatment plants in the Limpopo and Mpumalanga Provinces of South Africa Water SA Vol. 33 No. 2 :229 - 237.

Okamoto M, Kawabe T, Ohata K, Togo G, Hada T, Katamoto T, Tanno M, Matsumura M, Yamaji Y, Watabe H, Ikenoue T, Yoshida H, Omata M (2005). Amebic colitis in asymptomatic subjects with positive fecal occult blood test results: clinical features different from symptomatic cases. American Journal of Tropical Medicine and Hygiene, 73(5),934--935.

Olivier BJ, Bond RP, van Zyl WB, Delport M, Slavik T, Ziady C, Terhaar sive Droste JS, Lastovica A, van der Merwe SW (2006). Absence of Helicobacter pylori within the Oral Cavities of Members of a Healthy South African Community. J Clin Microbiol 44: 635–636.

Opintan JA, Newman MJ, Ayeh-Kumi PF, Affrim R, Gepi-Attee R, Sevilleja JE, Roche JK, Nataro JP, Warren CA, Guerrant RL (2010). Pediatric diarrhea in southern Ghana:

etiology and association with intestinal inflammation and malnutrition. *American Journal of Tropical Medicine and Hygiene,* 83(4), 936-43.

Orenstein JM (2003). Diagnostic pathology of microsporidiosis. *Ultrastruct Pathol* 27, 141-9.

Orenstein JM, Benator D, Kotler DP (1994). Microsporidia and HIV-related diarrhea. *Ann Intern Med* 120, 973-4.

Orenstein JM, Tenner M, Cali A, Kotler DP (1992). A microsporidian previously undescribed in humans, infecting enterocytes and macrophages, and associated with diarrhea in an acquired immunodeficiency syndrome patient. *Hum Pathol* 23, 722-8.

Pituch H, Obuch-Woszczatynski P, Luczak M, Meisel-Mikolajczyk F (2003). *Clostridium difficile* and enterotoxigenic *Bacteroides fragilis* strains isolated from patients with antibiotic associated Diarrhea. *Anaerobe* 9:161-3.

Potgieter N, Obi CL, Bessong PO, Igumbor EO, Samie A, Nengobela R (2005). Bacterial contamination of Vhuswa–a local weaning food and stored drinking-water in impoverished households in the Vhembe district of South Africa. Journal of Health, Population, and Nutrition, 23, 150–155.

Pulvirenti JJ, Mehra T, Hafiz I, DeMarais P, Marsh D, Kocka F, Meyer PM, Fischer SA, Goodman L, Gerding DN, Weinstein RA (2002). Epidemiology and outcome of *Clostridium difficile* infection and diarrhea in HIV infected inpatients. *Diagnostic Microbiology and Infectious Disease,* 44, 325-30.

Qadri F, Das SK, Faruque AS, Fuchs GJ, Albert MJ, Sack RB and Svennerholm AM, (2000). Prevalence of toxin types and colonization factors in enterotoxigenic *Escherichia coli* isolated during a 2-year period from Diarrheal patients in Bangladesh. *Journal of Clinical Microbiology,* 38, 27–31.

Quinn TC, Stamm WE, Goodell SE, Mkrtichian E, Benedetti J, Corey L, Schuffler MD, Holmes KK (1983). The polymicrobial origin of intestinal infections in homosexual men. N Engl J Med. 309(10):576-82.

Ramos F, Moran P, Gonzalez F, Garcia G, Ramiro M, Gomez A de Leon Mdel C, Melendro EI, Valadez A, Ximenez C (2005). *Entamoeba histolytica* and *Entamoeba dispar*: prevalence infection in a rural Mexican community. *Experimental Parasitology,* 110(3), 327--330.

Rappelli P,Maddau G, Mannu F,ColomboMM, Fiori PL,Cappuccinelli P (2001). Development of a set of multiplex PCR assays for the simultaneous identification of enterotoxigenic, enteropathogenic, enterohemorrhagic and enteroinvasive *Escherichia coli. New Microbiologica,* 24, 77–83.

Raymond J, Nguyen VB, Vidal-Trecan G, Kalach N (2005). *Helicobacter pylori* infection in children of developing countries. *Médecine tropicale,* 65, 383-8.

Reichardt C, Chaberny IF, Kola A, Mattner F, Vonberg RP, Gastmeier P (2007). [Dramatic increase of diarrhea associated with *Clostridium difficile* in Germany: has the new strain PCR-ribotype 027 reached us?] *Deutsche Medizinische Wochenschrift,* 132, 223-8.

Rivera WL, Santos SR, Kanbara H (2006). Prevalence and genetic diversity of *Entamoeba histolytica* in an institution for the mentally retarded in the Philippines. *Parasitology Research,* 98, 106-10.

Samie A, Barrett LJ, Bessong PO, Ramalivhana JN, Mavhandu LG, Njayou M, Guerrant RL (2010). Seroprevalence of *Entamoeba histolytica* in the context of HIV and AIDS: Case of the Vhembe district, Limpopo Province. *Annals of Tropical Medicine & Parasitology*, 104 (1), 55–63.

Samie A, Bessong PO, Obi CL, Sevilleja JEAD, Stroup S, Houpt E, Guerrant RL (2006) *Cryptosporidium species:* Preliminary descriptions of the prevalence and genotype distribution among school children and hospital patients in the Venda region, Limpopo Province, South Africa. *Experimental Parasitology*, 114, 314 – 322.

Samie A, Njayou M, Bessong PO, Obi CL, Mouchili F, Tuikue Ndam NG, Sabeta CT, and Mduluza T. (2006). Use of an immuno-peroxidase staining method for the detection of *Entamoeba histolytica* in stool samples in endemic areas. Journal of Tropical *Microbiology and Biotechnolology* 2: 10 – 18.

Samie A, Obi CL, Barrett LJ, Powell SM, Guerrant RL (2006) Prevalence of *Campylobacter* species, *Helicobacter pylori* and *Arcobacter* species in stool samples from the Vhembe district, Limpopo, South Africa: Studies using molecular diagnostic methods. *Journal of Infection*, 54(6), 558-66.

Samie A, Obi CL, Bessong PO, Stroup S, Houpt E, Guerrant RL (2006b). Prevalence and Species Distribution of E. *Histolytica* and E. *Dispar* In the Vhembe district, Limpopo, South Africa. *American Journal of Tropical Medicine and Hygiene*, 75, 565-71.

Samie A, Obi CL, Dillingham R, Pinkerton RC, Guerrant RL. (2007) Enteroaggregative *Escherichia Coli* in Venda, South Africa: Distribution of Virulence-Related Genes by Multiplex PCR in Stool Samples of HIV Positive and HIV Negative Individuals and Primary School Children. *American Journal of Tropical Medicine and Hygiene*, 77(1), 142-150.

Samie A, Obi CL, Franaziak J, Archbald-Pannone L, Bessong PO, Alcantara-Warren C, Guerrant RL (2008). PCR detection of *Clostridium difficile* triose phosphate isomerase (tpi), toxin A (tcdA), toxin B (tcdB), binary toxin (cdtA, cdtB) and tcdC genes in Vhembe district, South Africa: *American Journal Of Tropical Medicine and Hygiene*. 78, 577-585.

Samie A, Obi CL, Stroup S, Houpt E, Njayou M, Sabeta CT, Mduluza T, Guerrant RL (2008). Genetic diversity of *Entamoeba histolytica* from Africa based on the serine- rich gene polymorphism. *Experimental Parasitology*, 118(3), 354-61 .

Samie A, Obi CL, Tzipori S, Weiss LM, Guerrant RL. (2007). Microsporidiosis in South Africa: PCR detection in stool samples of HIV positive and HIV negative individuals and school children in the Vhembe district, Limpopo Province. *Transactions of the Royal Society of Tropical Medicine and Hygiene*, 101(6), 547-54.

Samie A, Obi LC, Bessong PO, Stroup S, Houpt E, Guerrant RL (2006) Prevalence And Species Distribution of E. *Histolytica* And E. *dispar* In The Venda Region, Limpopo, South Africa. *American Journal of Tropical Medicine and Hygiene*, 75(3), 565-71.

Samie A, Obi LC, Bessong PO, Stroup S, Houpt E, Guerrant RL (2006). Prevalence and Species Distribution of E. *Histolytica* and E. *Dispar* in the Vhembe district, Limpopo, South Africa. *American Journal of Tropical Medicine and Hygiene*, 75, 565-71.

Samie A, Ramalivhana J, Igumbor EO, Obi CL. (2007). Prevalence, Hemolytic and Hemagglutination Activities and Antibiotic Susceptibility Profiles of *Campylobacter spp* Isolated from Human Diarrheal Stools in the Vhembe District, South Africa. *Journal of Health Population and Nutrition*, 25 (4), 406 - 413.

Samie A., Obi CL, Barrett LJ, Powell SM, Guerrant RL (2007). Prevalence of *Campylobacter* species, *Helicobacter pylori* and *Arcobacter* species in stool samples from the Venda region, Limpopo, South Africa: Studies using molecular diagnostic methods. *Journal of Infection*, 54(6), 558-66.

Sarfati C, Bourgeois A, Menotti J, Liegeois F, Moyou-Somo R, Delaporte E, Derouin F, Ngole EM, Molina JM (2006). Prevalence of intestinal parasites including microsporidia in human immunodeficiency virus-infected adults in Cameroon: a cross-sectional study. *American Journal of Tropical Medicine and Hygiene*, 74, 162-4.

Scaletsky ICA, Fabbricotti SH, Aranda KR, Morais MB, and Fagundes-Neto U (2002). Comparison of DNA Hybridization and PCR Assays for Detection of Putative Pathogenic Enteroadherent *Escherichia coli Journal of Clinical Microbiology*, 40, 1254-1258.

Siddiqui U, Bini EJ, Chandarana K, et al. Prevalence and impact of diarrhea on health-related quality of life in HIV-infected patients in the era of highly active antiretroviral therapy. J Clin Gastroenterol 2007; 41:484.

Silva RC, Benati FJ, Pena GP, Santos N (2010). Molecular characterization of viruses associated with gastrointestinal infection in HIV-positive patients. Braz J Infect Dis. 14(6):549-52.

Simango C, Mutikani S (2004). Cryptosporidiosis in Harare, Zimbabwe. *Centl Afr J Med* 50, 52-54.

Snelling WJ, McKenna JP, Hack CJ, Moore JE, Dooley JS (2006). An examination of the diversity of a novel *Campylobacter* reservoir. *Arch Microbiol.* 186:31- 40.

Snijders F, van Deventer SJ, Bartelsman JF, den Otter P, Jansen J, Mevissen ML, van Gool T, Danner SA, Reiss P (1995). Diarrhea in HIV-infected patients: no evidence of cytokine-mediated inflammation in jejunal mucosa. *AIDS* 9, 367-73.

Speelman P, I Kabir and M Islam (1984). Distribution and spread of colonic lesion in Shigellosis: a colonoscopic study. *Journal of Infectious Diseases*, 50, 899-903.

Spigaglia P, and Mastrantonio P (2002). Molecular analysis of the pathogenicity locus and polymorphism in the putative negative regulator of toxin production (TcdC) among *Clostridium difficile* clinical isolates. *Journal of Clinical Microbiology*, 40, 3470-3475.

Stark D, Barratt JL, van Hal S, Marriott D, Harkness J, Ellis JT. Clinical significance of enteric protozoa in the immunosuppressed human population. *Clinical Microbiology Reviews*, 22(4), 634-50.

Steiner TS, Lima AAM, Nataro JP, Guerrant RL (1998). Enteroaggregative *Escherichia coli* produce intestinal inflammation and growth impairment and cause interleukin-8 release from intestinal epithelial cells. *Journal of Infectious Diseases*, 177, 88–96.

Steiner TS, Samie A, Guerrant RL (2006). Infectious diarrhea: new pathogens and new challenges in developed and developing areas. *Clinical infectious Diseases*, 43(4), 408-10.

Stubbs S, Rupnik M, Gibert M, Brazier J, Duerden B, Popoff M (2000). Production of actin-specific ADP-ribosyltransferase (binary toxin) by strains of *Clostridium difficile*. *FEMS Microbiology Letters*, 186, 307-12.

Sturbaum GD, Reed C, Hoover PJ, Jost BH, Marshall MM, Sterling CR (2001). Species-specific, nested PCR-restriction fragment length polymorphism detection of single

Cryptosporidium parvum oocysts. Applied Environmental Microbiology, 67(6), 2665-8.

Sulaiman IM, Hira PR, Zhou L, Al-Ali FM, Al-Shelahi FA, Shweiki HM, Iqbal J, Khalid N, Xiao L (2005). Unique endemicity of cryptosporidiosis in children in Kuwait. *Journal of Clinical Microbiology*, 43, 2805–2809.

Tadesse A, Kassu A (2005). Intestinal parasite isolates in AIDS patients with chronic diarrhea in Gondar Teaching Hospital, North West Ethiopia. *Ethiopian Medical Journal*, 43(2), 93--96.

Taniuchi M, Verweij JJ, Noor Z, Sobuz SU, Lieshout L, Petri WA Jr, Haque R, Houpt ER. High throughput multiplex PCR and probe-based detection with Luminex beads for seven intestinal parasites. *American Journal Of Tropical Medicine and Hygiene*, 84(2), 332-7.

Taylor AD, Ladd J, Yu Q, Chen S, Homola J, Jiang S (2006). Quantitative and simultaneous detection of four foodborne bacterial pathogens with a multi-channel SPR sensor. *Biosens Bioelectron* 22:752- 8.

Thielman NM, Guerrant RL (2004). Clinical practice. Acute infectious diarrhea. The New England Journal of Medicine, 350(1), 38-47.

Thomas JE, Gibson JR, Darboe MK (1992). Isolation of *Helicobacter pylori* from feces. *Lancet* 340: 1194- 1195.

Turner SM, Scott-Tucker A, Cooper LM, Henderson IR (2006). Weapons of mass destruction: virulence factors of the global killer enterotoxigenic *Escherichia coli*. FEMS *Microbiology Letters*, 263, 10-20.

Valenstein P, Pfaller M, Yungbluth M (1996). The use and abuse of routine stool microbiology: a College of American Pathologists Q-probes study of 601 institutions. *Archives of Pathology & Laboratory Medicine*, 120(2), 206-11.

Van Der Hulst RW, Keller JJ, Rauws EA, Tytgat GN (1996). Treatment of *Helicobacter pylori* infection: *a* review of the world literature. *Helicobacter* 1:6- 19.

Verweij JJ, Oostvogel F, Brienen EA, Nang-Beifubah A, Ziem J, Polderman AM, (2003). Short communication: Prevalence of *Entamoeba histolytica* and *Entamoeba dispar* in northern Ghana. *Tropical Medicine and International Health*, 8(12), 1153--1156.

Victora CG, Bryce J, Fontaine O, Monasch R (2000). Reducing deaths from diarrhoea through oral rehydration therapy. Bulletin of the World Health Organization, 78 (10), 1246-55.

Wang L, Calderon J, Stanley SL Jr (1997). Short report: identification of B-cell epitopes in the serine-rich *Entamoeba histolytica* protein. *American Journal Of Tropical Medicine and Hygiene*, 57, 723-6.

Wanke CA, Gerrior J, Blais V, Mayer H, Acheson D (1998b). Successful treatment of diarrheal disease associated with enteroaggregative *Escherichia coli* in adults infected with human immunodeficiency virus. *Journal of Infectious Diseases*, 178:1369-72.

Wanke CA, Mayer H, Weber R, Zbinden R, Watson DA, Acheson D (1998a). Enteroaggregative *Escherichia coli* as a potential cause of diarrheal disease in adults infected with human immunodeficiency virus. *Journal of Infectious Diseases*, 178, 185-190.

Wilcox MH (1996). Cleaning up *Clostridium difficile* infection. *Lancet* 348:767–8.

World Health Organization. World health report 2004: changing history. Geneva: World
    Health Organization, 2004. 200.
Wultanska D, Pituch H, Obuch-Woszczatynski P, Meisel-Mikolajczyk F, Luczak M (2005).
    [Profile of toxigenicity of *Clostridium difficile* strains isolated from paediatric
    patients with clinical diagnosis of antibiotic associated diarrhea (AAD)] *Medycyna
    Doswiadczalna I Mikrobiologia,* 57, 377-82.
Zaki M, Reddy SG, Jackson TF, Ravdin JI, Clark CG (2003). Genotyping of *Entamoeba* species
    in South Africa: diversity, stability, and transmission patterns within families.
    Journal of Infectious Diseases, 187, 1860-9.

6

The Sub-Saharan African HIV Epidemic - "Successes and Challenges"

Roos E. Barth and Andy I.M. Hoepelman
University Medical Centre Utrecht,
Department of Internal Medicine and Infectious Diseases,
The Netherlands

1. Introduction

The global impact of the human immunodeficiency virus (HIV) pandemic is enormous. To date, more than 25 million lives have been claimed by the acquired immunodeficiency syndrome (AIDS) and over 33 million people are currently estimated to be HIV-infected. Ninety-five percent of these people infected with HIV live in developing countries. Sub-Saharan Africa is the region that is hit hardest by the HIV pandemic.

During the quarter century since the first reports of a novel immunodeficiency syndrome in 1981, great advances have been made in HIV diagnosis, prevention and care. The first protease inhibitor (PI) was approved in 1996, marking the start of the highly active antiretroviral therapy (HAART) era. From then on, HIV-infections were no longer inevitably associated with AIDS and death, but could be viewed as a chronic condition [Merson, 2006; Sepkowitz, 2006]. Currently, the antiretroviral armamentarium includes over 20 different drugs and more are in the pipeline. The use of HAART can result in effective, long-term suppression of the virus with consequent recovery of the patient's immune system. Unfortunately, complete HIV eradication is still not feasible. Moreover, it is apparent that the virus generally resurges to pre-treatment levels within months after ART withdrawal. Patients therefore need a life-long commitment to their treatment.

The logistic and monetary costs associated with such long-term HIV-care are high. HIV monitoring and treatment was therefore initially only available in resource-rich countries. Great efforts and large funds were needed to make ART more widely available. This awareness and initiatives, such as the "United States' President's Emergency Plan for AIDS Relief" and the "Global fund for AIDS, TB and Malaria", resulted in an unprecedented roll-out of treatment since the turn of the millennium [United Nations]. The increase in HIV-infected individuals receiving ART has been especially large In Sub-Saharan Africa where over the last decade, many ART programs took off, treating millions of HIV-infected patients. Despite these impressive accomplishments however, monitoring and research facilities in low-income countries (LICs) still lag behind.

There are great differences between HIV care in resource-rich and LICs. First, due to limited resources, the number of clinics, health care providers and other necessities for quality health care are lower in LICs compared to high-income countries. Second, HIV is generally transmitted via heterosexual contact in African countries, whereas homosexual contacts and intravenous drug use are the main routes of transmission in western countries. Moreover, due to differences in genetic make up there may be different reactions to the virus and its treatment between different populations. Third, the virus itself differs between various geographical areas. While subtype B is the main HIV subtype in Europe and the United States, it is rarely seen in Sub-Saharan Africa, where subtype C is the prevailing HIV subtype.

The on-treatment HIV-RNA-level is associated with a patients' clinical outcome. Therefore, western guidelines recommend regular HIV-RNA monitoring in all patients receiving ART. Roll-out strategies in LICs on the other hand were initially mainly focused on providing as many patients with antiretroviral drugs (ARVs) as possible, thereby limiting the resources left for laboratory monitoring. As regular HIV-RNA testing is not feasible in many, Sub-Saharan African ART programs, treatment decisions are frequently solely based on clinical or immunological parameters. However, the correlation between these parameters and virological outcomes appears to be marginal [Kantor et al., 2009; Keiser et al., 2009; Reynolds et al., 2009b]. Moreover, making predictions on long-term treatment outcomes is difficult, as the virological effects of these programs are not clear and other surrogate markers for clinical outcomes are not available.

Despite the above mentioned difficulties, great progress has been made regarding HIV care in Sub-Sahara Africa. However, challenges remain. Both successes and challenges regarding prevention and treatment of HIV as well as viral resistance development and treatment of co-morbidities will be addressed in the following chapter.

2. Prevention

In 2007, the WHO announced that the HIV-epidemic seemed to be levelling off. Still, over 33 million people are estimated to be HIV-infected globally, with 2.6 million people becoming newly infected annually. The overall adult HIV prevalence in Sub-Saharan Africa is estimated to be over five percent, with prevalence rates up to twenty-five percent in some countries [UNAIDS, 2009]. This however means that the vast majority (more than ninety percent) is still HIV-negative. Keeping these people free from HIV, as well as preventing new generations from becoming infected, is a major challenge and should remain a priority on the HIV-care agenda.

2.1 Prevention of mother to child transmission

One of the great advances in HIV preventive-care has been the "prevention of mother to child transmission" (PMTCT) strategies. Testing pregnant women for the presence of HIV and subsequently providing those that are infected, as well as their new-born babies, with ARVs has the potential of reducing vertical HIV transmission rates to below one percent [Paintsil and Andiman, 2007; Paintsil and Andiman, 2009]. Short-course ARVs or single-dose nevirapine (SDNVP) are frequently used for PMTCT instead of complete ART regimens in low-income countries (LICs). Such regimens have shown to be efficacious in averting many infant-HIV infections. Still, with transmission rates ranging from one to above ten percent, results are lagging behind those observed in resource-rich settings [Boeke and Jackson, 2008; Chigwedere et al., 2008; Leroy et al., 2008; Palombi et al., 2007; Tonwe-Gold et al., 2007]. Moreover, administration of SDNVP can lead to the selection of non-nucleoside reverse transcriptase- (NNRTI-) associated resistance mutations. There is evidence that fewer mutations are selected when other ARVs are added to the SDNVP [Arrive et al., 2007; Chi et al., 2007a]. However, the optimal combination of drugs and best time for treatment initiation in order to create a feasible and effective PMTCT strategy for

LICs, still need to be defined [Chi et al., 2007b; Lockman et al., 2007]. In addition to improving the efficacy of PMTCT programmes, the PMTCT coverage needs to be expanded. Many resource-limited countries still have a limited PMTCT-coverage; in South Africa for example only sixty percent of HIV-infected pregnant women have access to this simple, cost-effective strategy and figures are worse for several other LICs [Abdool Karim et al., 2009; Paintsil and Andiman, 2009]. These data show that, even though much progress is made in the field of PMTCT, improvements are urgently needed to prevent even more infant-HIV infections and deaths.

2.2 Vaccines
Historically, vaccine development is one of the fields in health care where major progress is achieved. Many infectious diseases were effectively prevented and some nearly eradicated. Unfortunately, results of HIV vaccine research are unrelentingly negative. Many candidate vaccines were developed, but the results proved unsatisfactory and major vaccination studies were stopped [Johnston and Fauci, 2008]. Despite these failures, some vaccines are still being tested. Most of these are directed at stimulating the immune system [Fauci et al., 2008]. Still, finding an effective vaccine in the near future does not seem likely.

2.3 Circumcision
Several other preventive strategies were analyzed and implemented, resulting in variable success rates. Male circumcision was put forward to prevent heterosexual HIV transmission since a lower female HIV prevalence was observed in Sub-Saharan African countries with high levels of male circumcision [Auvert et al., 2005; Williams et al., 2006]. However, epidemiological evidence of a direct protective effect of male circumcision on women becoming infected with HIV is limited according to some [Weiss et al., 2009]. To date, most consider male circumcision to have a significant, albeit partial, efficacy in reducing heterosexual HIV transmission [Doyle et al.; Smith et al.]. To what extend expanding circumcision coverage will contribute to combating the global HIV epidemic, still needs to be determined.

2.4 Post- and pre-exposure prophylaxis
Post-exposure prophylaxis (PEP) is a successful prevention method after incidental needle or sex accidents. In Sub-Saharan Africa however, where heterosexual contact drives the HIV epidemic, PEP provision is limited and will not substantially influence the HIV statistics. Pre-exposure prophylaxis (PrEP) on the other hand may prove to be a promising strategy. An effective agent that can be used safely by women prior to sexual intercourse and without the need for agreement from a partner would be a major contributor to preventive HIV care [Al-Jabri and Alenzi, 2009]. However, until now trials of microbicide candidates have shown disappointing results; some even suggested a boosted risk of infection as more vaginal lesions were observed in treated patients [Al-Jabri and Alenzi, 2009; Wilson et al., 2008]. Possibly gels that incorporate ARVs will be more effective as PrEP. Studies are being set up and hopefully results will come available in the coming years [Grant et al., 2008].

2.5 Antiretroviral treatment as a preventive measure
In spite of these preventive strategies it is not likely that the high HIV incidence will change in the near future. Some strategies are only partly effective and many remain grossly

underused [USAID, UNAIDS, WHO, CDC and the POLICY project; Kerr et al.]. More importantly, the development of a preventive vaccine seems to be nearly impossible and HIV-eradication can not be realised with current treatment strategies. Still, provision of ART surpasses the obvious benefits it has on an individual level. Treating HIV can be used as an essential part of prevention efforts. For heterosexual contact and for mother-to-child-transmission a clear dose-response effect was found between HIV-RNA levels and risk of HIV transmission [Fang et al., 1995; Quinn et al., 2000; Tovanabutra et al., 2002]. As these are the main routes of HIV transmission in Sub-Saharan Africa, it seems likely that bringing down individual HIV-RNA levels can make a substantial contribution to reducing the number of new infections. Indeed, such positive effects were described previously, suggesting cost-saving effects of ART due to the reduction of HIV transmission, in addition to the clear benefits of such treatment on an individual basis [Granich et al., 2009; Mayer and Venkatesh; Montaner et al., 2006]. Up till now, the roll-out of ART has not clearly reduced HIV-incidence. If a preventive effect of ART becomes more apparent as treatment-coverage increases, and as patients receive care for longer periods of time, will largely depend on the number of patients experiencing virological failure.

2.6 Awareness
Creating awareness about the risks of unprotected sex and other potential transmission routes, as well as providing information on advances that have been made in HIV care, is of utmost importance in reducing the stigma's associated with HIV and in motivating people to do an HIV-test. An elevated level of awareness may lead to patients seeking care at a less advanced stage of disease. As a result, chances of a good clinical response to ART will be greater. Moreover, the period that patients will have high viral loads and therefore are highly infectious, will be shorter if patients have their HIV tested and treated at an earlier stage. Continued monitoring of HIV incidence, and possibly mathematical modelling studies, are needed to further calculate the preventive and cost-saving effects of ART expansion programmes.

3. Treatment

HIV leads to AIDS and death when left untreated. ART provides clear benefits for those infected and rendered HIV-infection a manageable chronic condition. Access to treatment increased considerably over the last decade. Still, by the end of 2008, less than half of the people in need of treatment in Sub-Saharan Africa actually received ART [UNAIDS 2009] and the United Nations endorsed target of "universal access by 2010" has not been met [WHO, 2006b]. It was recognized that access to treatment is especially limited for certain groups of people, such as those living in rural settings [Crowley et al., 2009]. Therefore, continued efforts are needed to increase the availability of ART even further.

3.1 When to start ART
When to start ART in HIV-infected individuals remains a controversial issue. Initially, treatment was deferred until CD4 counts dropped to below 200 cells/mm^3 in most LICs [Wood et al., 2005]. In western settings it is common practice to initiate ART earlier, when CD4 counts are less than 350 or even 500 cells/mm^3, as various studies suggest improved treatment outcomes at higher CD4 thresholds [Braithwaite et al., 2008; Emery et al., 2008; Kitahata; Sterne]. Benefits of an earlier treatment start may be even greater in LICs

compared to high-income countries, due to higher rates of opportunistic diseases and mortality there. However, the number of people eligible for ART will increase as CD4 treatment-initiation thresholds move up, putting extra pressure on the already fragile health care facilities and limited resources. A mathematical modelling study on the other hand reported that an increase of the CD4 treatment-initiation threshold (to 350 cells/mm^3) would reduce morbidity and mortality while remaining cost-effective, in the South African context [Walensky et al., 2009]. Moreover, the WHO recently adjusted its guidelines, recommending to start treatment at CD4 counts of 350 cells/mm^3 or less for all HIV-infected individuals [Crowley et al., 2009]. However, definite results from ongoing, international trials assessing when to initiate ART in resource-limited settings will not be available for several years.

3.2 Treatment outcomes

Overall, on-treatment, short-term outcomes of Sub-Saharan African ART programs that have access to HIV-RNA monitoring, are promising and similar to those initially observed in western settings. However, high early attrition (composed of all-cause mortality and patients being lost to follow up) is frequently observed, negatively influencing intention-to-treat results. Within a few years after treatment start, virological failure is observed in only fifteen percent of patients. It should be borne in mind though, that applied failure criteria are generally more lenient than those used in western settings [Barth RE, 2010b]. Long-term outcome data are still limited, but seem promising as well.

First-line ART regimens in Sub-Saharan Africa are generally NNRTI-based. Boosted PIs may also be used in treatment-naïve patients. Compared to an NNRTI-based first-line regimen this resulted in a slightly reduced treatment efficacy, but fewer resistance mutations [Riddler et al., 2008; von Wyl et al., 2007]. A review on clinical trials also showed that fewer nucleoside reverse transcriptase inhibitor- (NRTI)-associated resistance mutations were present in case of boosted PI-based regimen failure compared to NNRTI-based regimens [Gupta et al., 2008]. The answer to the question whether or not it is advisable to move to a PI-based first-line ART regimen in LICs will largely depend on the balance between costs, adverse events and resistance development profiles.

3.3 Adverse effects

Providing all those in need with ART is a daunting task. However, caring for those already receiving treatment poses many challenges as well. As HIV-infected people live longer, the long-term effects of the virus and its treatment become more evident. Simple, affordable treatment regimens facilitated the initial, extensive ART roll-out. However, the negative effects associated with these commonly used treatment options called for a reconsideration of widely applied treatment strategies. Mitochondrial toxicity causes neuropathy, lipodystrophy and lactic acidosis in many individuals receiving stavudine-containing ART. Therefore, it was recommended to move away from stavudine-based regimens to zidovudine or tenofovir (TDF) [Crowley et al., 2009; WHO, 2006a]. As yet, not all African countries have adopted TDF as a first-line regimen in their guidelines for financial reasons, but this may change during coming years. As TDF becomes more widely available, knowledge of its side-effects grows more important. TDF has potential nephrotoxic effects. Generally no negative effects on renal function are observed when TDF is used in a first-line ART regimen [Gallant and Moore, 2009], but little is known regarding the prevalence and nature of renal impairment in African cohorts. In one South African cohort the number of people with severe renal dysfunction was limited [Franey et al., 2009], but future studies will have to show what the long-term effects of TDF use in African patients are. Another concern with TDF use relates to the possible increased risk of bone disease. HIV-infected individuals have an increased risk of osteopenia compared to HIV-uninfected people. This risk is increased further by the use of TDF [Jacobson et al., 2008]. It is not yet clear whether patients receiving TDF also have an increased bone-fracture risk. The increased risk of cardiovascular disease and diabetes, associated with some antiretroviral drugs, will be discussed in more detail later. These and other negative effects of long-term ARV use in various populations have to be addressed in future studies.

3.4 Second line treatment

PIs are becoming more widely available in LICs since the advent of heat-stable drug formulations. They are typically used in second-line regimens, in case of treatment failure. As currently the vast majority of patients receiving ART in Sub-Saharan Africa are receiving a NNRTI-based, first-line regimen, limited data are available on the efficacy of PI-based regimens in African settings. Good, early, virological responses were reported, but a frequent occurrence of adverse events was also observed [Castelnuovo et al., 2009a; Hosseinipour et al.]. In a large trial performed in western countries (TITAN trial) over three quarters of treatment-experienced patients achieved an HIV-RNA less than 400 copies/mL after switching to either lopinavir/ritonavir or darunavir/ritonavir in combination with an optimized backbone regimen. Results were even better if patients with any prior PI-exposure were excluded from analysis [Madruga et al., 2007]. These data suggest that a boosted PI-based second-line regimen would be effective in the majority of African patients who experience treatment failure while receiving NNRTI-based first-line ART. However, the generalisability of these data is limited as defining an optimized backbone is hazardous in LICs, where fewer ARVs are available and resistance testing is not widely available. Long-term data regarding second-line efficacy in resource-limited settings are not yet available and should be a subject for future research.

3.5 New antiretroviral drugs

New drugs within traditional drug classes and new drug-classes were developed over the last years. In western countries drugs such as boosted darunavir and etravirine as well as drug-classes such as fusion and integrase inhibitors, CCR5-receptor antagonists and maturation inhibitors expanded the antiretroviral arsenal. Long-term care for HIV-infected patients frequently demands switching to third- or consecutive lines of ART. Moreover, an individualised- rather than a protocol-based approach is increasingly being used. Viral characteristics, such as HIV-subtype and presence of drug-resistance mutations, as well as host characteristics such as medical history, organ functions and genetic background, all contribute to the efficacy and toxicity of the various ARVs. Most HIV-related pharmacological research was done in resource-rich settings, where Caucasian, male patients, infected with a subtype-B virus, predominate. Important differences exist between western and non-western countries regarding both these viral- as well as these host-characteristics. Even though the new ARVs will not shortly become available on a large-scale in LICs, it will be interesting to analyse what effects such drugs have in different ethnic populations and on various HIV-subtypes. Such research hopefully provides more insight in the dynamics between drugs, viruses and hosts and increases therapeutic options for all

HIV-infected individuals in the future. Moreover, expansion of the ARV armamentarium for second- and consecutive- lines of treatment is needed to ensure treatment success in the future.

3.6 Paediatric HIV care

Ninety percent of the 2.1 million HIV-infected children worldwide live in LICs. Until recently it was estimated that few vertically HIV-infected children survived beyond the age of five years. However, despite high mortality-rates in HIV-infected infants, a substantial increase of older survivors of mother-to-child transmission is visible in Africa [Ferrand et al., 2009]. Caring for small, HIV-infected children is associated with specific challenges, such as drug-administration problems and weight-based dosing. Later, during adolescence, an increased fear for stigma and loss of social acceptance may lead to a decreased adherence to treatment. Still, paediatric ART can result in virological and immunological benefits which are comparable to those observed among children in more developed settings [Ciaranello et al., 2009]. Unfortunately, despite optimistic, initial outcomes, long-term paediatric ART is associated with frequent virological failure [Barth et al. 2010c]. Similar to adult patients, most children were receiving NNRTI-based ART. Paediatric treatment outcomes may improve when PI-based regimens are used, which have a higher genetic barrier and are therefore somewhat more forgiving in case of sub-optimal treatment adherence. However, the effects of a long-term HIV infection and many years of ART on growth and development are not yet known. Simplifying treatment regimens and limiting side effects will be crucial to retain children in care and achieve good, long-term clinical outcomes.

4. Drug-resistance development

First-line ART failure is generally caused by poor adherence to the drugs. Various issues are linked to poor adherence. Drug toxicity is a major contributor, but other factors such as co-morbidities, insufficient drug supply, stigma, pill burden and traditional beliefs can play a role in drug-adherence. Contrasting initial fears, observed adherence rates in African ART programmes are good [Mills et al., 2006]. Still, around 15 percent of patients receiving first-line treatment in Sub-Saharan Africa experience virological failure within a few years after treatment initiation [Barth RE, 2010b].

In western guidelines it is recommended to perform resistance testing in case of virological failure in order to determine an optimal second-line regimen with a sufficiently high genetic barrier. Regular resistance testing is not feasible in most African clinics. In western countries, most HIV-infected individuals are infected with HIV-1, subtype B. This is in stark contrast with Sub-Saharan African countries, were less than one percent of patients subtype-B virus. Various non-B subtypes are prevalent, with subtype-C being most prevalent. Therefore, treatment outcome data and genotypic resistance data from western studies can not simply be extrapolated to African settings.

Available resistance data of people experiencing virological failure in LICs typically show (multiple) NNRTI-associated mutations and the lamivudine-associated M184V mutation [Barth RE, 2010b; Barth et al., 2008; Hoffmann et al., 2009; Marconi et al., 2008]. With such drug-resistance profiles a PI-based second-line regimen will generally be effective. Actual second-line treatment outcomes may however be less good. As in many HIV-treatment programmes in LICs regular HIV-RNA testing is not feasible, and due to the delay before immunological and clinical decline becomes apparent, there may be a large number of people where virological failure remains unnoticed [Castelnuovo et al., 2009b; Kantor et al., 2009; Keiser et al., 2009; Reynolds et al., 2009b]. These people will continue their failing, first-line regimen. This is important, as a delay in treatment modification after virological failure is associated with an increased mortality [Petersen et al., 2008]. Moreover, an accumulation of drug-resistance mutations is observed in patients who continue first-line ARVs in spite of virological failure, limiting future treatment options [Cozzi-Lepri et al., 2007; Hoffmann et al., 2009; Reynolds et al., 2009a]. Empirically starting second-line ART in programmes with limited access to virological diagnostics, may therefore result in sub-optimal treatment outcomes, stressing the need for affordable, easy-access drug-resistance tests in LICs.

Drug-resistant HIV not only decreases the efficacy of new ART regimens in patients harbouring such a virus; transmission of resistant strains in the community may also limit first-line treatment outcomes of newly infected individuals [Barth et al., 2008; Kuritzkes et al., 2008; Wensing et al., 2005]. Fortunately, transmission of drug-resistant viruses is still limited in the African continent. Published primary resistance rates are generally well-below the WHO cut-off rate of five percent [Bartolo et al., 2009; Bussmann et al., 2005; Derache et al., 2008]. The prevalence of drug-resistant viruses will probably increase in LICs though, as ARVs become more widely available in those countries. Regular monitoring of primary resistance is needed to predict whether currently used treatment regimens will remain effective in the majority of patients.

5. Co-morbidities

Many other, both communicable and non-communicable, diseases can cause morbidity and mortality in HIV-infected individuals. Diagnosing and treating such co-morbidities are of utmost importance when caring for people with HIV. Below, a few of these diseases will be briefly addressed.

5.1 Tuberculosis

Concomitant with the HIV epidemic, South Africa has one of the worst TB epidemics of the world [Abdool Karim et al., 2009; WHO, 2009]. The HIV/TB co-infection rate is estimated to be as high as 70%, causing morbidity and mortality in many. However, making a definite TB diagnosis is hazardous, especially in HIV-infected individuals. In immuno-compromised patients, sputum-smear-negative and non-pulmonary TB are frequent, limiting the utility of commonly available TB diagnostics. Culturing mycobacterium tuberculosis, the golden standard when making a TB diagnosis, is often omitted due to the time and money needed for these tests. Therefore, there is a clear need for accurate, simple and low-cost diagnostic tests for the detection of TB infection.

The use of ART causes a great reduction in the risk of developing TB in the long term [Badri et al., 2002]. However, the incidence of TB increases soon after ART initiation, following the restoration of immune responses [Bonnet et al., 2006; Lawn et al., 2005; Moore et al., 2007]. As a result, TB is an important cause of the high mortality during the first months of ART, observed in many HIV treatment programmes [Brinkhof et al., 2007; Koenig et al., 2009; Lawn et al., 2008; Manabe et al., 2009].

The WHO declared that "urgent and extraordinary means" are needed in order to combat this massive disease burden, and it set targets for cure and case detection rates [WHO, 2009]. Unfortunately, in South Africa these targets are far from being met. Case detection rates are only 62% instead of the WHO minimum target of 70% and cure rates are only 58% instead of the intended 85% [Abdool Karim et al., 2009]. These worrying figures are partly due to the expansion of multi- and even extensively- drug-resistant TB (MDR and XDR). Case-fatality rates are much higher in case of drug-resistant TB, compared with sensitive mycobacterial infections. Exogenous, nosocomial re-infections are thought to drive the spread of drug-resistant TB. Drug-susceptibility testing is needed to identify those in need of stricter isolation and broader anti-tuberculosis treatment regimens. However, susceptibility testing is currently only done in a subgroup of re-treatment cases and even if such testing is performed, it often takes long before results are available. The development of cheap, fast HIV-tests was an important contribution to the massive scaling up of HIV-care. Such easy-access tests are also needed to make a rapid TB diagnosis and to differentiate drug-resistant from normally susceptible infections [Lawn et al.]. Hopefully efforts to optimize diagnostic and treatment strategies, combined with a better integration of HIV- and TB-care will eventually result in a reversal of the TB epidemic.

5.2 Hepatitis

Apart from TB, hepatitis B (HBV) and C (HCV) co-infections are commonly observed in HIV-infected individuals. As ART roll-out continues, life expectancy of HIV-infected individuals in resource-limited countries improves. As a result, long-term effects of such hepatitis co-infections, like liver cirrhosis and hepato-cellular carcinomas, become more evident. HBV as well as HCV are highly prevalent in African, HIV-infected individuals (15% and 7% respectively', but there is a wide geographical variation in HBV and HCV prevalence [Barth et al. 2010a].

In western countries HIV infection is strongly associated with an increased incidence of both HBV and HCV [Burnett et al., 2005; Rockstroh et al., 2005; Thio, 2009]. This association is attributed to shared routes of transmission: mostly (homo)sexual contact in the case of HBV and intravenous drug use (IVDU) for hepatitis C [Cooper et al., 2009; Lavanchy, 2004; Modi and Feld, 2007]. In African countries HBV acquisition is assumed to occur during early childhood. As the route of HIV transmission in Africa is mainly via heterosexual contact, at a later point in life, it can be expected that the association between both infections is limited. However, reliable data on the mode and age of HBV acquisition amongst HIV-infected individuals in Africa are lacking. The predominant mode of HCV transmission in Africa is not yet established. However, IVDU seems to be less influential as in western countries [Cooper et al., 2009; Lavanchy, 2004; Modi and Feld, 2007]. Due to the different times and modes of transmission, the observed association between HIV and the hepatic viruses is less evident in Sub-Saharan Africa. Still, the burden of HIV/hepatitis co-infections in that region is high, as all these viruses are highly endemic. According to WHO estimates, 22.5 million HIV-infected people lived in Sub-Saharan Africa by the end of 2007 [WHO, 2007]. When geographical variations in HBV and HIV prevalence are not taken into account, an HBV prevalence of 15% would mean that 3.4 million HBV/HIV co-infected people live in this region.

HIV accelerates the progression of HBV and HCV related liver disease. Evidence that such co-infections are also associated with an increased mortality came available only recently [Chen et al., 2009; Nikolopoulos et al., 2009]. It is to be expected that HBV and HCV related cirrhosis and malignancies will become even more evident during coming years, as ART roll-out carries on and life-expectancy for HIV-individuals improves.

Knowledge on a patients' HBV/HCV status can help clinicians interpret clinical problems and lab results. More importantly, such information can guide decisions on which ARVs can best be prescribed in co-infected patients. The vast majority of first-line ART regimens in Sub-Saharan Africa contain lamivudine. Lamivudine has long been approved for the treatment of chronic HBV. However, it has a poor resistance profile. Around half of HBV-isolates show drug-resistance mutations after 2-3 years of lamivudine use [Liaw et al., 2000; Lok et al., 2000]. Tenofovir is not yet widely available in Sub-Saharan Africa, but its use may increase during coming years. This nucleotide analogue has been approved for the treatment of HBV in 2008. Rates of HBV suppression in mono-infected patients are impressive and drug-resistance development seems to be limited [Marcellin et al., 2008]. Another problem regarding lamivudine use in HIV/HBV co-infected patients can arise when lamivudine is being stopped. A paradoxical HBV 'flare up' can occur, potentially causing liver tissue destruction [Lim et al., 2002].

Treating HCV infections is not feasible in most African settings due to the high costs and intensive monitoring associated with currently available therapies. Still, knowledge on a possible HCV co-infection is useful. Screening policies for liver cirrhosis and hepato-cellular carcinomas can be installed and the use of hepato-toxic agents can be minimized.

5.3 Non-communicable diseases

The unprecedented increase in ART roll-out which took place over the last decade shows what can be achieved with the joined efforts of international organisations, governments, non-governmental organisations and many enthusiastic, hard-working people. An extensive expansion of health care infrastructures was realized in many countries in order to reach and treat the millions of HIV-infected individuals. Large funds were made available to make ART free of charge for most patients. After being enrolled in an HIV-treatment programme, patients are frequently also provided with other medical care, like the diagnostics for and treatment of opportunistic infections. For HIV-negative persons on the other hand, medical care is frequently less readily available and costly. This may lead to disparities between individuals with HIV and those who are suffering from other (chronic) illnesses. Instead of increasing the gap between medical care that is available to HIV-infected and HIV-uninfected individuals, we should try to extend the benefits of the improved health care systems to other target groups. As in the established market economies, non-communicable disorders are the leading cause of death in adults in low- and middle-income countries. Ischemic heart disease and cerebrovascular accidents are the most frequent causes of death. Risk factors such as hypertension, diabetes, smoking and obesity are major contributors to this disease burden [Chopra et al., 2009; Gill et al., 2009; Lopez et al., 2006; Murray and Lopez, 1997; Sliwa and Mocumbi, 2009]. Sub-Saharan Africa includes countries with the highest non-communicable disease burden, such as South Africa. Poor people living in urban areas are affected most, but the burden is clearly rising in rural communities [Mayosi et al., 2009]. This rise is partly due to demographic changes; people grow older despite the negative effect of the HIV epidemic.

As ART roll-out continues, cardiovascular diseases will become even more evident due to a decline in HIV-related mortality. Moreover, an increased incidence of inflammatory circulatory disorders is observed in HIV-infected individuals and the use of PIs and certain NRTIs is associated with a greater risk of insulin resistance, lipodystrophy and dyslipidaemia [Friis-Moller et al., 2007; Grunfeld et al., 2009; Hsue et al., 2009]. Despite these worrying figures, attention for the prevention and treatment of non-communicable diseases in African countries has been limited because most efforts were directed at combating the

HIV and tuberculosis epidemics. However, there is a growing recognition that an integrated chronic care model is needed to combat both epidemics of communicable and non-communicable diseases in Sub-Saharan Africa. Surveillance, treatment and prevention strategies need to be improved [Unwin et al., 2001].

6. Finance

Over the last decade more funds have been raised to combat the HIV epidemic than have ever been made available for a single disease. The above described successes would never have been achieved without these funds. However, due to the number of HIV-infected people and the chronic nature of the disease, there remains a continued need for large amounts of money. Expansion of preventive strategies, earlier and wider access to ART, increased availability of laboratory testing, and improved health care facilities for both HIV-infected and HIV-uninfected individuals are all urgently needed, but costly. HIV-care is generally sponsor-based, making it sensitive to global economic instability. Currently, the economic crisis, and possibly donor fatigue, are negatively influencing the amount of money donors are willing to spend on the worldwide HIV epidemic [Ewing, 1990]. Therefore, using the available resources as efficiently as possible is of utmost importance. Prioritizing is needed when treatment capacity is limited, but leads to many difficult ethical and humanitarian dilemmas. Rather than considering the costs associated with expanding HIV care, we should consider the costs of not treating all HIV-infected individuals. A recent modelling study argues that by spending the available money wisely, but rapidly, eradication of AIDS will be feasible. Holding money in reserve now, could lead to extra, unnecessary infections and therefore extra costs in the future [Smith et al., 2009]. Moreover, the loss of large numbers of people who are in their working age and the resulting increase in HIV-related orphans has an enormous negative impact on economies and future generations. Therefore, continued attention and funds are still needed to control the HIV epidemic and to hopefully make HIV care more affordable in the future.

7. Conclusion

Since the start of the HIV epidemic, much progress has been made regarding global HIV-care. The joint efforts of people, organisations and governments around the world made it possible to reverse a previously fatal disease to a chronic condition and to prevent many from becoming newly infected. This is a great accomplishment. Still, the time to "sit back and relax" has by no means been reached. As in LICs large-scale ART has only been available for a couple of years, the long-term effects of HIV infections and their treatment in different groups of people are still unknown. Where initial programmes were mainly focussed on treating as many HIV-infected people as possible, future studies need to focus on the long-term care. There are important differences, both in host as in viral factors, between the western and African HIV epidemics. The long-term treatment effects, adverse events and viral resistance profiles in African ART programmes therefore need to be analyzed. In addition to the currently available strategies, new preventive methods and treatments are under development. Testing their efficacy and making them available in LICs should be another focus of future research. Moreover, by extending the focus beyond HIV-care and trying to improve the care for other important chronic diseases, HIV scale-up may generate substantial benefits for the broader health system in many countries.

8. Acknowledgement

We would like to thank Hugo Tempelman and all the people working at Ndlovu Medical Centre for their hard work in order to achieve a better standard of HIV care in Sub-Saharan Africa and for supporting research in a rural, South African setting.

9. References

United Nations. 2001. Declaration of Commitment on HIV/AIDS. "Global crisis - Global action."New York: United Nations, 2001. Accessed at: http://www.un.org/ga/aids/docs/aress262.pdf.

USAID, UNAIDS, WHO, CDC and the POLICY project. 2004. Coverage of selected services for HIV/AIDS prevention, care and support in low and middle income countries in 2003. Accessed at: http://www.who.int/hiv/pub/prev_care/en/coveragereport_2003.pdf.

Abdool Karim SS, Churchyard GJ, Abdool Karim Q, Lawn SD. 2009. HIV infection and tuberculosis in South Africa: an urgent need to escalate the public health response. Lancet 374(9693):921-933.

Al-Jabri AA, Alenzi FQ. 2009. Vaccines, virucides and drugs against HIV/AIDS: hopes and optimisms for the future. Open AIDS J 3:1-3.

Arrive E, Newell ML, Ekouevi DK, Chaix ML, Thiebaut R, Masquelier B, Leroy V, Perre PV, Rouzioux C, Dabis F. 2007. Prevalence of resistance to nevirapine in mothers and children after single-dose exposure to prevent vertical transmission of HIV-1: a meta-analysis. Int J Epidemiol 36(5):1009-1021.

Auvert B, Taljaard D, Lagarde E, Sobngwi-Tambekou J, Sitta R, Puren A. 2005. Randomized, controlled intervention trial of male circumcision for reduction of HIV infection risk: the ANRS 1265 Trial. PLoS Med 2(11):e298.

Badri M, Wilson D, Wood R. 2002. Effect of highly active antiretroviral therapy on incidence of tuberculosis in South Africa: a cohort study. Lancet 359(9323):2059-2064.

Barth RE, Huijgen Q, Taljaard J, Hoepelman AI. 2010a. Hepatitis B/C and HIV in sub-Saharan Africa: an association between highly prevalent infectious diseases. A systematic review and meta-analysis. Int J Infect Dis 14(12):e1024-1031.

Barth RE SvdLM, Schuurman R, Hoepelman AIM, Wensing AJM. 2010b. Virological follow up of adult patients in antiretroviral treatment programmes in Sub-Saharan Africa: a Review. Lancet Infect Dis: 10(3):155-166.

Barth RE, Tempelman HA, Smelt E, Wensing AM, Hoepelman AI, Geelen SP. 2010c. Long-Term Outcome of Children Receiving Antiretroviral Treatment in Rural South Africa: Substantial Virologic Failure on First-Line Treatment. Pediatr Infect Dis J.

Barth RE, Wensing AM, Tempelman HA, Moraba R, Schuurman R, Hoepelman AI. 2008. Rapid accumulation of nonnucleoside reverse transcriptase inhibitor-associated resistance: evidence of transmitted resistance in rural South Africa. Aids 22(16):2210-2212.

Bartolo I, Rocha C, Bartolomeu J, Gama A, Fonseca M, Mendes A, Cristina F, Thamm S, Epalanga M, Silva PC, Taveira N. 2009. Antiretroviral drug resistance surveillance among treatment-naive human immunodeficiency virus type 1-infected individuals in Angola: evidence for low level of transmitted drug resistance. Antimicrob Agents Chemother 53(7):3156-3158.

Boeke CE, Jackson JB. 2008. Estimate of infant HIV-free survival at 6 to 8 weeks of age due to maternal antiretroviral prophylaxis in Sub-Saharan Africa, 2004-2005. J Int Assoc Physicians AIDS Care (Chic Ill) 7(3):133-140.

Bonnet MM, Pinoges LL, Varaine FF, Oberhauser BB, O'Brien DD, Kebede YY, Hewison CC, Zachariah RR, Ferradini LL. 2006. Tuberculosis after HAART initiation in HIV-positive patients from five countries with a high tuberculosis burden. Aids 20(9):1275-1279.

Braithwaite RS, Roberts MS, Chang CC, Goetz MB, Gibert CL, Rodriguez-Barradas MC, Shechter S, Schaefer A, Nucifora K, Koppenhaver R, Justice AC. 2008. Influence of alternative thresholds for initiating HIV treatment on quality-adjusted life expectancy: a decision model. Ann Intern Med 148(3):178-185.

Brinkhof MW, Egger M, Boulle A, May M, Hosseinipour M, Sprinz E, Braitstein P, Dabis F, Reiss P, Bangsberg DR, Rickenbach M, Miro JM, Myer L, Mocroft A, Nash D, Keiser O, Pascoe M, van der Borght S, Schechter M. 2007. Tuberculosis after initiation of antiretroviral therapy in low-income and high-income countries. Clin Infect Dis 45(11):1518-1521.

Burnett RJ, Francois G, Kew MC, Leroux-Roels G, Meheus A, Hoosen AA, Mphahlele MJ. 2005. Hepatitis B virus and human immunodeficiency virus co-infection in sub-Saharan Africa: a call for further investigation. Liver Int 25(2):201-213.

Bussmann H, Novitsky V, Wester W, Peter T, Masupu K, Gabaitiri L, Kim S, Gaseitsiwe S, Ndungu T, Marlink R, Thior I, Essex M. 2005. HIV-1 subtype C drug-resistance background among ARV-naive adults in Botswana. Antivir Chem Chemother 16(2):103-115.

Castelnuovo B, John L, Lutwama F, Ronald A, Spacek LA, Bates M, Kamya MR, Colebunders R. 2009a. Three-year outcome data of second-line antiretroviral therapy in Ugandan adults: good virological response but high rate of toxicity. J Int Assoc Physicians AIDS Care (Chic Ill) 8(1):52-59.

Castelnuovo B, Kiragga A, Schaefer P, Kambugu A, Manabe Y. 2009b. High rate of misclassification of treatment failure based on WHO immunological criteria. Aids 23(10):1295-1296; author reply 1296.

Chen TY, Ding EL, Seage Iii GR, Kim AY. 2009. Meta-analysis: increased mortality associated with hepatitis C in HIV-infected persons is unrelated to HIV disease progression. Clin Infect Dis 49(10):1605-1615.

Chi BH, Sinkala M, Mbewe F, Cantrell RA, Kruse G, Chintu N, Aldrovandi GM, Stringer EM, Kankasa C, Safrit JT, Stringer JS. 2007a. Single-dose tenofovir and emtricitabine for reduction of viral resistance to non-nucleoside reverse transcriptase inhibitor drugs in women given intrapartum nevirapine for perinatal HIV prevention: an open-label randomised trial. Lancet 370(9600):1698-1705.

Chi BH, Sinkala M, Stringer EM, Cantrell RA, Mtonga V, Bulterys M, Zulu I, Kankasa C, Wilfert C, Weidle PJ, Vermund SH, Stringer JS. 2007b. Early clinical and immune response to NNRTI-based antiretroviral therapy among women with prior exposure to single-dose nevirapine. Aids 21(8):957-964.

Chigwedere P, Seage GR, Lee TH, Essex M. 2008. Efficacy of antiretroviral drugs in reducing mother-to-child transmission of HIV in Africa: a meta-analysis of published clinical trials. AIDS Res Hum Retroviruses 24(6):827-837.

Chopra M, Lawn JE, Sanders D, Barron P, Abdool Karim SS, Bradshaw D, Jewkes R, Abdool
    Karim Q, Flisher AJ, Mayosi BM, Tollman SM, Churchyard GJ, Coovadia H. 2009.
    Achieving the health Millennium Development Goals for South Africa: challenges
    and priorities. Lancet 374(9694):1023-1031.
Ciaranello AL, Chang Y, Margulis AV, Bernstein A, Bassett IV, Losina E, Walensky RP. 2009.
    Effectiveness of pediatric antiretroviral therapy in resource-limited settings: a
    systematic review and meta-analysis. Clin Infect Dis 49(12):1915-1927.
Cooper CL, Mills E, Wabwire BO, Ford N, Olupot-Olupot P. 2009. Chronic viral hepatitis
    may diminish the gains of HIV antiretroviral therapy in sub-Saharan Africa. Int J
    Infect Dis 13(3):302-306.
Cozzi-Lepri A, Phillips AN, Ruiz L, Clotet B, Loveday C, Kjaer J, Mens H, Clumeck N,
    Viksna L, Antunes F, Machala L, Lundgren JD. 2007. Evolution of drug resistance in
    HIV-infected patients remaining on a virologically failing combination
    antiretroviral therapy regimen. Aids 21(6):721-732.
Crowley S, Rollins N, Shaffer N, Guerma T, Vitoria M, Lo YR. 2009. New WHO HIV
    treatment and prevention guidelines. Lancet.
Derache A, Maiga AI, Traore O, Akonde A, Cisse M, Jarrousse B, Koita V, Diarra B,
    Carcelain G, Barin F, Pizzocolo C, Pizarro L, Katlama C, Calvez V, Marcelin AG.
    2008. Evolution of genetic diversity and drug resistance mutations in HIV-1 among
    untreated patients from Mali between 2005 and 2006. J Antimicrob Chemother
    62(3):456-463.
Doyle SM, Kahn JG, Hosang N, Carroll PR. The impact of male circumcision on HIV
    transmission. J Urol 183(1):21-26.
Emery S, Neuhaus JA, Phillips AN, Babiker A, Cohen CJ, Gatell JM, Girard PM, Grund B,
    Law M, Losso MH, Palfreeman A, Wood R. 2008. Major clinical outcomes in
    antiretroviral therapy (ART)-naive participants and in those not receiving ART at
    baseline in the SMART study. J Infect Dis 197(8):1133-1144.
Ewing T. 1990. AIDS programme faces donor fatigue. Nature 346(6285):595.
Fang G, Burger H, Grimson R, Tropper P, Nachman S, Mayers D, Weislow O, Moore R,
    Reyelt C, Hutcheon N, Baker D, Weiser B. 1995. Maternal plasma human
    immunodeficiency virus type 1 RNA level: a determinant and projected threshold
    for mother-to-child transmission. Proc Natl Acad Sci U S A 92(26):12100-12104.
Fauci AS, Johnston MI, Dieffenbach CW, Burton DR, Hammer SM, Hoxie JA, Martin M,
    Overbaugh J, Watkins DI, Mahmoud A, Greene WC. 2008. HIV vaccine research:
    the way forward. Science 321(5888):530-532.
Ferrand RA, Corbett EL, Wood R, Hargrove J, Ndhlovu CE, Cowan FM, Gouws E, Williams
    BG. 2009. AIDS among older children and adolescents in Southern Africa:
    projecting the time course and magnitude of the epidemic. Aids 23(15):2039-2046.
Franey C, Knott D, Barnighausen T, Dedicoat M, Adam A, Lessells RJ, Newell ML, Cooke
    GS. 2009. Renal impairment in a rural African antiretroviral programme. BMC
    Infect Dis 9:143.
Friis-Moller N, Reiss P, Sabin CA, Weber R, Monforte A, El-Sadr W, Thiebaut R, De Wit S,
    Kirk O, Fontas E, Law MG, Phillips A, Lundgren JD. 2007. Class of antiretroviral
    drugs and the risk of myocardial infarction. N Engl J Med 356(17):1723-1735.
Gallant JE, Moore RD. 2009. Renal function with use of a tenofovir-containing initial
    antiretroviral regimen. Aids 23(15):1971-1975.

Gill GV, Mbanya JC, Ramaiya KL, Tesfaye S. 2009. A sub-Saharan African perspective of diabetes. Diabetologia 52(1):8-16.

Granich RM, Gilks CF, Dye C, De Cock KM, Williams BG. 2009. Universal voluntary HIV testing with immediate antiretroviral therapy as a strategy for elimination of HIV transmission: a mathematical model. Lancet 373(9657):48-57.

Grant RM, Hamer D, Hope T, Johnston R, Lange J, Lederman MM, Lieberman J, Miller CJ, Moore JP, Mosier DE, Richman DD, Schooley RT, Springer MS, Veazey RS, Wainberg MA. 2008. Whither or wither microbicides? Science 321(5888):532-534.

Grunfeld C, Delaney JA, Wanke C, Currier JS, Scherzer R, Biggs ML, Tien PC, Shlipak MG, Sidney S, Polak JF, O'Leary D, Bacchetti P, Kronmal RA. 2009. Preclinical atherosclerosis due to HIV infection: carotid intima-medial thickness measurements from the FRAM study. Aids 23(14):1841-1849.

Gupta R, Hill A, Sawyer AW, Pillay D. 2008. Emergence of drug resistance in HIV type 1-infected patients after receipt of first-line highly active antiretroviral therapy: a systematic review of clinical trials. Clin Infect Dis 47(5):712-722.

Hoffmann CJ, Charalambous S, Sim J, Ledwaba J, Schwikkard G, Chaisson RE, Fielding KL, Churchyard GJ, Morris L, Grant AD. 2009. Viremia, resuppression, and time to resistance in human immunodeficiency virus (HIV) subtype C during first-line antiretroviral therapy in South Africa. Clin Infect Dis 49(12):1928-1935.

Hosseinipour MC, Kumwenda JJ, Weigel R, Brown LB, Mzinganjira D, Mhango B, Eron JJ, Phiri S, van Oosterhout JJ. Second-line treatment in the Malawi antiretroviral programme: high early mortality, but good outcomes in survivors, despite extensive drug resistance at baseline. HIV Med 11(8):510-518.

Hsue PY, Hunt PW, Wu Y, Schnell A, Ho JE, Hatano H, Xie Y, Martin JN, Ganz P, Deeks SG. 2009. Association of abacavir and impaired endothelial function in treated and suppressed HIV-infected patients. Aids 23(15):2021-2027.

Jacobson DL, Spiegelman D, Knox TK, Wilson IB. 2008. Evolution and predictors of change in total bone mineral density over time in HIV-infected men and women in the nutrition for healthy living study. J Acquir Immune Defic Syndr 49(3):298-308.

Johnston MI, Fauci AS. 2008. An HIV vaccine--challenges and prospects. N Engl J Med 359(9):888-890.

Kantor R, Diero L, Delong A, Kamle L, Muyonga S, Mambo F, Walumbe E, Emonyi W, Chan P, Carter EJ, Hogan J, Buziba N. 2009. Misclassification of first-line antiretroviral treatment failure based on immunological monitoring of HIV infection in resource-limited settings. Clin Infect Dis 49(3):454-462.

Keiser O, MacPhail P, Boulle A, Wood R, Schechter M, Dabis F, Sprinz E, Egger M. 2009. Accuracy of WHO CD4 cell count criteria for virological failure of antiretroviral therapy. Trop Med Int Health 14(10):1220-1225.

Kerr T, Kaplan K, Suwannawong P, Jurgens R, Wood E. 2004. The Global Fund to Fight AIDS, Tuberculosis and Malaria: funding for unpopular public-health programmes. Lancet 364(9428):11-12.

Kitahata MG, S: Moore, R. North American AIDS Cohort Collaboration on Research and Design. Initiating rather than deferring HAART at a CD4+ count >500cells/mm3 is associated with imporved survival [Abstract 71]. Montreal, Quebec, Canada, 8-11 February 2009.

Koenig SP, Riviere C, Leger P, Joseph P, Severe P, Parker K, Collins S, Lee E, Pape JW, Fitzgerald DW. 2009. High mortality among patients with AIDS who received a diagnosis of tuberculosis in the first 3 months of antiretroviral therapy. Clin Infect Dis 48(6):829-831.

Kuritzkes DR, Lalama CM, Ribaudo HJ, Marcial M, Meyer WA, 3rd, Shikuma C, Johnson VA, Fiscus SA, D'Aquila RT, Schackman BR, Acosta EP, Gulick RM. 2008. Preexisting resistance to nonnucleoside reverse-transcriptase inhibitors predicts virologic failure of an efavirenz-based regimen in treatment-naive HIV-1-infected subjects. J Infect Dis 197(6):867-870.

Lavanchy D. 2004. Hepatitis B virus epidemiology, disease burden, treatment, and current and emerging prevention and control measures. J Viral Hepat 11(2):97-107.

Lawn SD, Badri M, Wood R. 2005. Tuberculosis among HIV-infected patients receiving HAART: long term incidence and risk factors in a South African cohort. Aids 19(18):2109-2116.

Lawn SD, Edwards DJ, Wood R. Reducing the burden of tuberculosis presenting during the initial months of antiretroviral therapy in resource-limited settings. Clin Infect Dis 50(1):124-125; author reply 125.

Lawn SD, Harries AD, Anglaret X, Myer L, Wood R. 2008. Early mortality among adults accessing antiretroviral treatment programmes in sub-Saharan Africa. Aids 22(15):1897-1908.

Leroy V, Ekouevi DK, Becquet R, Viho I, Dequae-Merchadou L, Tonwe-Gold B, Rouet F, Sakarovitch C, Horo A, Timite-Konan M, Rouzioux C, Dabis F. 2008. 18-month effectiveness of short-course antiretroviral regimens combined with alternatives to breastfeeding to prevent HIV mother-to-child transmission. PLoS One 3(2):e1645.

Liaw YF, Leung NW, Chang TT, Guan R, Tai DI, Ng KY, Chien RN, Dent J, Roman L, Edmundson S, Lai CL. 2000. Effects of extended lamivudine therapy in Asian patients with chronic hepatitis B. Asia Hepatitis Lamivudine Study Group. Gastroenterology 119(1):172-180.

Lim SG, Wai CT, Rajnakova A, Kajiji T, Guan R. 2002. Fatal hepatitis B reactivation following discontinuation of nucleoside analogues for chronic hepatitis B. Gut 51(4):597-599.

Lockman S, Shapiro RL, Smeaton LM, Wester C, Thior I, Stevens L, Chand F, Makhema J, Moffat C, Asmelash A, Ndase P, Arimi P, van Widenfelt E, Mazhani L, Novitsky V, Lagakos S, Essex M. 2007. Response to antiretroviral therapy after a single, peripartum dose of nevirapine. N Engl J Med 356(2):135-147.

Lok AS, Hussain M, Cursano C, Margotti M, Gramenzi A, Grazi GL, Jovine E, Benardi M, Andreone P. 2000. Evolution of hepatitis B virus polymerase gene mutations in hepatitis B e antigen-negative patients receiving lamivudine therapy. Hepatology 32(5):1145-1153.

Lopez AD, Mathers CD, Ezzati M, Jamison DT, Murray CJ. 2006. Global and regional burden of disease and risk factors, 2001: systematic analysis of population health data. Lancet 367(9524):1747-1757.

Madruga JV, Berger D, McMurchie M, Suter F, Banhegyi D, Ruxrungtham K, Norris D, Lefebvre E, de Bethune MP, Tomaka F, De Pauw M, Vangeneugden T, Spinosa-Guzman S. 2007. Efficacy and safety of darunavir-ritonavir compared with that of lopinavir-ritonavir at 48 weeks in treatment-experienced, HIV-infected patients in TITAN: a randomised controlled phase III trial. Lancet 370(9581):49-58.

Manabe YC, Breen R, Perti T, Girardi E, Sterling TR. 2009. Unmasked tuberculosis and tuberculosis immune reconstitution inflammatory disease: a disease spectrum after initiation of antiretroviral therapy. J Infect Dis 199(3):437-444.

Marcellin P, Heathcote EJ, Buti M, Gane E, de Man RA, Krastev Z, Germanidis G, Lee SS, Flisiak R, Kaita K, Manns M, Kotzev I, Tchernev K, Buggisch P, Weilert F, Kurdas OO, Shiffman ML, Trinh H, Washington MK, Sorbel J, Anderson J, Snow-Lampart A, Mondou E, Quinn J, Rousseau F. 2008. Tenofovir disoproxil fumarate versus adefovir dipivoxil for chronic hepatitis B. N Engl J Med 359(23):2442-2455.

Marconi VC, Sunpath H, Lu Z, Gordon M, Koranteng-Apeagyei K, Hampton J, Carpenter S, Giddy J, Ross D, Holst H, Losina E, Walker BD, Kuritzkes DR. 2008. Prevalence of HIV-1 drug resistance after failure of a first highly active antiretroviral therapy regimen in KwaZulu Natal, South Africa. Clin Infect Dis 46(10):1589-1597.

Mayer KH, Venkatesh KK. Antiretroviral therapy as HIV prevention: status and prospects. Am J Public Health 100(10):1867-1876.

Mayosi BM, Flisher AJ, Lalloo UG, Sitas F, Tollman SM, Bradshaw D. 2009. The burden of non-communicable diseases in South Africa. Lancet 374(9693):934-947.

Merson MH. 2006. The HIV-AIDS pandemic at 25--the global response. N Engl J Med 354(23):2414-2417.

Mills EJ, Nachega JB, Buchan I, Orbinski J, Attaran A, Singh S, Rachlis B, Wu P, Cooper C, Thabane L, Wilson K, Guyatt GH, Bangsberg DR. 2006. Adherence to antiretroviral therapy in sub-Saharan Africa and North America: a meta-analysis. Jama 296(6):679-690.

Modi AA, Feld JJ. 2007. Viral hepatitis and HIV in Africa. AIDS Rev 9(1):25-39.

Montaner JS, Hogg R, Wood E, Kerr T, Tyndall M, Levy AR, Harrigan PR. 2006. The case for expanding access to highly active antiretroviral therapy to curb the growth of the HIV epidemic. Lancet 368(9534):531-536.

Moore D, Liechty C, Ekwaru P, Were W, Mwima G, Solberg P, Rutherford G, Mermin J. 2007. Prevalence, incidence and mortality associated with tuberculosis in HIV-infected patients initiating antiretroviral therapy in rural Uganda. Aids 21(6):713-719.

Murray CJ, Lopez AD. 1997. Mortality by cause for eight regions of the world: Global Burden of Disease Study. Lancet 349(9061):1269-1276.

Nikolopoulos GK, Paraskevis D, Hatzitheodorou E, Moschidis Z, Sypsa V, Zavitsanos X, Kalapothaki V, Hatzakis A. 2009. Impact of hepatitis B virus infection on the progression of AIDS and mortality in HIV-infected individuals: a cohort study and meta-analysis. Clin Infect Dis 48(12):1763-1771.

Paintsil E, Andiman WA. 2007. Care and management of the infant of the HIV-1-infected mother. Semin Perinatol 31(2):112-123.

Paintsil E, Andiman WA. 2009. Update on successes and challenges regarding mother-to-child transmission of HIV. Curr Opin Pediatr 21(1):94-101.

Palombi L, Marazzi MC, Voetberg A, Magid NA. 2007. Treatment acceleration program and the experience of the DREAM program in prevention of mother-to-child transmission of HIV. Aids 21 Suppl 4:S65-71.

Petersen ML, van der Laan MJ, Napravnik S, Eron JJ, Moore RD, Deeks SG. 2008. Long-term consequences of the delay between virologic failure of highly active antiretroviral therapy and regimen modification. Aids 22(16):2097-2106.

Quinn TC, Wawer MJ, Sewankambo N, Serwadda D, Li C, Wabwire-Mangen F, Meehan MO, Lutalo T, Gray RH. 2000. Viral load and heterosexual transmission of human immunodeficiency virus type 1. Rakai Project Study Group. N Engl J Med 342(13):921-929.

Reynolds SJ, Kityo C, Mbamanya F, Dewar R, Ssali F, Quinn TC, Mugyenyi P, Dybul M. 2009a. Evolution of drug resistance after virological failure of a first-line highly active antiretroviral therapy regimen in Uganda. Antivir Ther 14(2):293-297.

Reynolds SJ, Nakigozi G, Newell K, Ndyanabo A, Galiwongo R, Boaz I, Quinn TC, Gray R, Wawer M, Serwadda D. 2009b. Failure of immunologic criteria to appropriately identify antiretroviral treatment failure in Uganda. Aids 23(6):697-700.

Riddler SA, Haubrich R, DiRienzo AG, Peeples L, Powderly WG, Klingman KL, Garren KW, George T, Rooney JF, Brizz B, Lalloo UG, Murphy RL, Swindells S, Havlir D, Mellors JW. 2008. Class-sparing regimens for initial treatment of HIV-1 infection. N Engl J Med 358(20):2095-2106.

Rockstroh JK, Mocroft A, Soriano V, Tural C, Losso MH, Horban A, Kirk O, Phillips A, Ledergerber B, Lundgren J. 2005. Influence of hepatitis C virus infection on HIV-1 disease progression and response to highly active antiretroviral therapy. J Infect Dis 192(6):992-1002.

Sepkowitz KA. 2006. One disease, two epidemics--AIDS at 25. N Engl J Med 354(23):2411-2414.

Sliwa K, Mocumbi AO. 2009. Forgotten cardiovascular diseases in Africa. Clin Res Cardiol.

Smith DK, Taylor A, Kilmarx PH, Sullivan P, Warner L, Kamb M, Bock N, Kohmescher B, Mastro TD. Male circumcision in the United States for the prevention of HIV infection and other adverse health outcomes: report from a CDC consultation. Public Health Rep 125 Suppl 1:72-82.

Smith RJ, Li J, Gordon R, Heffernan JM. 2009. Can we spend our way out of the AIDS epidemic? A world halting AIDS model. BMC Public Health 9 Suppl 1:S15.

Sterne. When to start consortium. When should HIV-1infected infected persons initiate ART? Collaborative analysis of HIV cohort studies [Abstract 72LB]. Montreal, Quebec, Canada, 8-11 February 2009.

Thio CL. 2009. Hepatitis B and human immunodeficiency virus coinfection. Hepatology 49(5 Suppl):S138-145.

Tonwe-Gold B, Ekouevi DK, Viho I, Amani-Bosse C, Toure S, Coffie PA, Rouet F, Becquet R, Leroy V, El-Sadr WM, Abrams EJ, Dabis F. 2007. Antiretroviral treatment and prevention of peripartum and postnatal HIV transmission in West Africa: evaluation of a two-tiered approach. PLoS Med 4(8):e257.

Tovanabutra S, Robison V, Wongtrakul J, Sennum S, Suriyanon V, Kingkeow D, Kawichai S, Tanan P, Duerr A, Nelson KE. 2002. Male viral load and heterosexual transmission of HIV-1 subtype E in northern Thailand. J Acquir Immune Defic Syndr 29(3):275-283.

UNAIDS. 2005a. Financing the expanded response to AIDS: HIV vaccine and microbicide research and development. Accessed at:

http://data.unaids.org/UNAdocs/financingresdevvaccinemicrobicide_report_en.pdf.

UNAIDS. 2005b. Resource needs for an expanded response to AIDS in low- and middle-income countries. Accessed at:
http://data.unaids.org/pub/Report/2005/jc1239_resource_needs_en.pdf.

UNAIDS. 2009. AIDS epidemic update.
http://www.unaids.org/en/media/unaids/contentassets/dataimport/pub/report/2009/jc1700_epi_update_2009_en.pdf.

Unwin N, Setel P, Rashid S, Mugusi F, Mbanya JC, Kitange H, Hayes L, Edwards R, Aspray T, Alberti KG. 2001. Noncommunicable diseases in sub-Saharan Africa: where do they feature in the health research agenda? Bull World Health Organ 79(10):947-953.

von Wyl V, Yerly S, Boni J, Burgisser P, Klimkait T, Battegay M, Furrer H, Telenti A, Hirschel B, Vernazza PL, Bernasconi E, Rickenbach M, Perrin L, Ledergerber B, Gunthard HF. 2007. Emergence of HIV-1 drug resistance in previously untreated patients initiating combination antiretroviral treatment: a comparison of different regimen types. Arch Intern Med 167(16):1782-1790.

Walensky RP, Wolf LL, Wood R, Fofana MO, Freedberg KA, Martinson NA, Paltiel AD, Anglaret X, Weinstein MC, Losina E. 2009. When to start antiretroviral therapy in resource-limited settings. Ann Intern Med 151(3):157-166.

Weiss HA, Hankins CA, Dickson K. 2009. Male circumcision and risk of HIV infection in women: a systematic review and meta-analysis. Lancet Infect Dis 9(11):669-677.

Wensing AM, van de Vijver DA, Angarano G, Asjo B, Balotta C, Boeri E, Camacho R, Chaix ML, Costagliola D, De Luca A, Derdelinckx I, Grossman Z, Hamouda O, Hatzakis A, Hemmer R, Hoepelman A, Horban A, Korn K, Kucherer C, Leitner T, Loveday C, MacRae E, Maljkovic I, de Mendoza C, Meyer L, Nielsen C, Op de Coul EL, Ormaasen V, Paraskevis D, Perrin L, Puchhammer-Stockl E, Ruiz L, Salminen M, Schmit JC, Schneider F, Schuurman R, Soriano V, Stanczak G, Stanojevic M, Vandamme AM, Van Laethem K, Violin M, Wilbe K, Yerly S, Zazzi M, Boucher CA. 2005. Prevalence of drug-resistant HIV-1 variants in untreated individuals in Europe: implications for clinical management. J Infect Dis 192(6):958-966.

WHO. 2006a. antiretroviral therapy for HIV infection in adults and adolescents: recommendations for a public health approach. p accessed at:
http://www.who.int/hiv/pub/guidelines/artadultguidelines.pdf.

WHO. 2006b. Global access to HIV therapy tripled in past two years, but significant challenges remain. p Accessed at:
http://www.who.int/hiv/mediacentre/news57/en/index.html.

WHO. 2007. AIDS epidemic update.
http://www.unaids.org/en/KnowledgeCentre/HIVData/EpiUpdate/EpiUpdArchive/2007/.

WHO. 2009. Global Tuberculosis control report. p Accessed at:
http://www.who.int/tb/publications/global_report/2009/update/tbu_2009.pdf.

Williams BG, Lloyd-Smith JO, Gouws E, Hankins C, Getz WM, Hargrove J, de Zoysa I, Dye C, Auvert B. 2006. The potential impact of male circumcision on HIV in Sub-Saharan Africa. PLoS Med 3(7):e262.

Wilson DP, Coplan PM, Wainberg MA, Blower SM. 2008. The paradoxical effects of using antiretroviral-based microbicides to control HIV epidemics. Proc Natl Acad Sci U S A 105(28):9835-9840.

Wood E, Hogg RS, Harrigan PR, Montaner JS. 2005. When to initiate antiretroviral therapy in HIV-1-infected adults: a review for clinicians and patients. Lancet Infect Dis 5(7):407-414.

7

Infection for *Mycobacterium tuberculosis* and Nontuberculous Mycobacteria in the HIV/AIDS Patients

Lilian María Mederos Cuervo
National Reference Laboratory TB/Mycobacteria Collaborate Center PAHO/WHO
Tropical Medicine Institute Pedro Kourí (IPK)
Cuba

1. Introduction

Tuberculosis (TB) is a disease also know as consumption, wasting disease, and the white plague, it has affected humans for centuries. Until the mid-1800s, people thought that tuberculosis, or TB, was hereditary. They did not realize that it could be spread from person to person through the air. Also, until the 1940s and 1950s there was no cure for TB. For many people, a diagnosis of TB was a slow death sentence [1-4].

In 1865 a French surgeon, Jean-Antoine Villemin, proved that TB was contagious, and in 1882 a german scientist named Robert Koch discovered the bacteria causes TB, denominated as *Mycobacterium tuberculosis*. Yet half a century passed before drugs were discovered that could cure TB, until then, many people with TB were sent to sanatoriums, special rest homes where they followed a prescribed routine every day. A breakthrough came in 1943, an american scientist, Selman Waksman discovered a drug that could kill TB bacteria. Between 1943 and 1952, two more drugs were found, after these discoveries, many people with TB were cured and the death rate for TB in the United States dropped dramatically, and fewer and fewer people got TB [5].

A global health emergency [6,7]:

- Someone in the world is newly infected with TB bacilli every second.
- Overall, one-third of the world's population is currently infected with the TB bacillus.
- 5-10 % of people who are infected with TB bacilli become sick or infectious at some time during their life.

TB program activities, reinforced by successful chemotherapy, resulted in a pronounced reduction of infection and death rates. The disease became greatly controlled but it never quite disappeared. Then, in around 1985, cases of TB began to rise again in industrialized countries. Several inter-related forces drove this resurgence, including increase in prison populations, homelessness, injection drug use, crowded housing and increased immigration from countries where TB continued to be endemic. Above all, the decline in TB control activities and the human immunodeficiency virus/acquired immunodeficiency syndrome (HIV/AIDS) epidemic were two major factors fuelling each other in the re-emergence of TB. People with HIV and TB infection are much more likely to develop TB. The HIV/AIDS epidemic has produced a devastating effect on TB control worldwide. While one out of ten immunocompetent people infected with *M. tuberculosis* will fall sick in their lifetimes, among those with HIV infection, one in ten per year will develop active TB. In developing countries, the impact of HIV infection on the TB situation, especially in the 20-35 age groups, is overwhelming. While wealthy industrialized countries with good public health care systems can be expected to keep TB under control, in much of the developing world a catastrophe awaits. In poorly developed countries, TB remains a significant threat to public health, as incidences remain high, even after the introduction of vaccination and drug treatment. The registered number of new cases of TB worldwide roughly correlates with economic conditions: highest incidences are seen in the countries of Africa, Asia, and Latin America with the lowest gross national products. Supervised treatment, including sometimes direct observation of therapy (DOT), was proposed as a means of helping patients to take their drugs regularly and complete treatment, thus achieving cure and preventing the development of drug resistance [5-7].

2. Transmission and pathogenesis

TB is spread from person through the air. When a person with pulmonary or laryngeal TB coughs, sneezes, speaks, or sings, droplet nuclei containing *Mycobacterium tuberculosis* are expelled into the air. Depending on the environment, these tiny particles (1-5 microns in diameter) can remain suspended in the air for several hours. If another person inhales air containing droplet nuclei, transmission may occur. The probability that TB will be transmitted depends on these factors [4, 5]:

- The infectiousness of the person with TB (the number of organisms expelled into the air).
- The environment in which exposure occurred.
- The duration of exposure and the virulence of the organism.

The best way to stop transmission is to isolate patients with infectious TB immediately and start effective TB therapy. Infectiousness declines rapidly after adequate therapy is started, as long as the patient adheres to the prescribed regimen. Persons at the highest risk of becoming infected with *Mycobacterium tuberculosis* are close contacts, the persons who had prolonged, frequent, or intense contact with a person with infectious TB. Close contacts may be family members, roommates, friends, coworkers, or others. Data collected by CDC since 1987 show that infection rates have been relatively stable, ranging form 21-23% for the contacts of infectious TB patients [6-9]. Some people with infection develop TB disease. This disease develops when the immune system cannot keep the tubercle bacilli under control and the bacilli begin to multiply rapidly. The risk that TB disease will develop is higher for some people than for others [3, 10-12]. Among contacts of persons with drug-resistant TB, infection rates seem to be similar. However, because they may have a poor response to treatment persons with drug-resistant disease are often infectious for longer periods and therefore have the potential to infect more contacts [10-13].

Extra pulmonary TB is rarely contagious; however, transmission from extrapulmonary sites has been reported during aerosol-producing procedures, such as autopsies and tissue irrigation [14-16].

3. Pathogenesis

The tubercle bacilli that alveoli are ingested by alveolar macrophages, the majority of these bacilli are destroyed or inhibited. A small number multiply intracellulary and are released when the macrophages die. These bacilli can spread through the lymphatic channels to regional lymph nodes and then through the bloodstream to more distant tissues and organs, including areas in which TB disease is most likely to develop: the apices of the lung, the kidneys, the brain, and bone.   Extracellular bacilli attract macrophages form the bloodstream. The immune response kills most of the bacilli, leading to the formation of a granuloma. At this point the person has TB infection, which can be detected by using the tuberculin skin test. It may take 2-10 weeks for the infected person to develop a positive reaction to the tuberculin skin test. Immune responses soon develop to kill the bacilli. Within 2-10 weeks after infection, the immune system is usually able to halt the multiplication of the tubercle bacilli, preventing further spread [4, 17-19].

In persons infected with *Mycobacterium tuberculosis* but that don't have TB disease cannot spread the infection to other people. TB infection in persons who does not have TB disease is not considered a case of TB and referred to as "latent TB infection". In some persons, TB bacilli overcome the defenses or the immune system and begin to multiply, resulting in the progression from TB infection to TB disease. This process may occur soon after or many years after infection. Some study demonstrated that approximately 5% of person who have been infected with *Mycobacterium tuberculosis* will develop TB disease in the first year or two after infection and another 5% will develop disease some time later in life. Recent infection (with the past 2 years) with *Mycobacterium tuberculosis* is therefore an important risk factor for progression to TB disease and in approximately 10% of persons with normal immune system who are infected with *Mycobacterium tuberculosis* , TB disease will develop at some point [5-7].

Some medical conditions increase the risk that TB infection will progress to disease. Some studies suggest that the risk is mayor in inmmunosuppressed patients, for example persons with Diabetes mellitus, prolonged therapy with corticosteroids, immunosuppressive therapy, certain types of cancer, severe kidney disease, injection of illicit drugs, and infection with Human Immunodeficient Virus (HIV) [2,3,12].

TB disease most commomly affects the lung, 73% of TB cases are exclusively pulmonary, and however, TB is a systemic disease and may also commonly occur in the following ways; as pleural effusion in the central nervous, lymphatic, or genitourinary systems, as disseminated disease (military TB). Also the infection for *Mycobacterium tuberculosis* can occur in the other body sites; in the breast, skin, or peritoneum [16,20-23]. Extrapulmonary TB is more common in immunosuppressed persons and in young children; meningoencephalitis TB, lymphatic TB and military disease are particularly common in immunosuppressed persons, in some case the extrapulmonary TB is often accompanied by pulmonary TB [3, 8, 16-23].

4. Epidemiology of TB

TB infection is one of the most common infections in the world. It is estimated that 30-60% of adults in developing countries have TB infection. Annually about 8-10 million people develop TB disease and 2-3 million people die of the disease. TB disease is the leading cause of death due to infectious disease around the world [24, 25]. When the health department learns about a new case of TB, it should take steps to ensure that the person receives appropriate treatment. Is very important that the health authorities should also start a contact investigation, this means interviewing a person who has TB disease to determinate who may have been exposed to TB, this person are screened for TB infection and disease [8, 26-28].

In order to the decrease in the number of TB cases reported annually is very important to comply three factors [29]:

- To increase federal resources for TB control and other public health efforts.
- To improve prevention and TB control programs in state and local health department.
- To Increase attention to ensuring that patients complete drug therapy through directly observed therapy (DOT).

In the control of TB disease is also important to know the Groups at High Risk for TB [29, 30]:

People at Higher Risk for Exposure or Infection:

- Close contacts of people with infectious TB disease.
- People born in areas of the world where TB is common.
- Elderly people.
- Low-income groups with poor access to health care, including homeless people.
- People who inject illicit drugs.
- People who live or work in residential facilities (Example: nursing correctional facilities).
- Other people who may be exposed to TB on the job.
- People in other groups as identified by local public health officials.

People at Higher Risk for TB disease:

- People with other medical conditions that can increase the risk for TB.
- People recently infected with *Mycobacterium tuberculosis*.
- People with chest x-ray suggestive of previous TB disease.
- People who inject illicit drugs.
- People with HIV infection.

Infection with HIV makes people susceptible to rapidly progressive tuberculosis; over 10 millions peoples are infected with both HIV and *Mycobacterium tuberculosis* [8].

TB in Children:

The occurrence of TB infection and disease in children provide important information about the spread of TB in homes and communities. When a child has TB infection or disease is important to learn if [29-31]:

- Recent TB transmition.
- Other adults and children in the household or community have probably been exposed to TB; if they are infected, they may develop TB disease in the future.

4.1 Drug-resistant tuberculosis

Drug-resistant TB is transmitted in the same way as drug-susceptible TB. The earlier outbreaks of multidrugs-resistant (MDR) TB support the findings that drug-resistant TB is no less infectious than drug-susceptible TB, although prolonged periods of infectiousness that often occur in the patients with drug-resistant TB may facililate transmission. Drug resistance was divided in two types; primary resistance and secondary or acquired resistance. Primary resistance develops in persons who are initially infected, with resistant organisms. Second resistance, or acquired resistance develops during TB therapy, either because the patient was treated with an inadequate regimen or because the patient did not take the prescribed regimen appropriately [27, 29, 32]. The MDR-TB are resistant to rifampicin and isoniazid drugs. Recently drug-resistant tuberculosis (XDR-TB) is defined as tuberculosis caused by a *Mycobacterium tuberculosis* strain that is resistant to at least rifampicin and isoniazid among the first-line antitubercular drugs (MDR-TB) in addition to resistance to any fluroquinolones and at least one of three second-line drugs, namely amikacin, kanamycin and/or capreomycin. Current studies have described XDR-TB strains from all continents. Worldwide prevalence of XDR-TB is estimated in 6.6% in all the studied countries among MDR-TB strains. The emergence of XDR-TB strains is a reflection of poor tuberculosis management, and controlling its emergence constitutes an urgent global health reality and a challenge to tuberculosis control activities in all parts of the world, especially in developing countries and those lacking resources and as well as in countries with increasing prevalence of HIV/AIDS [32-34].

5. Diagnosis of tuberculosis

The systemic symptom of Tuberculosis include fever, chills, night sweats, appetite loss, weigh loss, and easy fatigability, the symptoms of pulmonary TB are productive and prolonged cough (>14-21 week) , chest pain and in some case the patient present hemoptysis. It is important to ask persons suspected of having tuberculosis about their history of TB exposure, infection, or disease. The clinicians may also contact the local health department for information about whether a patient has received tuberculosis treatment in the past, if the drug regimen was inadequate or if the patient may did not adhere to therapy, this disease may recur and may be drug resistant. Also is important to consider demographic factors; country of origin, age, ethnic or racial group and occupation, this factors may increase the patient's risk for exposure to TB or drug-resistant TB disease. Clinicians should determinate whether the patient has medical conditions, especially HIV infection, because this infection increases the risk for TB disease. All patients who do not know their current HIV status should be referred for HIV counseling and testing [26, 27].

The tuberculin skin test and the chest radiography, are two probes that help in the diagnostic for TB disease. Tuberculin skin testing useful for [29]:

- To examine a person who is not ill but may be infected with *Mycobacterium tuberculosis*, such as a person who has been exposed to someone who has TB. This test is the only way to diagnose tuberculosis infection before it has progressed to tuberculosis disease.
- To determine how many people in group are infected with *Mycobacterium tuberculosis*.
- To examine person who has symptoms of TB.

A negative reaction to the tuberculin skin test does not exclude the diagnosis of TB, especially for patients with severe TB illness or infection with HIV. Some persons may not react to the tuberculin skin test if they are tested too soon after being exposed to the infection. Generally it takes 2-10 week after infection for a person to develop an immune response to tuberculin. In children younger than 6 months of age may not react to the tuberculin skin test because their immune systems are not yet fully developed [32].

5.1 Chest radiography
The chest radiography is for:
- To detect abnormalities often seen in apical or posterior segments of upper lobe or superior segments of lower lobe.
- To detect atypical images in immunosuppressed persons an in HIV-positive persons.

In HIV-infected persons, pulmonary TB may appear in the chets radiograph. For example; TB disease may cause infiltrates without cavities in any lung zone, or it may cause mediastinal or hiliar lymphadenophaty with or without accompanying infiltrates and/or cavities. In HIV-positive persons, almost any abnormality on a chest radiographic may indicate TB. In fact, the radiograph of an HIV-positive person with TB disease may even appear entirely normal. Abnormalities on chest radiographs may be suggestive of, but are never diagnostic of TB. However, chest radiographic may be used to rule out the possibility of pulmonary TB in a person who has a positive reaction to the tuberculin skin test and no symptoms of disease [29, 31, 32, 34].

Summarizing the possibility of TB should be considered in persons who have these symptoms, person suspected of having this disease should be referred for a medical evaluation, which should include a medical history, a physical examination, a Mantoux tuberculin skin test or tuberculosis purified protein derivate (PPD) skin test, a chest radiograph. Also, it is very important any appropriate bacteriologic or histological examinations in this patients, principally in all inmmunosuppressed patients, of course including the HIV patients [29].

Person with symptoms of TB pulmonary disease should have at least three sputum specimens examined by smear and culture. The bets way would be to get serial specimens collected early in the morning on 3 consecutive days. A health care worked should be prepared and directly supervise at least during the first time sputum collection. This personal should give properly instructed in how to produce a good specimen, the patients should be informed that sputum is the material brought up form the lungs and that mucus from the nose or throat and saliva are not good specimens [35, 36].

Recommends for Specimen Collection:

- Get 3 sputum specimens for smear examination and culture.
- In persons unable to cough up sputum, induce sputum, bronchoscopy or gastric aspiration.
- Before chemotherapy and drug therapy is started.
- To use clean, sterile, one-use, plastic, disposable containers that have been washed with dichromate sulfuric acid and sterilized.
- To transport specimens to the laboratory as soon as possible.

5.2 Laboratory examination

Detection of acid-fast bacilli (AFB) in stained smears examined microscopically may provide the first bacteriologic of TB. The traditional method for to detect AFB is the Zielh-Neelsen coloration, it is a method more economic. There are other methods that increased sensitivity as fluorescent methods. Smear examination is an easy and quick procedure, because the results should be available within 24 hours of specimen collection. However, smear examination permits only the presumptive diagnosis of TB because many TB patients have negative AFB smears. The sensitivity of smear examination may be reduced if the directed inflammatory response and relative absence of cavitary lesions results in fewer organisms expectorated in sputum. There has been concern that the utility of sputum acid-fast smears may be reduced in HIV-infected populations [36, 37].

5.3 Extrapulmonary TB disease

This disease is not taking in account as causative agent of an extrapulmonary disease because the chest radiography is normal or tuberculin skin test is negative, or both. Mycobacteria may infect almost any organ in the body, the laboratory should expect to receive a variety of extrapulmonary specimens: aseptically collected body fluids, surgically excised tissue, aspirated or draining pus, and urine. Others ascetically collected specimens are the body fluids as spinal, pleural, pericardial, synovial, ascetic, blood, pus, and bone marrow are aseptically collected by the physician using aspiration techniques or surgical procedure. Acid-fast bacilli may be difficult to isolate from some of these specimens because they often are diluted by the large fluid volume [16-19, 37-39].

The identification of TB can be done by traditional culture materials include egg-based solid media, such as Löwenstein-Jensen medium, and synthetic solid media as Middlebrook 7H10 and 7H11 agars. The identification depends on the visualization of mycobacterial colonies and is limited by the slow growth rate of these organisms. A major advance in laboratory diagnosis of TB has been the development of systems based on detecting growth in liquid media with the use of radiometric methods as Bactec System. In this, the medium contains palmitic acid labeled with carbon-14. The metabolism of this fatty acid by growing mycobacteria liberates radioactive carbon dioxide, periodic sampling of the gasses in the culture-containing flask permits rapid detection of mycobacterial growth [40-41].

Species identification was accomplished with biochemical test that often involved additional diagnostic delays. Others techniques, currently being evaluated in a number of clinical settings include identification based on chromatography techniques for the studies of some specific lipids present in the wall of Mycobacterium [42, 43]. Also genetic probes are now availed for the identification of Mycobacterium tuberculosis and several other common mycobacterial species. These probes recognize species-specific sequences of ribosomal RNA. Theoretically, genetic probe as polymerase chain reaction (PCR), may permit diagnosis directly form patients specimens, eliminating the need for culture of organism. In practice, the utility of PCR has been limited by problems with the sensitivity and particularly, the specificity of results. In some laboratories, the sensitivity and specificity have been reported to exceed 85%. However, in several laboratories, false-positive rates ranged from 3% to 20%, and in one, 77% of positive results were false. In the last time the Genotype Mycobacteria Direct Assay (GTMD), a novel commercial assay based on nucleic acid sequence-based amplification technology, was evaluated for detection of Mycobacterium tuberculosis complex and some atypical mycobacterial species from clinical samples, and your sensitivity, specificity, positive predictive, and negative predictive were evaluated and these results were more better [44-46].

6. Nontuberculous mycobacteria in the environment

Environmental opportunistic mycobacteria are those that are recovered form natural and human influenced environments and can infect and cause disease in humans, animals, and birds. Other names for these mycobacteria are nontuberculous, however, they cause tuberculous lesions, also other name is atypical mycobacterial, it distinguish from "typical" Mycobacterium tuberculosis, and them nontuberculous mycobacteria (NTM). The environmental opportunistic mycobacteria are normal inhabitants of natural waters, drinking water, and soils. They can be isolated from biofilms, aerosol, and dusts. The distribution of NTM and the incidence of disease caused by them is perhaps are not fully understood in most parts of the world. NTM are widely distributed in nature and have been isolated from natural water, rap water, tap water, and water used in showers and surgical solutions [47-51].

It is common observation that environmental mycobacteria cause disease in individuals who offer some opportunity due to altered local or systemic immunity. Chronic obstructive pulmonary diseases, emphysema, pneumoconiosis, bronchiectasis, cystic fibrosis, thoracic scoliosis, aspiration due to esophageal disease, previous gastrectomy and chronic alcoholism are some of conditions which have been linked to disease due to NTM. While the reasons may be less clear in conditions like adenitis in children, such factors may be quite obvious in other conditions like bronchiectasis, surgical procedures, injections, break in skin surface due to wounds and generalized immune deficiency states like AIDS, use of immunosuppressive agents as used in transplant patients, etc [50, 51].

6.1 Pathogenesis

The mechanisms of pathogenesis of NTM are not very clear and have not been adequately investigated. Very low CD4 counts and defective cytokine response have been linked to severe infections in AIDS patients [50].

Nontuberculous mycobacteria have been reported to cause localized or disseminated disease depending on local predisposition and/or degree of immune deficit. In non-HIV patients, different NTM may cause localized pulmonary disease, adenitis, soft tissue infections, infections of joints and bones, bursae, skin ulcers and generalized disease in individuals like leukemia, transplant patients, etc. In AIDS patients the manifestations may range from localized to disseminated disease. Clinical features will include local organ specific signs and symptoms to persistent high grade fever, night sweats, anemia and weight loss in addition to nonspecific symptoms of malaise, anorexia, diarrhea, myalgia and occasional painful adenopathy [52-57].

7. Epidemiology of human infection with nontuberculous mycobacteria

The frequency of NTM pulmonary disease has been reported to be increasing on several continents. Changing patient populations, most notably from infection with HIV, have greatly increased the numbers of people at risk [57-60]. Studies addressing the epidemiology of NTM infection may be broadly divided into three types: cutaneous delayed-type hypersensitivity to NTM antigens has been used to study large samples of people in many countries. These studies have the strength of providing information regarding simple infection in large groups of people but suffer from the lack of information regarding the prevalence of disease. Another drawback of this study type reflects the relatively poor specificity of the skin test, as well as overlap in reactivity among various Mycobacterial species. The second useful type of epidemiologic study of NMT infection includes investigations reviewing consecutive isolates from a mycobacterial laboratory. In the presence of adequate laboratory protocols to avoid contamination with environmental organisms, these studies provide unequivocal evidence of infection but have the obvious shortcoming of a lack of clinical data, preventing the assessment regarding the presence or absence of disease. The final and most useful study type combines information from the mycobacterial laboratory and the clinician's assessment [55-62].

A true increase in rates of infection and disease could be related to the host, the pathogen, or some interaction between the two. Host changes leading to increased numbers of susceptibility could play an important role, with increased numbers of patients with inadequate defenses from diseases such as HIV infection, malignancy, or simply advanced age. Many investigations have observed decreasing rates of TB concomitant with the increases in NTM. Finally, an interaction between the host and pathogen could involve a major increase in pathogen exposure or potential inoculum size [63-67].

7.1 Clinical manifestations

Environmental opportunist or nontuberculous mycobacteria (NMT) include both slowly and rapidly growing. The range of infections caused by environmental opportunist mycobacteria is quite broad [8, 51].

7.2 Pulmonary infections

Mycobacterium avium-intracellulare complex (MAC) strains have been a major cause of pulmonary and other infections, principally in the HIV patients. MAC infections were commonly seen in chronic obstructive airway disease and in the in the geriatric patients too. *Mycobacterium kansasii and Mycobacterium scrofulaceum* have been considered an important cause of pulmonary infections. *Mycobacterium xenopi*, an unusual specie has been encountered as a pathogen in patients with other underlying lung diseases. Others species of slow grown as *Mycobacterium simiae (Mycobacterium 'habana'), Mycobacterium szulgai, Mycobacterium malmoense* and *Mycobacterium fortuitum* of rapid grown are other pathogens reported to be associated with pulmonary infections [51, 65-68].

7.3 Cutaneous infection

Mycobacterium szulgai, Mycobacterium marinum, Mycobacterium ulcerans and *Mycobacterium vaccae* have been reported to be a cause of skin infectious. *Mycobacterium marinum*, specie has been recognized as a causative organism of swimming pool granuloma or fish tank granuloma. It causes papular lesions in the extremities and may be confused with sporotricosis. *Mycobacterium ulcerans* is established cause of buruli ulcer, *Mycobacterium vaccae* has also been reported to be a cause of skin infections [51-56].

7.4 Wound infection bone, joints and bursae and sepsis

Mycobacterium fortuitum causes pyogenic lesions in the soft tissue, joints, bursae and injection abscesses, while *Mycobacterium chelonae abscessus* is a well known cause of wound infections, a new related species *Mycobacterum immunogenum* has been recently been recognized as a cause of sepsis. *Mycobacterium marinum* also causes infections of bones, joints, tendon sheaths especially in AIDS patients. *Mycobacterium smegmatis,* and more recently *Mycobacterium wolinskyi* and *Mycobacterium thermoresistible* have been reported to cause wound infection and also bacteraemia. *Mycobacterium terrae* complex *(Mycobacterium terrae, Mycobacterium nonchromogenicum* and *Mycobacterium triviale)* may be associated with mycobacterial disease. Also occasionally *Mycobacterium nonchromogenicum* and *Mycobacterium chelonae* have been identified as causes of acupuncture induced infections. *Mycobacterium septicum* a new rapidly growing species has been reported to be associated with catheter related bacteremia [49, 51, 57,58].

7.5 Lymphadenitis

Infection of the submaxillar, cervical, inguinal or preauricular lymph nodes is the most common presentation of NTM lymphadenitis. The involved lymph nodes are generally unilateral (95%) and not tender [54-57]. The nodes may enlarge rapidly, and even rupture, with formation of sinus tracts that result in prolonged local drainage. Other nodal groups outside of the head and neck may be involved occasionally. Distinguishing tuberculous from nontuberculous lymphadenitis is key because the former requires drug therapy and public health tracking, whereas the latter does not. A definitive diagnosis of NTM lymphadenitis is made by recovery of the causative organism form lymph node cultures. A simple diagnostic biopsy or incision and drainage of the involved lymph nodes should be avoided, since most of these procedures will be followed by fistulae formation with chronic drainage. However, even with excised nodes with compatible histopathology, only about 50% will yield positive cultures, because in some case these smear-positive, culture-negative cases may be due to fastidious species such as *Mycobacterium haemophilum* or *Mycobacterium genavence*. Approximately 80% of culture-proven cases of NTM lymphadenitis are due to MAC. It´s predominance is due to a change approximately from 20-30 years ago, when most geographic areas reported *Mycobacterium scrofulaceum* as the most common etiologic agent, only about 10% of the culture-proved mycobacterial cervical lymphadenitis in children is due to *Mycobacterium avium* complex and *Mycobacterium scrofulaceum*. Also *Mycobacterium haemophilum*, *Mycobacterium malmoense*, *Mycobacterium fortuitum* and others have been isolated from cases of lymphadenitis including HIV patients. In contrast, in adults more than 90% of the culture-proven mycobacterial lymphadenitis is due to *Mycobacterium tuberculosis* [8, 67, 70-76].

7.6 Disseminated disease in immunocompromized individuals

Disseminated disease due to NTM in AIDS patients usually occurs only in those with very advanced immunosuppressant, because these patients frequently have other complications, the diagnosis of mycobacterial infection may be confused or delayed. The diagnosis is exceedingly rare in person with >100 CD4 cells, and it should usually be suspected only in persons with <50 CD4 cells [53]. MAC have been found to be more commonly isolated from HIV-positive and HIV-negative patients, in their the portal of entry mainly through the gut [31] [67,69]. Persistent high grade fever, night sweats, anemia and weight loss in addition to nonspecific symptoms of malaise, anorexia, diarrhoea, myalgia and occasional painfuladenopathy are common signs and symptoms associated with MAC disease in AIDS cases. Others pulmonary and extrapulmonary mycobacterial infections in AIDS patients are for *Mycobacterium kansasii* , *Mycobacterium scrofulaceum*, *Mycobacterium xenopi*, *Mycobacterium simiae*, *Mycobacterium fortuitum-Mycobacterium chelonei* complex, *Mycobacterium malmoense*, *Mycobacterium szulgai*, and more recently *Mycobacterium genavense*, *Mycobacterium haemophilum* and *Mycobacterium celatum* [74-82].

8. Identification of nontuberculous mycobacteria

Traditional identification of NTM, as well as *Mycobacterium tuberculosis*, has relied upon statistical probabilities of presenting a characteristic reaction pattern in battery biochemical test. The niacin test was the most useful for separating NTM and *Mycobacterium tuberculosis* because the former is usually negative, whereas isolates of *Mycobacterium tuberculosis* are positive. Runyon devised the first good scheme for grouping NTM based on growth rates and colony pigmentation. For the diagnostic of NTM is very important to know the growth rates and colony pigmentation, and biochemical test such as, niacin production, nitrate reduction, tween-80 hydrolysis, arylsulphatase, urease, tellurite reduction, catalase qualitative and quantitative, grown on MaConkey agar, sodium chloride tolerance, etc, are adequate to identify majority of clinically relevant mycobacteria. This strategy is very necessary and important for the diagnostic of NTM, however, some time consuming and is not conclusive for many isolates with variable characters. For this reason others alternative diagnostic techniques are recommended, for example, the analysis of the mycolic acids of mycobacteria by thin layer chromatography (TLC) and high performance liquid chromatography (HPLC), and more recently the identification and characterization of NTM by molecular methods, based on new knowledge about the gene sequences of mycobacteria many gene probes for the identification of isolates as well as amplification of specific gene fragments from the lesions and mycobacterial culture isolates have been developed; gene probes, polymerase chain reaction (PCR) techniques, DNA fingerprinting techniques, etc, [35-40, 43,44,48, 83, 84]

9. *Mycobacterium tuberculosis* and nontuberculous mycobacteria diseases in the HIV/AIDS patients

After years of worldwide decline of tuberculosis (TB), this disease has returned as a big problem in the Public Health. The resurgence of TB in the past decades is closely linked to acquired immunodeficiency syndrome (AIDS) pandemic. The high susceptibility of patients infected with the human immunodeficiency virus (HIV) to TB and others mycobacterial infections is unique, creating a lot of diagnostic and therapeutic challenges for clinicians [12,32,24]. Pulmonary tuberculosis is the most common manifestation of tuberculosis in adults infected with HIV [53,85,86].

HIV/TB co-infection occurs in various stages of HIV infection, with the clinical pattern correlating with the patient's immune status. In the early stages of HIV infection, when immunity is only partially compromised, the features are more typical of tuberculosis, commonly with upper lobe cavitations, and the disease resembles that seen in the pre-HIV era. HIV-infected patients present with atypical pulmonary disease due to immune deficiency advances, resembling primary tuberculosis or extra pulmonary and disseminated disease, commonly with hilar adenopathy and lower lobe infection [87].

9.1 Clinical symptoms in pulmonary tuberculosis
The clinical symptoms are severally similar in HIV-infected and HIV-negative patients. However, cough is reported less frequently by HIV-infected patients, probably because there is less cavitations, inflammation and endobronchial irritation as a result of a reduction in cell-mediated immunity. Similarly, haemoptysis, which results from caseous necrosis of the bronchial arteries, is less common in HIV-infected patients [87,88].

In general, the traits that characterize HIV-TB co-infection include the potential for rapid progression from primary infection to disseminated disease, atypical radiographic features of pulmonary disease, increased frequency of extrapulmonary disease and involvement of unusual sites of infection. All of these atypical features seem to occur more commonly with more advance stages of immunosuppression and the paradigm that emerges is one of typical TB early in the course of HIV infection and atypical manifestation with advanced HIV disease, in this case the atypical features included lower lobe alveolar opacities, multifocal alveolar opacities, interstitial infiltrates, mediastinal adenopathy and pleural effusions [24,30,67,69,89].

9.2 Clinical symptoms in extrapulmonary tuberculosis

The main manifestation of extrapulmonary tuberculosis in AIDS patients are lymphadenopathy, pleural effusion, meningitis, pericardial effusion and miliary tuberculosis. This diagnostic is often difficult because the patients with HIV are prone to all of the usual bacterial and viral infection that affect a non-HIV infected patients, so, the presentation of extrapulmonary tuberculosis in HIV-infected patients is generally no different [8, 69].

9.3 Nontuberculous mycobacterial infection in HIV/AIDS patients

The clinical relevant of NMT infection in HIV/AIDS patients are very frequent, this infection can be pulmonary and extrapulmonary and their symptoms are the same that *Mycobacterium tuberculosis* [51-54, 69]. Recently, the nontuberculous mycobacterial are also denominated as environmental opportunist mycobacterial. Normally, they live as environmental saprophytes and they cause opportunist disease in human. Many cases of NTM are associated with some form of immune deficiency in special HIV/AIDS patients. In this group of patients is frequently to find this mycobacterial species as etiological agent for this reason is very important their microbiology diagnostic which is different to *Mycobacterium tuberculosis* [90, 91].

Disseminate *Mycobacterium avium complex* (MAC) diseases was one of the first opportunist infections recognized in the syndrome of AIDS since 20 years ago. The interest of the diagnostic of disseminated MAC and others species of nontuberculous mycobacteria infection have been increased as a result of the HIV pandemic. The prevention and treatment in nontuberculous mycobacteria are life long because cure of them were not achievable in AIDS patients with profound immune suppression. The precise immune defect predisposing HIV/AIDS patients to disseminated diseases is unknown [92].

The main manifestation of pulmonary and extrapulmonary infections for *Mycobacterium tuberculosis* and nontuberculous mycobacterial are the same affecting lung, pleura, skin, lymphatic system and producing dissemination infection (**Figure 1, Figure 2**), (**Figure 3A-3B-3C, Figure 4A-4B**) [8, 63,69]. For this reason is very important the highly active antiretroviral therapy (HAART) for treatment of AIDS patients that has been associated with a market reduction in the incidence of most opportunistic infection [82,89,92].

So, is very important that the mycobacteriology laboratory should give a definitive diagnostic, because in immunosuppressed patients is important to find resistant alcohol acid bacillus in order to detect the co-infection with *Mycobacterium tuberculosis* which is the most frequently agent found. Nevertheless, others species of mycobacteria may be causing infection and should be search for.

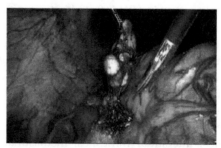

Fig. 1. Messenteric lymph nodes for *Mycobacterium tuberculosis* in AIDS patients.

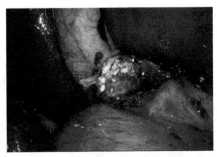

Fig. 2. Biopsy of liver pedicle lymph nodes for *Mycobacterium tuberculosis* in AIDS patients.

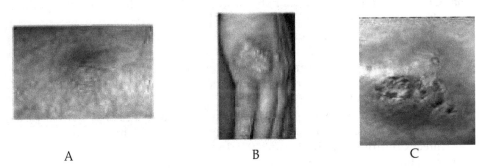

Fig. 3. AIDS patients with skin lesions from *Mycobacterium avium complex* (**Figure 3A, Figure 3B**) and *Mycobacterium fortuitum* (**Figure 3C**)

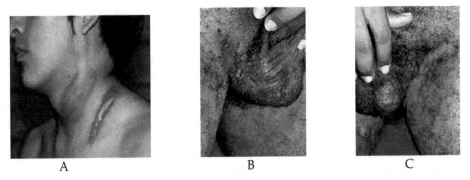

Fig. 4. Lymphadenitis cervical from *Mycobacterium tuberculosis* (**Figure 4A**), inguinal-testes lesions from *Mycobacterium avium complex* in lymphatic system (**Figure 4B, Figure 4C**).

10. References

Center for Disease Control and Prevention. A strategic plan for the elimination of tuberculosis from the United States. MMWR 1989;38 (Suppl No. S-3).

American Thoracic Society and Center for Disease Control and Prevention. Treatment of tuberculosis and tuberculosis infection in adults and children. Am J Respir Crit Care Med1994;149:1359-1374.

Center for Disease Control and Prevention, National Center for HIV, STD, and

TB Prevention Division of Tuberculosis Elimination. Trans mission and Pathogenesis of Tuberculosis. CDC 1995:8-19.

Center for Disease Control and Prevention. Tuberculosis elimination revisited: obstacles, opportunities, and renewed commitment. MMWR 1999;48(No. RR-9).

Benedek TG. The history of gold therapy for tuberculosis. J Hist Med Allied Sci 2004; 59: 50-89.

Daniel TM. The history of tuberculosis. Respir Med 2006; 100: 1862-70.

Hutton MD, Stead WW, Cauthen GM, Bloch AB, Ewing WM. Nosocomial transmission of tuberculosis associated with a draining abscess. J Infect Dis 1990;161:286-295.

Kumar V, Abbas AK, Fausto N, Aster JC. Robbins and Cotran, Pathologic basis of disease. Professional Edition, Eigth Edition, Ed Saunders/Elsevier 2010;Chapter 8: 366-372.

Cosma CL, Sherman DR, Ramakrishnan L. The secret lives of the pathogenic Mycobacteria. Annu Rev Microbiol 2003;57:641-671.

Lundgren R, Norrman E, Asberg I. Tuberculosis infection transmitted at autopsy. Tubercle 1987;68:147-150.

Tuberculosis and Human Immunodeficiency Virus Infection: Recommendations of the Advisory Committee for the Eliminations of Tuberculosis (ACET). MMWR Morb Mortal Wkly Rep 1989;23:250-4.

Ussery XT, Bierman JA, Valway SE. Transmission of multidrug-resistant *Mycobacterium tuberculosis* among persons exposed in a medical examiner's office, New York. Infect Control Hosp Epidemiol 1995;16:160-165.

Selwyn PA, Hartel D, Lewis VA. A prospective study of the risk of tuberculosis among intravenous drug users with human immunodeficiency virus infection. N Engl J Med 1989;320:545-550.

Selwyn PA, Sckell BM, Alcabes P. High risk of active tuberculosis in HIV-infected drugs users with cutaneous anergy. JAMA 1992;268:504-509.

Rieder HL, Snider DE Jr, Cauthen GM. Extrapulmonary tuberculosis lymphadenitis in the United States. Am Rev Respir Dis 1990;141:347-51.

Shriner KA, Mathisen GE, Goetz MB. Comparison of mycobacterial lymphadenitis among persons infected with human immunodeficiency virus and seronegative controls. Clin Infect Dis 1992;15:601-5.

Artesntein AW, Kim JH, Williams WJ, Chungg RC. Isolated peripheral tuberculous lymphadenitis in adults: current clinical and diagnostic issues. Clin Infect Dis 1995; 20:876-82.

Rojas A, La Cruz H, Salinas P, Rangel D, Hernández M. Adenitis tuberculosa inguinal. Reporte de um caso. MedULA, 2006;15:37-9.

Al Soub H, Al Alousi FS, Al-Khal AL. Tuberculoma of the cavernous sinus. *Sand J Infect Dis* 2001; 33: 868-70.

Donald PR. Schoeman JF. Tuberculous Meningitis. *Tehe New England Journal of Medicine* 2004; 351:1719-1720.

Karande S, Gupta V, Kulkarni M. Tuberculous Meningitis and HIV. *Indian Journal of Pediatric* 2005;72:7-9.

Kaplan JB, Masur H, Holmes KK. Guidelines for preventing opportunistic infections among HIV infected persons. Recommendations of the US Public Health Service and the Infectious Diseases Society of America MMWR 2002;51(RR-8):1-52.

Mederos LM, Banderas JF, Valdés L, Capó V, Fleites G, Martínez MR, Montoro EH. Meningitis y diseminación tuberculosa en paciente con el síndrome de inmunodeficiencia humana (sida). AVFT 2010;29:35-38.

Rieder HL, Cauthen GM, Comstock GW, Snider DE. Epidemiology of tuberculosis in the Unites States. Epidemiol Rev 1989;11:79-98.

Center for Disease Control and Prevention, National Center for HIV, STD, and TB Prevention Division of Tuberculosis Elimination. Epidemiology of Tuberculosis. CDC 1995:3-23.

Center for Disease Control and Prevention. Tuberculosis morbility- United States, 1996. MMWR 1997;46:695-70.

World Health Organization, Geneva. Toman´s Tuberculosis. Case detection, treatment, and monitoring: questions and answers. Ed. Frieden T, Second Edition, 2004.

Department of Health and Human Services, Center for Disease Control and Prevention, Center for Disease Control and Prevention, National Center for HIV, STD, and TB Prevention Division of Tuberculosis Elimination. Core Curriculum on Tuberculosis. CDC, Fourth Edition, 2000: 15-21.

World Health Organization. WHO Report. Global Tuberculosis Control. Surveillance, Planning, Financing, 2005.

American Academic of Pediatrics. Tuberculosis. In: Peter G, ed. 1997 Red Book: Report of the Committee on Infectious Diseases. 24 th ed. Elk Grove Village, IL: American Academy of Pediatrics;1997:541-563.

Center for Disease Control and Prevention. Prevention and treatment of tuberculosis among patients infected with human immunodeficiency virus: principles of therapy and revised recommendations. MMWR 1998;47(No. RR-20).

Jain A, Mondal R. Extensively drug-resistant tuberculosis: current challenges and threats. FEMS Immunol Med Microbiol 2008;53:145-150.

Jassal M, Bishai WR. Extensively drug-resistant tuberculosis. www.thelancet.com/infection Vol 9, January 2009.

Cohen R, Muzaffar S, Capellan J, Azar H, Chinikamwala M. The validity of classic symptoms and chest radiographic configurations in predicting pulmonary tuberculosis. Chest 1996;109:420-23.

Kent PT, Kubica GP. Public Health Mycobacteriology. A Guide for the Level III Laboratory. Department of Health and Human Services, Public Health Service, Centers for Disease Control, Atlanta, Georgia, 1985: 21-27.

Tenover FC, Crawford JT, Huebner RE, Geiter LJ, Horsburgh LR, Good RC. The resource of tuberculosis: Is your laboratory ready?. J Clin Microbiol 1993:31:767-770.

Crawford JT. New Technologies in the diagnosis. Semin Respir Infect 1994;9:62-70.

Shinnick TN, Good RC. Diagnostic mycobacteriology laboratory practices. Clin Infect Dis 1995;21:291-9.

Organización Panamericana de la Salud. Manual para el diagnostic bacteriológico de la Tuberculosis. Normas y Guía Técnicas. Parte II, Cultivo, 2008.

Ruiz P, Zerolo FJ, Casal M. Comparison of susceptibility of *Mycobacterium tuberculisis* using the ESP Culture System II with that using the BACTEC Method. J Clin Microbiol 2000;38:4663-4664.

Valero-Guillén PL, Martín-Luengo F, Larsson L, Jiménez J, Juhlin I, Portaels F. Fatty and mycolic acids of *Mycobactarium malmoense* . L Clin Microbiol 1988;26:153-154.

Leite CQF, Souza CWO, Leite SRA. Identification of Mycobacteria by thin layer chromatographic analysis of mycolic acid and conventional biochemical method: Four years of experience. Mem Inst Oswaldo Cruz 1998;93:801-805.

Mederos LM, Frantz JL, Perovani MA, Sardiñas M, Montoro EH. Identificación de Micobacterias no tuberculosas en pacientes VIH/SIDA por métodos convencionales y de fracciones de ácidos micólicos. Rev Soc Venezolana de Microbiología 2007;27:50-53.

Forbes SA, Hicks KE. Direct detection of *Mycobacterium tuberculosis* in respiratory specimens in clinical laboratory by polymerase chain reaction. J Clin Microbiol 1993;31:1688.

Noordhoek GT, Kolk AH, Bjune G et al. Sensitivity and specificity of PCR for detection of *Mycobacterium tuberculosis*: a blind comparison study among seven laboratories. J Clin Microbiol 1994;32:277.

Franco-Alvarez F, Ruiz P, Gutierrez J, Casal M. Evaluation of the GenoType Mycobacteria Direct Assay for detection *Mycobacterium tuberculosis* complex and Four Atypical Mycobacterial Species in clinical samples. J of Clin Microbiol 2006;44:3025-3027.

Wolinsky E. Nontuberculous mycobacteria and associated disease. Am Rev Respir Dis 1979;119:107-159.

Wallace RJ Jr, O´Brein R, Glassroth J, Raleigh J, Dutta A. Diagnosis and treatment of disease caused by nontuberculous mycobacteria. Am Rev Respir Dis 1990;142:940- 953.

DeVita VT, Hellman S, Rosenberg SA. AIDS Etiology, Diagnosis, Treatment and Prevention. Fourth Edition, Chapter: Tuberculosis and Human Inmmunodeficiency Virus Infection 1997: 245-257, Lippincott-Raven Publishers, Philadelphia, New York.

Murphy SM, Brook G, Birchall MA. HIV Infection and AIDS. Churchill Livinsgstone-ELSEVIER, Second Edition, Chapter: Tuberculosis 2000: 23-24, 63,71,119-120.

Katoch VM. Infections due to non-tuberculous mycobacteria (NTM). Indian J Med Res 2004;120:290-304.

García-Río I, Fernádez-Peñas P, Fernández-Herrera J, Gracía-Díez A. Infección cutánea por *Mycobacterium chelonae*. Revisión de seis casos. Clin Microbiol & Infection 2002;8:125-127.

Guía Práctica Clínica de Dermatología Tropical. Colegio Ibero Latinoamericano de Dermatología (CILAD), Madrid, J´Editor Prof. Vilata JJ, Editora ¨adalia¨ , 2009; Capítulo ¨Micobacteriosis Atípica¨: 11-14.

Saggese D, compadretti GC, Burnelli R. Nontuberculous mycobacterial adenitis in children: Diagnostic and therapeutic management. Am J Otolaryngol 2003; 24:79-84.

Panesar J, Higgins K, Daya H, Forte V, Allen U. Nontuberculous mycobacterial cervical adenitis: a ten-year retrospective review. Laryngoscope 2003; 113:149-54.

Barr KL, Lowe L, Su LD. *Mycobacterium marinum* infection simulating interstitial granuloma annulare: a report of two case. Am J Dermatopathol 2003;25:148-151.

American Thoracic Society. Diagnosis and treatment of disease cause by nontuberculous mycobacteria. Am J Respir Crit Care Med 1997;156:S1-19.

Moore JE, Kruijshaar ME, Ormerod LP, Drobniewski F, Abubakar I. Increasing reports of non-tuberculous mycobacteria in England, Wales and Norther Ireland, 1995-2006. BMC Public Health 2010;10:612, Article URL: http://www.biomedcentral.com/1471-2458/10/612.

O'Brien RJ, Geiter LJ, Snider Jr. DE. The epidemiology of nontuberculous mycobacterial diseases in the United States. Results from a national survey. Am Rev Respir Dis 1987;135:1007-1014.

Tsukamura, M, Kita N, Shimoide H, Arakawa H, Kuze A. Studies on the epidemiology of nontuberculous mycobacteriosis in Japan. Am Rev Respir Dis 1988;137:1280-1284.

Frappier-Davignon L, Fortin R, Desy M. Sensitivity to "atypical" mycobacteria in high school children in two community health departments. Canadian J of Public Health 1989;80:335-338.

Sackett DL. Bias in analytic research. J Chronic Dis 1979;32:51-63.

de Armas Y, Capó V, González I, Mederos LM, Díaz R, de Waard JH, Rodríguez A, García Y, Cabanas R. Concomitant *Mycobacterium avium* infection and Hodgkin's disease in lymph node from an HIV-negative child. Pathol Oncol Res 2011;17:139-140.

Marras TK, Daley CL. Epidemiology of human pulmonary infection with nontuberculous mycobacteria. Clin Chest Med 2002;23:553-567.

Chakrabarti A, Sharma M, Dubey ML. Isolation rates of different mycobacterial species from Chandinarh (north India). Indian J Res 1990;111-4.

Levy-Frebaulth V, Pangon B, Bure A, Katima C, Marche C, David HL. *Mycobacterium simiae, Mycobacterium avium-intrecellulare* mixed infection in AIDS. J Clin Microbiol 1987;25:154-157.

Wagner D, Young LS. Nontuberculous mycobacterial infections: a clinical review. Infection. 2004; 130: 257-70.

Gupta AK, Nayar M, Chandra M. Critical appraisal cytology of fine needle aspiration cytology in tuberculosis lymphadenitis. Acta Cytol 1992;36:391-94.

Ioachim HL, Medeiros LJ. Lymph Node Pathology. 2009;Chapter 21- Section III:130-135, and Chapter 23-Section III:137-143, Fourth Edition, Lippincott William & Wilkins, Wolters Kluwer Health.

Mederos LM, González D, Pérez D, Paneque A, Montoro EH. Linfadenitis causada por *Mycobacterium malmoense* en paciente infectado con el virus de inmunodeficiencia humana. Rev Chil Infect 2004;21: 229-31.

Mederos LM, González D, Montoro EH. Linfadenitis ulcerativa por *Mycobacterium fortuitum* en un paciente con sida. Enferm Infecc Microbiol Clin 2005;23:573-77.

Mederos LM, Rodríguez ME, Mantecón B, Sardiñas M, Montoro EH. Adenitis submaxilar en niño causada por *Mycobacterium fortuitum* . Folia Dermatológica Cubana 2007;1:6-10.

Nightingale SD, Byrd LT, Southern PM, Jockusch JD, Cal SX, Wynne BA. Incidence of *Mycobacterium avium-intracellulare*complex in humans immunodeficiency virus- positive patients. J Infetc Dis 1990;165:1082-1085.

Horsburgh CR. *Mycobacterium avium* complex in deficiency syndrome infection in the acquired immuno. N Engla J Med 1991;324:1332-1338.

Maloney JM, Gregg CM, Stephens DS, Manian FA, Rimland D. Infections caused by *Mycobacterium szulgai* in human. Rev Infect Dis 1987;9:1120-1126.

Corti M, Palmero D. *Mycobacterium avium* complex infection in HIV/AIDS patients. Expert Rev Anti Infect Ther 2008;6:351-563.

Mederos LM, Pomier O, Trujillo A, Fonseca C, Montoro EH. Micobacteriosis sistémica por *Mycobacterium avium* en paciente con SIDA. AVFT 2009;28:61-63.

Lawn SD, Checkley A, Wansbrough MH. Acute bilateral parotiditis caused by *Mycobacterium scrofulaceum*: immune reconstruction disease in a patient with AIDS. Sex Trasm Infect 2005;5:361-73.

Botteger EC, Teske A, Kirschner P, Bost S, Chang HR, Beer V. Disseminated *Mycobacterium genavense* infection in patients with AIDS. Lancet 1992;340:76-80.

Dever LL, Martin JWm Seaworth B, Jorgense JH. Varied presentation and responses to treatment of infections caused by *Mycobacterium haemophilum* in patients with AIDS. Clin Infect Dis 1992;32:1195-2000.

Jones D, Havlir DV. Nontuberculous mycobacteria in the HIV infected patient. Clin in Chest Med 2002;23: 312-24.

Olalla J, Pombo M, Aguado JM, Rodríguez E, Palenque E, Costa JR, Riopérez. *Mycobacterium fortuitum* complex endocarditis-case report and literature review. Clin Microbiol & Infect 2002;8:197-201.

Casal MM, Casal M. Las micobacterias atípicas como patógenos emergentes. Enf Emerg 2000;2:220-230.

Zumla A, Grange J. Infection and disease caused by environmental mycobacteria. Curr Opin Pulm Med 2002;8:166-172.

Lanjewar DN, Duggal RP. Pulmonary pathology in patients with AIDS: an autopsy study from Mumbai. HIV Med 2001; 2:266-271.

Escombe AR, Moore DA, Gilman RH, Pan W, Navincova M, Ticona E, Martínez C, Caviedes L, Sheen P, Gonzalez A, Noakes CJ, Friedland JS, Evans CA. The Infectiousness of Tuberculosis Patients Coinfected with HIV. PLoS Med 2008;5: 188.

Nunes EA, De Capitani EM, Coelho E, Panunto AC, Joaquim AO, Ramos Mde C. *Mycobacterium tuberculosis* and nontuberculous mycobacterial isolates among patients with recent HIV infection in Mozambique. J Bras Pneumol 2008;34:822-828.

Buchacz K, Baker RK, Palella FJ, Chmiel JS, Lichtenstein KA, Novak RM, Wood KC, Brooks JT. AIDS-defining opportunistic illnesses in US patients, 1994-2007: a cohort study. AIDS 2010; 10:1549-1459.

Browth-Elliot BA, Griffith DE, Wallace RJ. Diagnosis of nontuberculous mycobacterial infections. Clin Lab Med 2002;22:911-915.

Catanzaro A. Diagnosis, differentiating colonization, infection, and disease. Clin Chest Med 2002;23:599-601.

Horsburgh CJJr, Selik RM. Th epidemiology of disseminated nontuberculous mycobacterial infectio in the Acquired Immunodeficiency Syndrome (AIDS). Am Rev Respir Dis 1989;99:1-132.

Dos Santos RP, Scheid K, Goldani LZ. Disseminated nontuberculous mycobacterial disease in patients with acquired immune deficiency syndrome in the south of Brazil. Trop Doct 2010;40:211-213.

8

Human Immunodeficiency Virus Transmission

Goselle Obed Nanjul[1, 2]
[1]*School of Biological Sciences, Bangor University*
[2]*Applied Entomology and Parasitology Unit, Department of Zoology, University of Jos,*
[1]*UK*
[2]*Nigeria*

1. Introduction

Human Immunodeficiency Virus (HIV) is the causative organism of AIDS which has become one of the greatest public health challenges faced by mankind. AIDS was first identified in 1981 in Los Angeles, USA. Two types of HIV exist presently- HIV-1 and HIV-2 (Alizon et al., 2010; Adoga et al., 2010). HIV-1 was first isolated in the early 1980s (Barre-Sinoussi et al., 1983) and linked as causative agent of AIDS (Gallo et al., 1984). HIV-2 which is similar to HIV-1 was later identified in the developing world (Clavel, 1987, Clavel et al., 1986), but found to be less virulent and can differ in its response to antiretroviral agents. HIV-1 is classified into three groups [M, N and O] based on the genetic diversity. Group M (major) has 10 subtypes (A-J), and Group O (outlier) represents a number of highly divergent strains (Carr et al., 1998; Jassens et al., 1997 Chen et al., 2010). Francois Simon and his group reported a group N of HIV-1. Despite the phenotypic classification of HIV-1 into subtypes, the number of sequenced isolates remains limited (Sharp et al., 1994). Both strains are spread in the same way and have the same AIDS causing consequences. While HIV-1 has been reported to have a shorter incubation period of 7-10years, HIV-2 is considerably longer and often less severe (Barre-Sinoussi, 1996; WHO, 1989).

HIV infection is usually followed by a chronic progressive destruction of the immune and neurologic system (Price, 1996), which if not managed leads to the possible invasion and establishment of multiple opportunistic infections.(Lindo et al., 1998; Pozio et al., 1997) and malignancy (Schulz et al., 1996). Although on average, an infected individual spends several years without manifesting the disease, AIDS has always been certain. The time from infection to AIDS varies widely between individuals, from a few months to as many as 20 years with existing evidences accepting that 50% of individuals progress to AIDS in 7-10years and this has been accepted as the incubation period of the virus (Del Amo et al., 1998; WHO, 1994).

2. Portals of HIV transmission

The concentration of virus in a body fluid and the extent of exposure to body fluids determine to a great extent the transmission of a virus. Jaffe and McMahon-Pratt (1983) first indicated in their Epidemiological studies conducted in 1981 and 1982 that the major channel of transmission of AIDS were intimate sexual contact and contaminated blood. Gottlieb et al (1981); Masur et al (1981); Siegal et al (1981); Callazos et al (2010); van

Griensven and de Lin van Wijngaarden (2010) all described the syndrome in homosexual and bisexual men and, intravenous drug users, while Harris et al (1983); Padian et al (1991); Cameron et al (1989); Quinn et al (2000) and Decker et al (2010) recognised their mode of transmission through heterosexual activity. Evidences later showed that transmission recipients and haemophiliacs could contract the illness from blood or blood products (CDC, 1982; Peterson, 1992; CDC, 2010) and newborn infants get infected from their mothers' (Ammann et al., 1983; Scarlatti, 1996; Brookmeyer, 1991; Landesman, et al., 1996; Goedert et al., 1989; Mackelprang et al., 2010). Brookmeyer (1991); Stoneburner et al (1990) all agreed that the three principal means of transmission – blood, sexual contact and mother-to-child have not changed which could be attributed to a greater degree to the relative amount of the virus in various body fluids.

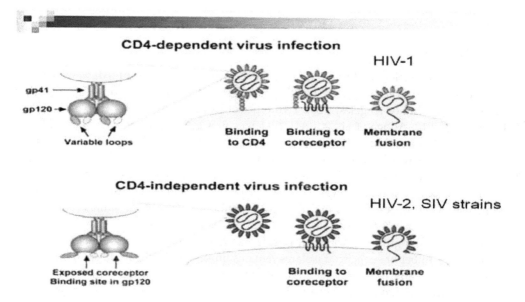

Fig. 1. Diagrammatic representation of HIV-1 and HIV-2 showing their dependent and independence on CD4+ [Courtesy-]

HIV is present in semen (including pre-seminal fluid), vaginal/cervical secretions and blood, breast milk expressed through feeding; organ donations; sharing infected objects (needles, tattoos and piercing) which are the main vehicles through which the virus is transmitted (Kim et al., 2010; Yu et al., 2010; Suligoi et al., 2010; Pruss et al., 2010 and Baggaley et al., 2010). The virus may also be present in saliva, tears, urine, cerebrospinal fluid and infected discharges, but these are not vehicles of which HIV is spread. Epidemiological survey do not support transmission through water or food, sharing eating utensils, coughing or sneezing, vomiting, toilets, swimming pools, insect bites, shaking of hands or other casual contacts, hence there is no public health reason for discrimination and or restrictions.

A study of French hospital patients by Grabar et al (2009) found that approximately 0.5% of HIV-1 infected individuals retain high levels of CD4+ T-cells and a low or clinically undetectable viral load without anti-retroviral treatment. These individuals are classified as HIV controllers or long-term non-progressors.

For conveniences, we will share the mode of infections into: Sexual and Non-sexual.

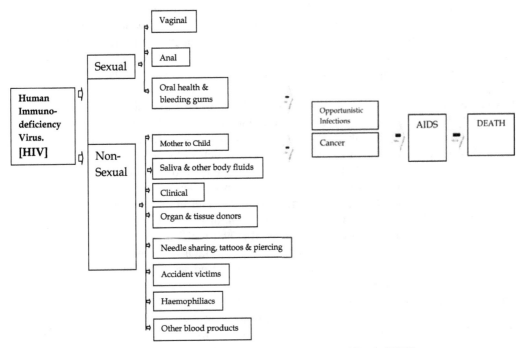

Fig. 2. Routes of Transmission of Human Immuno-deficiency Virus. [HIV]

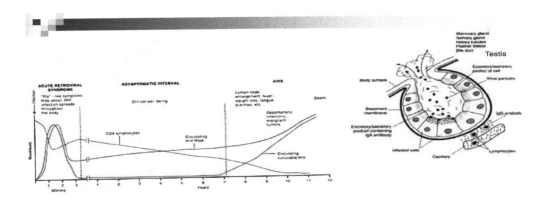

Low HIV plasma load,
but high semen load

Fig. 3. Levels of HIV load in semen [Courtesy:...]

3. Vertical or Mother To Child Tranmission (MTCT)

The major source of paediatric infection of Human immunodeficiency virus one (HIV-1) is from mother to child. Since the first reported case of HIV-1 transmission in children in 1983, the global pandemic has had a serious impact on the health and survival of children. Transmission rates have been reported to be about 14% in industrialised countries and about 35-45% in developing countries especially in Africa (Bryson, 1996; Reinhardt et al., 1995).

It was estimated that MTCT accounts for over 1.5million HIV infection in children (Burton, 1996) with the WHO projecting between 5-10million child infections through MTCT during the next decade. HIV-2 though is related to HIV-1 is less readily transmitted from mother to child, this could be attributed to their differences which influences pathogenecity, natural history and therapy so that their susceptibility to antiretroviral therapy (ART) follows different mutation pathways to develop drug resistance (Mamata and Merchant, 2010).

According to Wollinsky et al (1992) as quoted by Pasquier et al (1998), the transmission of HIV-1 from mother to child occur *utero, intrapartum*, or postnatally by breastfeeding and a fourth dimension as reported by Pasquier et al (1998) which involves the transmission of multiple maternal variants to the infant and a rapid, fatal outcome in the child and the development of an HIV-based clinical disease in children seems to be correlated with the timing of the vertical transmission.

Infection in about two-thirds of children are thought to have occurred at the terminal end of pregnancy or at delivery with the disease progressing slowly; while in one-thirds, it is thought to progress rapidly to AIDS with increased indices of viral replication (De Rossi et al., 1998), these children appear to have been infected during pregnancy.

Infected children with slow progression to AIDS have a higher viral diversity than children who progress rapidly as evidenced in molecular variability studies (Halapi et al., 1996; Strunnikora et al., 1995) as reported in Adults (Delwart et al., 1997; Pasquier et al., 1998).

Although progress has been made in recent years in the curbing of MTCT, the mechanisms and timing of transmission remains uncertain and the relative contributions of each of the three modes of transmission is still not well defined. Bryson et al (1992) proposed that in most non-breastfeeding population; the lack of detection of virus in the child at birth might indicate that contamination took place at or shortly before delivery while detection of virus at birth indicates *utero* contamination. Evidences for both early and late utero transmission have been documented (Peckham and Gibb, 1995; Kuhn and Stein, 1995). Most prior estimates and hypothesis seem to agree that transmission usually occur during the *intrapartum* HIV exposure just as premature infants.

Perinatal or *Antepartum* HIV transmission has been documented as a route of infection estimated to occur in 13-30% of infants delivered to HIV-1 infected mothers (Andiman et al., 1990).

High proviral DNA/ or RNA concentration of virus is a risk factor for the transmission of HIV-1 from an untreated mother to infant. The reduction in such transmission after zidovudine is only partly explained by the reduction in plasma levels of viral RNA. To prevent HIV-1 transmission initiating maternal treatment with zidovudine is recommended regardless of the plasma level of HIV-1 RNA or the CD4+ Count (Sperling et al., 1996). Because of the different mutation pathways to develop drug resistance, pregnant women with detectable HIV-2 should be ideally managed using a Highly Active antiretroviral therapy (HAART) regimen to which the virus is sensitive. Non-nucleoside Reverse

Transcriptase Inhibitor (NNRTIs) and Fusion Inhibitor Enfuvirtide have no activity against HIV-2 and in the light of the current albeit limited data, zidovudine mono-therapy should not be used. These factors make it crucial that proper selection of and adherence to the first antiretroviral combination regimen is in place in order to achieve a successful treatment response. Though of recent, a combination of Combivir and nevarapine is given to mothers to prevent transmission of HIV to children. The Emergency Lower Segment Caesarian Section (ELSCS) could be planned at 38 weeks of gestation with regards to the mode of delivery if the viral load is undetectable or the mother is either symptomatic or has low CD4 cell count. HIV is present in breast milk and postnatal transmission via breastfeeding is an important component of MTCT in Sub-Saharan Africa (Kreiss, 1997). World-wide, an estimated one in three of vertical transmission may be due to breastfeeding with above 12months of age carrying higher risk (Bulterys et al., 1995). Kuhn and Stein (1997) demonstrated that under certain conditions prevailing in specific settings in developing countries, breast feeding for six months would be preferable to breast feeding beyond this age. Breastfeeding has been reported to account for 5-15% of infants becoming infected with HIV-1 after delivery (ECS 1991; Ryder et al., 1989; Mok et al., 1989). Although the placental entry of some infections is a critical aspect of these infections, the role of placental cells and the mechanism by which pathogens pass from the maternal to the foetal circulation varies. The placenta provides a barrier that prevents transmission of some viruses, but allows others to reach the foetal circulation. Mother to foetus placental transmission of some viruses occurs through transcytosis across placental cells. The placenta may also act as a reservoir in which virus replicates before reaching the foetus. Placental transmission of HIV-1 is a complex incompletely understood process which requires advanced studies (Al-husaini, 2009). The antiretroviral therapy, zidovudine (ZDV) is metabolized into its active form in the placenta (Qian et al., 1994). ZDV inhibits HIV replication within placental cells. To reach the foetal circulation, HIV-1 should cross the trophoblastic placental barrier (cytotrophoblasts and syncitiotrophoblasts). Blood borne maternal pathogens that arrive at the uteroplacental circulation and intervillous space may reach the foetus through the villous capillaries. HIV-1 has been detected on both the maternal and the foetal parts of the placenta. HIV-1 experiences replication in the placenta. The virus may cross the trophoblastic barrier by endocytosis, or by an injured villous surface. However, superficial breaks in syncytiotrophoblast cells do not radically affect the vertical transmission of viruses (Burton et al., 1996). The reverse transcriptase enzyme of HIV-1 is important in the life cycle of the virus by converting the single-stranded RNA genome into double-stranded DNA that integrates into the host chromosome. There is a lower degree of viral heterogeneity in transmitting mothers compared with nontransmitting mothers (Sundaravaradan et al., 2005).

Human chorionic gonadotropin (hCG) has been shown in vitro to inhibit reverse transcriptase and to block viral transmission between virus-carrying lymphocytes and placental trophoblasts (Bourinbaiar and Lee-Huang, 1995). However, role of hCG in protecting the foetus from vertical transmission HIV-1 needs to be studied. In summary, the restricted heterogeneity of HIV-1 in the infected mothers is more likely associated with lack of vertical transmission (Al-husaini, 2009).

As access to services for preventing the mother-to-child transmission of HIV has increased, the total number of children being born with HIV has also decreased. An estimated 370 000 [230 000–510 000] children were newly infected with HIV in 2009 (a drop of 24% from five years earlier)[UNAIDS, 2010].

4. Risk factors for vertical transmission of HIV

Documented evidence primarily based on PCR and virus culture studies or co-culture studies but short of serology which revealed maternal antibodies present in infants at birth showed that transmission of HIV from mother to child appears to occur in 11-60% of children delivered by HIV-positive mothers but reasons for the wide variations in virus transmission and sources of virus in newborn which could have provided approach to prevention are not known (Ades et. al., 1991; Courgnaud et. al., 1991; Lindgren et. al., 1991; Newell et. al., 1992; Scarlatti et. al., 1991; Tovo and Martino, 1988; Oxtoby, 1990; Rogers et. al., 1991).

Maternal, viral, obstetric, foetal, infant factors all affect transmission making it essentially multifactorial. Frequency of sexual activity, 'hard' drug ingestion during pregnancy, unprotected sexual intercourse, cigarette smoking during pregnancy, lack of adherence to drugs, HIV disease, degraded maternal immunocompetence or prolonged rupture of the amniotic membranes before delivery (Havens et al., 1997; Turner et al., 1996; Bryson, 1996; John and Kreiss, 1996; Lambert, 1996; Glenn and Dietrich, 1993).

The maternal factors involve transmission through the placenta to the unborn child, at the time of labour and delivery, or through breast-feeding. (CDC HIV/AIDS surveillance, October, 1989), seroconversion during pregnancy, advanced stage of the disease with high viral load and low immunity, concomitant malnutrition, micronutrient deficiencies, sexually transmitted diseases, no or suboptimal therapy; in the intranatal period, risk factors for increased transmission are mode of delivery, prolonged contact with maternal blood or cervicovaginal secretions, prolonged rupture of membranes, chorioamnionitis, invasive procedures like episiotomy, foetal scalp electrode, instrumental delivery; thin skin, susceptible mucous membranes, immature immune functions and low levels of maternal antibodies make prematurity a risk factor for increased transmission. In the postnatal period, risk factors are breast feeding, feeding with cracked nipples/mastitis, mixed feeding, new seroconversion of the mother, high viral load, low CD4 cell count; In the absence of any intervention, rates of MTCT of HIV-1 can vary from 15 to 30% in developed countries and increase to 30 to 45% in developing countries, the difference mainly attributable to infant feeding practices that comprise almost universally of breastfeeds for prolonged duration (De Cock et al., 2000 as quoted by Mamata and Merchant, 2001).

The foetus and mother circulatory systems though different, there still exists tiny mixing of blood that could serve as portal for the flow of infected maternal white blood cells or the AIDS virus in the maternal serum to be transmitted to the foetus with a confirmation found in the foetal tissues affirming such spread (CDC HIV/AIDS surveillance, October 1989; Glenn and Dietrich, 1993).

Bruising, abrasions and local swelling could occur to the baby and mother during labour owing to a great deal of trauma which produces visible and microscopic openings that could allow the virus to penetrate blood stream of infant. Another means of infection could be experienced or seen when the mother's perineum tears or if she receives an episiotomy which might lead to a large amounts of blood ingested by the baby or might get into the baby's mouth, eyes, rectum or vagina.

Glenn et al (1993) reported that breastfeeding is another means of risks exposure and it has been confirmed in the spread of hepatitis B from mother to infant and hepatitis B and AIDS as well which are thought to occur when the infant ingests the mothers blood through a cracked and bleeding nipples.

Other known correlates include high maternal plasma viremia, advanced clinical HIV disease, degraded maternal immunocompetence or prolonged rupture of the amniotic membranes before delivery. Others include vaginal delivery process and prematurity of low birth weight of the neonate (Bryson, 1996; John and Kreiss, 1996; Lambert, 1996).

High frequency of sexual activity and "hard" drug injection during pregnancy had previously been identified, along with unprotected sexual intercourse during pregnancy as certain behavioural risk factors for mother-to-child-transmission (Bulterys et al., 1997; Bulterys and Goedert, 1996). Firstly, unprotected intercourse might increase the concentration of strain diversity of HIV-1, particularly in the birth canal where ejaculated virus could be partially sequestered. Secondly, frequent intercourse might increase inflammation of the cervix or vagina either micro abrasion or if unprotected, by STDs. Third, frequent intercourse might increase the risk of chorioamnionitis or otherwise alter the integrity of the placenta (Bulterys and Goedert, 1996). Matheson et al (1997) found that continued drug users had significantly higher mother-to-child-transmission rates in maternal drug use during pregnancy. However, this was confounded by other variables such as premature delivery, prolonged membrane rupture, zidovudine non-use and unprotected sexual intercourse.

In the USA, cigarettes' smoking during pregnancy has been identified as independent risk factor for mother-to-child-transmission. The effect was greatest among women with critical evidence of more advanced HIV disease (Turner et al., 1996). Intensive nurse care management in supporting zidovudine use in women with HIV infection and their infants is a proven effective method in decreasing mother-to-child-transmission (Havens et al., 1997).

MTCT of HIV is influenced by multiple factors. Known correlates include high maternal plasma viremia, advanced clinical HIV disease, degraded maternal immunocompetence or prolonged rupture of the amniotic membranes before delivery. Others include vaginal delivery process and prematurity of low birth weight of the neonate (Bryson 1996; John and Kreiss, 1996; Lambert, 1996).

Results from zidovudine therapy to bridge MTCT have improved understanding of the pathophysiology of MTCT. First, the reduction in plasma viremia and MTCT (from 25.5% to 8.3%) by treating the mother and neonates suggests that relatively small changes in maternal viral load might have substantial effects on MTCT (Bulterys and Godert 1996; CDC, 1994). Secondly, cleaning of birth canal with chlorhexidine had no overall effect yet apparently did reduce MTCT for one subgroups of high-risk deliveries; those after 4hrs of membrane rupture (Scarlatti, 1996).

Maternal immunologic and virologic factors such as quantitative HIV-1 RNA (though insufficient) are strongly correlated with Mother-to-child-transmission. When stratified by the stage of HIV disease, the only group with significant association between viral load and mother-to-child-transmission were AIDS-free women with high CD4+ Counts. The interactions of virus burden and maternal immune status has also demonstrated that CD4+, CD8+ cell subsets are percentages of CD8+ cell subsets (e.g. activation markers CD8/CD38 and CD8/DR) were all associated with vertical transmission. Women in the highest CD4+ cell percentage quartile or the lowest CD8+ cell percentage quartile had only less than or equal to 4 percent of mother-to-child-transmission (Njoku, 2004).

5. Parental, saliva and other body fluids

Prior to Groopman and Greenspan (1996) report of oral manifestation of AIDS which increases the potentials of HIV transmission through several lesions which form exists for virus into the saliva, it was assumed that about 10% of both free virus and infected cells report in saliva were not very important in the spread of HIV (Groopman et al., 1984).

Dean et al (1988) and Mundy et al (1987) reported none or low level of pathogens in urine, sweat, breast milk, branchoalvolar lavage fluid, amniotic fluid, synovial fluid, faeces and tears which were not thought to be important source in virus transmission (Fujikawa et al., 1985), but this assumption has also changed with the report of Groopman and Greenspan (1996); Amory et al. (1992); Scarlatti (1996); van da Perre et al. (1991). Though not a natural source of HIV transmission, cerebrospinal fluid (CSF) in neurologic patients have been shown to contain large amount of virus when compared to other body fluids (Hollander and Levy, 1987; Ho et al., 1989).

6. Organs, blood, tissue donors and occupational health workers

Prior to 1985 (PPHS/MMWR, 1985; MMWR, 1985), when screening of blood, organ and tissue donors for HIV-1 antibody became available, several reports have documented the transmission of HIV-1 by transplantation of kidney (MMWR, 1987; Kumar et al., 1987; Erice et al., 1991; Schwartz et al., 1987; Prompt et al., 1985; L'age-Stehr et al., 1985; Neumayer et al., 1987; Quarto et al., 1989; Carbone et al., 1988), liver (MMWR, 1987; Kumar et al., 1987; Erice et al., 1991; Schwartz et al., 1987; Prompt et al., 1985; L'age-Stehr et al., 1985; Neumayer et al., 1987; Quarto et al., 1989; Carbone et al., 1988; Samuel et al., 1988), heart (Erice et al., 1991; Dummer et al., 1989), pancreas (Erice et al., 1991), bone (MMWR, 1988a) and possibly skin(Clarke, 1987) and In most cases involving donors whose serum had not been tested for HIV-1 antibody (MMWR, 1987; Kumar et al., 1987; Erice et al., 1991; Schwartz et al., 1987; Prompt et al., 1985; L'age-Stehr et al., 1985; Neumayer et al., 1987; Quarto et al., 1989; Carbone et al., 1988; Samuel et al., 1988; Dummer et al., 1989; MMWR, 1988a; Clarke, 1987).

As proposed by Simonds et al (1992), approaches to prevention could include: the screening of prospective donors and laboratory markers for HIV1 infection (MMWR, 1985); the inactivation of HIV-1 in allograft through processing techniques (Hilfenhaus et al., 1990; Kitchen et al., 1989; Wells et al., 1986) and the quarantining of tissues from living donors until repeated antibody testing more definitely excludes the possibility of subsequent seroconversion in the donor (MMWR, 1988a ; MMWR, 1988b).

The U.S. Centers for Disease Control and Prevention (2002) reported that in the health care industry there have been 57 confirmed cases and an additional 139 possible cases of health care workers in the U.S. who have become HIV positive from exposure to HIV in the work place. The Canadian HIV/AIDS Legal Network (2001) has also reported two of such cases in the laboratory workers and one health-care provider in Canada.

7. Horizontal (heterosexual) transmission

These could be through unprotected and protected sexual process. Ma et al (2010) reported that the probability of unprotected heterosexual transmission may vary with population and be influenced by many factors, these could include: the type of sex (Mastro et al., 1994: De Vincenzi, 1994; Varghese et al., 2002); bleeding during intercourse (Royce et al., 1997), semen viral load (Gupta et al., 1997; Tachet et al., 1999; Kalichman et al., 2008; Butler et al., 2008), stage of HIV infection (Mastro et al., 1994; Fauci et al., 1996; Wawer et al., 2005), co-morbid sexually transmitted diseases (Royce et al., 1997), vaginal or anal canal, co-occurring psychosocial risk factors (Safren et al., 2010).

Sexual forms of transmission are seen as a major portal of entry of HIV as 10-30% of seminal/vaginal fluids have transmissible virus (Royce et al., 1997; Henin et al., 1993).

In semen viral load, the males HIV-1 infected cells forms about 10^4 of the 10^6 leucocytes per ejaculation (Winkelstein et al., 1987), which confirms AIDS first association with sexual route, with the high prevalence in homosexual men. The virus subsequently became synonymous with heterosexual activity and is now attributed to the AIDS pandemic (UNAIDS 1986; Nkowane 1991; Stoneburner et al., 1990). Bouvier et al (1997) believes that vaginal pH neutralization by semen is a co-factor of HIV transmission.

The chances of transmission also depends on the type of sexually transmitted infections (STI), as co-infection with genital ulcers have been reported to increase the chances of transmission by increasing the susceptibility to HIV infection which also depends on HIV subtypes efficient (Gray et al., 2001; Mahiane et al., 2009; Limpakarnianarat et al., 1993; Wang, 2009; Xu, 2009).

Male circumcision have been documented to decrease the chances of HIV transmission (Mahiane et al., 2009; Lavreys et al., 1999; Gray et al., 2000; Reynolds et al., 2004; Gray et al., 2007; Donoval et al., 2006), but this also depends on the country (Ben et al., 2008; Sullivan et al., 2009; Ruan et al., 2009; Wawer et al., 2009).

The high level of heterosexual spread of HIV in Sub-Saharan Africa and developing countries where genital ulcers from existing venereal diseases (e.g. Chanchroid Chlamydia, Syphilis or Herpes virus infections) are aligned with increased HIV seroprevalence (UNAIDS, 1998, Hook et al., 1992; Plummer et al., 1991) could be tight to abrasions at the site of entry in the vagina or anal canal. Heise et al (1991) however reported that HIV could directly infect the bowel mucosa and perhaps cervical epithelium without the need for ulcerations which gave clue to the relatively low risk of the mucosal lining of the foreskin, urethral canal and oral genital contact (through minimal) to be implicated (Winkelstein et al., 1987).

Men having Sex with Men (MSM) have been reported as one of the first way of transmission of HIV. Various authors have showed evidence that the involvement of MSM could be traced to psychosocial behaviour (PB). These PB are said to be depression, violent victimisation, substance abuse, alcohol, psychiatric disorders, psychological distress, lower perceived social support (Berlan et al., 2010; King et al., 2008; Meyer , 2003; Cochran et al., 2003; Cochran and Mays, 2000; Gilman et al., 2001., Marshal et al., 2008; Mimiaga et al., 2009a; b; Safren and Heimberg, 1999; Stall et al., 2001; Chesney et al., 2003; The EXPLORE Study Team, 2004; Herbst et al., 2005). Although some studies have shown how substance use and high risk of HIV transmission are correlated (Stall et al., 2001; Hirshfield et al., 2004), most recent studies are now focussing on how 'syndemic'- a situation where these diverse psychosocial issues could interact to enhance HIV risky behaviour among MSM (Mustanski et al., 2007; 2010; Stall et al., 2008; Centers for Disease Control and Prevention, 2010). However, varieties of cognitive behavioural interventions have been studied and validated for the treatment of mood and anxiety disorders (Barlow, 2008) behavioural activation therapy and HIV risk reduction counselling in MSM who abuse crystal methamphetamine (Mimiaga et al., 2010).

Addressing co-occurring psychosocial behaviour is a means to increase the effective size of current HIV prevention intervention and allow for more effective uptake by MSM, since they have been reported to be more than 44 times more likely to be newly diagnosed with HIV than other men (Purcell et al., 2010) and the focus on ameliorating disparities in HIV infection is essential for enhancing the health of MSM at the population level (Sanfren et al., 2010).

The Centers for Diseases Control and Prevention (CDC, 2007) reported the prevalence rate among heterosexual African American (AA) women and men with data indicating that more heterosexual AA women having a 74% HIV/AIDS prevalence as compared to the 27% in their male counterpart.

Myths and misperceptions of HIV/AIDS such as HIV being a genocide, suspicion of government information, belief that it is possible to identify risky partners by odour and appearance, belief that partners reported histories are accurate, misperceptions about the meaning of safe sex and the believe that specific classes of people (not one self) are at risk of HIV that resulted from sexual risk contributes to the risky behaviours of HIV transmission (Essien et al.,2002; Catania et al.,1994; Smith et al., 2000; Coleman et al., 2010; Coleman and Ball, 2007; Coleman, 2007).

The increase in the number of sexual partners also increases HIV transmission (Stranford, 1999; Coleman, 2007; Catania et al., 1994; Smith et al., 2000; Coleman et al., 2010; Coleman and Ball, 2007) with most under the influence of alcohol or drugs.

Unprotected oral and vaginal sex have been reported as a risk factor in the transmission of HIV especially where it is carried out in high risk settings, having sex more often under the influence of alcohol and/or drugs (Milam et al., 2006; Catania et al., 1994; Smith et al., 2000).

Even under protection for example the use of condoms, many cases has been reported where the barrier has failed especially where risky behaviours are undertaken. A case in study which made the People Living With HIV/AIDS (PLWHA) in Nigeria to sue the Federal Government of Nigeria to Court for promotion of condoms (Ogundele, 2010).

Though Tenofovir gel has been advocated for women to prevent HIV transmission (Karim et al., 2010).

The nature of HIV transmission from anecdotal records has not changed neither is a new means of transmission of the virus recorded. In view of this development, it is the earnest desire of this write up to bring to fore genealogical reports of the transmission of HIV and to also continue to write on the various modes of transmission as a way of curtailing the spread of the dreaded virus.

8. References

Adoga M .P., Nimzing, L., Mawak, J. D., Agwale, S. M. (2010). Human Immunodeficiency Virus Types 1 and 2: Sero-prevalence and Risk Factors Among a Nigerian Rural Population of Women of Child-bearing Age. *Shiraz E-Medical Journal* Vol. 11, No. 1: (29-33), Januar y, 2010. http://semj.sums.ac.ir/vol11/jan2010/87068.htm.

Ades, A.E., Newell, M.L., and Peckham, C.S., (1991). Children born to women with HIV-1 infection: natural history and risk of transmission. *Lancet*, 337: 253-260.

Andiman, W.A. et al. (1990). *American Journal of Diseases of Children*, 144:75.

Al-husaini, A.M. (2009). Role of placenta in the vertical transmission of HIV. *Journal of Perinatology*, 29:321-326.

Alizon, S., von Wyl, V., Stadler, T., Kouyos, D.R., Yerly, S., Hirschel, B., Boni, J., Shah, C., Klimkait, T., Furrer, H., Rauch, A., Vernazza, L. P., Bernasconi, E., Battegay, M., Burgisser, P., Telenti, A., Gunthard, F. H., Boenhoeffer, S., the Swiss HIV Cohort study (2010). Phylogenetic approach reveals that virus genotype largely determines HIV set-point viral load. *PLOS pathogens*, volume 6 issue 9, e1001123.

Ammann, A.J., Cowan, M.J., Wara, D.W., Weintrup, P., Dritz, S., Goldman, H. and Perkins, H.A. (1983). Acquired Immunodeficiency in an infant: possible transmission by means of blood products. *Lancet i:* 956-958.

Amory, J., Martin, N., Levy, J.A and Wara, W.W. (1992). The large molecular weight glycoprotein (MGI) a component of human saliva inhibits HIV-1 infectivity. *Clinical Research*, 40:51A (Abstract).

Andiman, W.A. et al. (1990). *American Journal of Diseases of Children*, 144:75.

Baggaley, R.F., White, R.G. and Boily, M. (2010). HIV transmission risk through anal intercourse: systematic review, meta-analysis and implifications for HIV prevention. *International Journal of Epidemiology*, 39: 1048-1063.

Barlow DH, ed. Clinical Handbook of Psychological Disorders: A Step-by-Step Treatment Manual. 4th ed. New York, NY: Guilford Press; 2008.

Barre-Sinoussi, F., Cherman, J.C., Rey, F., Nugeyre, M.T., Chamaret, S., Gruest, J., Dauguet, C., Axler-Blin, C., Vezinet-Brun, F., Rouzioux, W., Rozenbaum, W. and Montagnier, L. (1983). Isolation of a T-lymphotrophic retrovirus from a patient at risk for AIDS. *Science*, 220:868-871.

Barre-Sinoussi, F. (1996). HIV as the cause of AIDS. *Lancet*, 348:31-35.

Ben, K., Xu, J., Lu, L., Yao, J.P., Min, X.D., Li, W.Y., Tao, J., Wang, J., Li, J.J., Cao, X.M. (2008). Promoting male circumcision in China for preventing HIV infection and improving reproductive health. *National Journal of Andrology* 14(4), 291-297. (In Chinese-English version read).

Berlan, E.D., Corliss, H.L., Field, A.E., Goodman, E., Bryn Austin, S. (2010). Sexual orientation and bullying among adolescents in the Growing up Today Study. *Journal of Adolescence Health*; 46:366-371.

Brookmeyer, R. (1991). Reconstruction and future trends of the AIDS epidemic in the United States. *Science*, 253:37-42.

Bourinbaiar, A.S., Lee-Huang, S.(1995). Anti-HIV effect of beta subunit of human chorionic gonadotropin (beta hCG) in vitro. *Immunology Letters*; 44(1): 13-18.

Bouvier, P., Rougemont, A., Breslow, N., Doumbo, O., Delley, V., Dicko, A., Diakite, M.., Mauris, A., Robert, C. (1997). Seasonality and malaria in a West African village: does high parasite density predict fever incidence? *American Journal of Epidemiology*, 145:850-857.

Brabin, B.J. (1983). An analysis of malaria in pregnancy in Africa. *Bulletine of World Health Organisation*, 61:1005-1016.

Bryson, Y. J. (1996). Perinatal HIV-1 transmission: recent advances and therapeutic interventions. *AIDS*, 10:S33–S42.

Bryson, Y. J., Luzuriaga, K., Sullivan, J.L. and Wara, D.W. (1992). Proposed definitions for in utero versus intrapartum transmission of HIV-1. *New England Journal of Medicine*, 327:1246–1247.

Bulterys, M.., Chao, A., Dushimimana, A. and Saah, A. (1995). HIV-1 seroconversion after 20months of age in a cohort of breastfed children born to HIV-1 infected women in Rwanda (letter). *AIDS*, 9:93-94.

Bulterys, M. and Goedert, J.M. (1996). From biology to sexual behaviour-towards the prevention of mother to child transmission of HIV/AIDS. *AIDS*, 10:1287-1289.

Bulterys, M.., Landesman, S., Burns, D.N., Rubin-Stein, A. and Goedert, J.J. (1997). Sexual behaviour and injection drug use during pregnancy and vertical transmission of HIV-1. *Journal of Acquired Immunodeficiency Syndrome and Human Retrovirology*, 15:76-82.

Butler, D. M., Smith, D. M., Cachay E. R., Edward, R., Hightower, G. K., Nugent, C. T., Richman, D. D., Little, S. J. (2008). Herpes simplex virus 2 serostatus and viral loads of HIV-1 in blood and semen as risk factors for HIV transmission among men who have sex with men. *AIDS*, 22(13), 1667-1671.

Burton, G.J., O'Shea, S., Rostron, T., Mullen, J.E., Aiyer, S., Skepper, J.N., Smith, R. and Banatvala, J.E. (1996). Significance of placental damage in vertical transmission of human immunodeficiency virus. Journal of Medical Virology, 50: 237–243.

Catania, J. A., Coates, T. J., Golden, E., Dolcini, M. M., Peterson, J., Kegeles, S., Siegel, D., Fullilove, M.T. (1994). Correlates of condom use among Black, Hispanic, and White heterosexuals in San Francisco: The AMEN longitudinal survey. *AIDS Education and Prevention*, 6(1), 12–26.

Canadian HIV/AIDS Legal Network. (2001). Testing of persons believed to be the source of an accidental occupational exposure to HBV, HCV, or HIV: A backgrounder (Health Canada, Canadian Strategy on HIV/AIDS Information Sheet). Retrieved September 1, 2007, from http://www.aidslaw.ca/maincontent/issues/testing.htm.

Cameron, D.W., D'Costa, L.J., Maitha, G. M., Cheang, Piot, P., M., Simonsen, J.N., Ronald, A.R., Gakinya, M.N., Ndinya-Achola, J.L., Brunham, R.C. and Plummer, F.A. (1989). Female to male transmission of human immunodeficiency virus type 1: risk factors for seroconversion in men. *Lancet*, volume 334, issue 8660: 403-407.

Carr, J.K., Suleiman, M.O., Albert, J., Sanders-Buell, E., Gotte, D., Bird, D.L. and McCutchan, F.E. (1998). Full genome sequences of HIV-1 subtypes G and A/G heterotype recombinants. *Journal of Virology*, 247:22-31.

Carbone, L.G., Cohen, D.J., Hardy, M.A., Benvenisty, A.I., Scully, B.E., Appel, G.B. (1988). Determination of AIDS after renal transplantation. *American Journal of Kidney Diseases*, 11:387-92.

Centers for Disease Control (1982). *Pneumocystis carini* pneumonia among persons with haemophilia. *Morbidity and Mortality Weekly Report*, 31:365-367.

Centers for Disease Control, "HIV/AIDS Surveillance", October 1989.

Centres for Disease Control and Prevention (1994). Zidovudine for the prevention of HIV transmission from mother to infant. *Morbidity and Mortality Weekly Report*, 43:285-287.

Centers for Disease Control and Prevention (CDC) HIV/AIDS Surveillance Report. (2007). Atlanta: US Department of Health and Human Services, (17), 1–54. Coleman, C. L. (2007). Health beliefs and high risk sexual behaviour among HIV infected African American men. *Applied Nursing Research*, 20, 110–115.

Centers for Disease Control and Prevention (2010). HIV transmission through transfusion-Missouri and Colorado, (2008). *Morbidity and Mortality Weekly Report,* 59 (41): 1335-9.

Chen, J.H., Wong, k., Chen, Z., Chan, K., Lam, H., To, S. W., Cheng, C., Yuen, K., Yam, W. (2010). Increased genetic diversity of HIV-1 circulating in Hong Kong. *PLOS one,* volume 5, issue 8, e12198.

Chesney, M.A., Koblin, B.A., Barresi, P.J., Husnik, M.J., Celum, L.C., Colfax, G., Mayer, K., McKirnan, D., Judson, N.F., Huang, Y., Coates, J.T.(2003). An individually tailored intervention for HIV prevention: baseline data from the EXPLORE study. *American Journal of Public Health,* 93:933–938.

Clavel, F., Guetard, D., Brun-Vezinet, F., Chamaret, S., Rey, M.A., Santos-Ferreira, M.O., Laurent, A.G., Danduet, C., Klatzmann, D., Champalimand, and Montagnier, (1986). Isolation of a new human retrovirus from West African patients with AIDS. *Science,* 233: 343-346.

Clavel, F. (1987). The West African AIDS virus. *AIDS,* 1:135-140.

Clarke, J.A. (1987). HIV transmission and skin grafts. *Lancet,* 1:983.

Collazos, J., Asensi, V., Carton, J.A. (2010). Association of HIV transmission categories with sociodemographic, viroimmunological and clinical parameters of HIV- infected patients. *Epidemiology and Infection,* 138(7): 1016-1024.

Cochran, S.D., Mays, V.M. (2000). Lifetime prevalence of suicide symptoms and affective disorders among men reporting same-sex sexual partners: Results from NHANES III. *American Journal of Public Health,* 2000; 90:573–578.

Cochran, S.D., Sullivan, J.G., Mays, V.M. (2003). Prevalence of mental disorders, psychological distress, and mental services use among lesbian, gay, and bisexual adults in the United States. Journal of Consulting and Clinical Psychology,. 2003; 71: 53–61.

Coleman, C. L. (2007). Health beliefs and high risk sexual behaviour among HIV infected African American men. *Applied Nursing Research,* 20, 110–115.

Coleman, C. L. and Ball, K. (2007). Determinants of perceived barriers to use condoms among HIV infected African American men middle-aged and older. *Journal of Advanced Nursing,* (60), 368–376.

Coleman, C.L. and Ball, K. (2010). Sexual diversity and HIV risk among older heterosexual African American males who are seropositive. *Applied Nursing Research,* 23: 122-129.

Contag, C. H., Ehrnst, A., Duda, J., Bohlin, A.B., Lindgren, S., Learn, G.H. and Mullins, J.I. (1997). Mother-to-infant transmission of human immunodeficiency virus type 1 involving five envelope sequence subtypes. *Journal of Virology,* 71:1292-1300.

Courgnard, V., Laure, F., Brossard, A., Goudeau, A., Barin, F., and Brechot, C. (1991). Frequent and early *in utero* HIV-1 infection. *AIDS Research on Human Retroviruses,* 7:337-341.

Dean, N.C., Golden, J.A., Evans, L., Wornock, M.L., Addison, T.E., Hopewell, P.C. and Levy, J.A. (1998). HIV recovery from bronchoalveolar lavage fluid in patients with AIDS. *Chest,* 93:1173-1176.

Decker, M.R., McCauley, H.L., Phuengsamram, D., Janyam, S., Seage, G. R. and Silverman, J.G. (2010). Violence victimisation, sexual risk and sexually transmitted infection symptoms among female sex workers in Thailand. *Sexually Transmitted Infections*, 86(3): 236-240.

De Cock, K.M., Fowler, M.G., Mercier, E., de Vincenzi, I., Saba, J., Hoff, E., Alnwick, J.D., Rogers, M., Shaffer, N. (2000). Prevention of mother-to-child HIV transmission in resource-poor countries: translating research into policy and practice. Journal of American Medical Association, 283(9):1175–82.

Del Amo, J., Petruckevitch, A., Philips, A., Johnson, A.M., Stephenson, J., Desmond, N., Hanscheid. T., Low, N., Newell, A., Obasi, A., Paine, K., Pym, A., Theodore, C.M. and De Cock, K.M. (1998). Disease progression and survival in HIV-1 infected Africans in London. *AIDS*, 12 (10): 1203-1209.

Delwart, E. L., Pan, H., Sheppard, H.W., Wolpert, D., Neumann, A.U., Korber, B. and Mullins. J.I. (1997). Slower evolution of human immunodeficiency virus type 1 quasispecies during progression to AIDS. *Journal of Virology*, 71: 7498–7508.

De Vincenzi , I. (1994). A longitudinal study of human immunodeficiency virus transmission by heterosexual partners. *New England Journal of Medicine*, 331(6), 341-346.

De Rossi, A., Masiero, S., Giaquinto, C., Ruga, E., Comar, M., Giacca, M. and Chieco-Bianchi, L. (1996). Dynamics of viral replication in infants with vertically acquired human immunodeficiency virus type 1 infection. *Journal of Clinical Infections*. 2:323–330.

Donoval, B. A., Landay, A. L., Moses, S., Agot, K., Ndinya-Achola, J.O., Nyagaya, E.A., MacLean, I., Bailey, R.C. (2006). HIV-1 target cells in foreskins of African men with varying histories of sexually transmitted infections. *American Journal of Clinical Pathology* 125(3), 386-391.

Dummer, J.S., Erb, S., Breinig, M.K., Ho, M., Rinaldo, C.R. Jr., Gupta, P., Ragni, M.V., Tzakis, A., Makowka, L., Van Thiel D. (1989). Infection with HIV in the Pittsburg transplant population: a study of 583 donors and 1043 recipients, 1981-1986. *Transplantation*, 47: 134-40.

Essien, E. J., Meshack, A. F., & Ross, M. W. (2002). Misperceptions about HIV transmission among heterosexual African-American and Latino men and women. *Journal of the National Medical Association*, 94(5), 304–312.

Erice, A., Rhame, F.S., Heussner, R.C., Dunn, D.L., Balfour, H.H. Jr. (1991). HIV infection in patients with solid organ transplants: report of five cases and review. *Rev Infectious Diseases*, 13:537-47.

European Collaborative Study (1991). *Lancet*, 337:253.

Fauci A S, Pantaleo G, Stanley S., Weissman, D. (1996). Immunopathogenic mechanisms of HIV infection. *Annals of Internal Medicine* 124(7), 654-663.

Fujikawa, L.S., Salahuddin, S.Z., Palestine, A.G., Nussenblatt, R.B., and Gallo, R.C. (1985). Isolation of human T-lymphotropic virus type III from the tears of a patient with acquired immunodeficiency syndrome. *Lancet*, ii: 529-530.

Gallo, R.C., Salahuddin, Z., Popovic, M., Shearer, G.M., Kaplan, M., Haynes, B.F., Palker, T.J., Redfield, R., Oleske, J. and Satai, B. (1984). Frequent detection and isolation of cytopathic retroviruses HTLV-III) from patients with HIV and at risk for AIDS. *Science*, 224:500-503.

Glenn, W.G. and Dietrich, E. John.(1993). *The AIDS Epidemic, Balancing Comparison and Justice*. Multnomah, Oregon, U.S.A. *Multnomah* Press, 1990. .... 1990 Inter-Varsity

Christian Fellowship of the *U.S.*, PO Box 7985, Madison, WI, 53707-7895. 800-828-2100

Gilman, S.E., Cochran, S.D., Mays, V.M., Hughes, M., Ostrow, D., and Kessler, R.C.(2001). Risk of psychiatric disorders among individuals reporting same-sex sexual partners in the National Comorbidity Survey. *American Journal of Public Health*, 2001;91:933–939.

Goedert, J.J., Drummond, E.J., Minkoff, L.H., Stevens, R., Blattner, A.W., Mendez, H., Robert-Guroff, M., Holman, S., Rubinstein, A., Willoughby, A. and Landesman, H.S. (1989). Mother-to-infant transmission of HIV-1: association with prematurity or low anti-gp120. *Lancet*, vol. 3342, issue 8679: 1351-4.

Gottlieb, M.S. Shcroff, R., Schanker, H., Weisman, J.D., Fan, P.T., Wolf, R.A., and Saxon, A. (1981). *Pneumocystis carinii* pneumonia and mucosal candidiasis in previously healthy homosexual men. *New England Journal of Medicine*, 305:1425-1430.

Grabar, S., Selinger-Leneman, H., Abgrak, S., Pialoux, G., Weiss, L. and Costagliola, D. (2009). Prevalence and comparative characteristics of long-term non-progressors and HIV controller patients in French hospital database on HIV. *AIDS*, 23(9):1163-1169. Doi.10.1097/QAD.obo13e32832644c8PMD19444075.

Gray, R H, Kiwanuka N, Quinn T C, *et al.* (2000). Male circumcision and HIV acquisition and transmission: cohort studies in Rakai, Uganda. *AIDS*, 14(15), 2371-2381.

Gray R H, Wawer M J, Brookmeyer R, *et al.* (2001). Probability of HIV-1 transmission per coital act in monogamous, heterosexual, HIV-1-discordant couples in Rakai, Uganda. *The Lancet*, 357(9263), 1149-1153.

Gray, R. H., Kigozi, G., Serwadda, D., Makumbi, F., Watya, S., Nalugoda, F., Kiwanuka, N., Moulton , H.L., Chaudhary, A.M.., Chen, M.Z., Sewankambo, N.K., Wabwire-Mangen , F., Bacon, M.C., Williams, F.MC., Opendi, P., Reynolds, S.J., Laeyendecker, O., Quinn , T.C., Wawer, M.J. (2007). Male circumcision for HIV prevention in men in Rakai, Uganda: a randomised trial. *The Lancet*, 369(9562), 657-666.

Groopman, D. and Greenspan, J.S. (1996). HIV-related oral disease. *Lancet*, 348: 729-733.

Groopman, J.E., Salahuddin, S.Z., Sarngadharan, M.G., Markham, D., Gonda, M., Sliski, A. and Gallo, R.C. (1984). HTLV-III in saliva of people with AIDS. Sexual men at risk for AIDS. *Science*, 226:447-449.

Gupta, P., Mellors, J., Kingsley, L., Riddler, S., Singh, M.K., Schreiber, S., Cronin, M. and Rinaldo, C.R. (1997). High viral load in semen of human immunodeficiency virus type 1-infected men at all stages of disease and its reduction by therapy with protease and nonnucleoside reverse transcriptase inhibitors. *Journal of Virology*, 71(8), 6271-6275.

Halapi, E., Gigliotti, D., Hodara, V., Scarlatti, G., Tovo, P.A., DeMaria, A., Wigezll, H. and Rossi, P. (1996). Detection of CD8 T-cell expansions with restricted T-cell receptor V usage in infants vertically infected by HIV-1. *AIDS*, 10: 1621–1626.

Harris, C., Small, C.B., Klein, R.S., Friedland, G.H., Moll, B., Emeson, E.E., Spigland, I. and Steigbigel, N.H. (1983). Immunodeficiency in female sexual partners of men with the AIDS. *New England Journal of Medicine*, 308:1181-1184.

Havens, P.L., Cuene, B.E., Hand, J.R., Gern, J.E., Sullivan, B.W. and Chusid, M.J. (1997). The puzzle of HIV-1 subtypes in Africa. *AIDS*, 11:705-712.

Heise, C., Dandekar, S., Kumar, P., Duplantie, R., Donovan, R.M. and Halsted, C.H. (1991). HIV infection of enterocytes and monuclear cells in human jejuna mucosa. *Gastroenterology*, 100:1521-1527.

Henin, Y., Mandelbrot, L., Henrion, R., Pradinaud, R., Couland, J. and Montagnier, L. (1993). Virus excretion in the cervicovaginal secretions of pregnant and non-pregnant HIV-infected women. *Journal of Acquired Immunodeficiency Syndrome*, 6: 72-75.

Herbst, J.H., Sherba, R.T., Crepaz, N., DeLuca J.B., Zohrabyan L, Stall, R.D., Lyles, C.M. (2005). HIV/AIDS Prevention Research Synthesis Team A meta-analytic review of HIV behavioral interventions for reducing sexual risk behaviour of men who have sex with men. *Journal of Acquired Immune Deficiency Syndrome*, 2005; 39:228-241.

Hilfenhaus, J.W., Gregersen, J.P., Mehdi, S., Volk, R. (1990). Inactivation of HIV-1 and HIV-2 by various manufacturing procedures for human plasma proteins. *Cancer Detection and Prevention Journal*, 14:369-75.

Hirshfield, S., Remien, R., Humberstone, M., Walavalkar, I., Chiasson, M. (2004). Substance use and high-risk sex among men who have sex with men: A national online study in the USA. AIDS Care 2004; 16:1036-1047.

Hollander, H. and Levy, J.A. (1987). Neurologic abnormalities and recovery of HIV from cerebrospinal fluid. *Annals of Internal Medicine*, 106: 692-695.

Ho, D.D., Rota, T.R., Schooley, R.T., Kaplan, J.C., Allan, J.D., Groopman, J.E., Resnick, L., Felsenstein, D., Andrews, C.A. and Hirsch, M.S. (1995). Isolation of HTLV-III from cerebrospinal fluid and neural tissues of patients with neurologic syndromes related to the AIDS. *New England Journal of Medicine*, 313:1493-1497.

Hook, E.W., Cannon, R.O., Nahmias, A.J., Lee, F.F., Campbell, C.H., Glasser, D. and Quian, T.C. (1992). Herpes simplex virus infection as a risk factor for the HIV infection in heterosexuals. *Journal of Infectious Diseases*, 165:251-255.

Human immunodeficiency virus infection transmitted from an organ donor screened for HIV antibody-North Carolina. *MMWR* 1987; 36:306-8.

Jaffe, C.L. and McMahon-Pratt, D. (1983). Monoclonal antibodies specific for *Leishmania tropica*: characterization of antigens associated with stage and species-specific determinants. *Journal of Immunology*, 131:1987-1993.

Jassens, W., Bure, A., Nkengasong, J.N. (1997). The puzzle of HIV-1 subtypes in Africa. *AIDS*, 11: 705-712.

John, G.C. and Kreiss, J. (1996). Mother-to-child transmission of HIV type 1. *Epidemiological Reviews*, 18:149-157.

Landesman, H.S., Kalish, A.L., Burns, N.D., Minkoff, H., Fox, E.H., Zorrilla, C., Garcia, P., Fowler, G.H., Mofenson, L. and Toumala, R. (1996). Obstetrical factors and the transmission of HIV-1 from mother to child. *New England Journal of Medicine*, 334; 1617-23.

Karim, Q.A., Karim, S.S.A., Frohlich, J.A., Grobler, C.A., Baxter, C., Mansoor, E.L., Kharsany, A.B.M., Sibeko, S., Mlisana, P.K., Omar, Z., Gengiah, N.T., Maarschalk, S., Arulappan, N., Mlotshwa, M., Morris, L., Taylor, D. (2010). Effectiveness and safety of Tenofovir gel and antiretroviral microbicide, for the prevention of HIV infection in women. CAPRISA 004 Trial Group. *Science*, 3rd Sept vol. 329:1168-1174.

Kalichman, S. C., Berto, G. D. and Eaton L (2008). Human immunodeficiency virus viral load in blood plasma and semen: review and implications of empirical findings. *SexuallyTransmitted Diseases* 35(1), 55-60.

Kitchen, A.D., Mann, G.F., Harrison, J.F., Zuckerman, A.J. (1989). Effect of gamma irradiation on the HIV and human coagulation proteins. *Vox Sang*, 56: 2323-9.

Kim, K.A., Yolamanova, M., Zirafi, O., Roan, N.R., Staendker, L., Forssmann, W.G., Burgener, A., Dejucq-Rainsford, N., Hahn, B.H., Shaw, G.M., Greene, W.C., Kirchhoff, F., Munch, J. (2010). Semen-mediated enhancement of HIV infection is donor-dependent and correlates with the levels of SEVI *Retrovirology*, 7: Article 55. doi: 10.1186/1742-4690-7-55

King M, Semlyen J, Tai SS, et al. (2008).A systematic review of mental disorder, suicide, and deliberate self harm in lesbian, gay, and bisexual people. *BMC Psychiatry*, 2008; 18:70. doi: 10.1186/1471-244X-8-70.

Kuhn, L. and Stein, Z.A. (1995). Mother-to-infant HIV transmission: timing risk factors and prevention. *Paediatric Perinatal Epidemiology*, 9:1-29.

Kumar, P., Pearson, J.E., Martin, D.H., Leech, S.H., Buisseret, P.D. , Bezbak, H.C., Gonzalez, F.M., Royer, J.R., Streicher, H.Z., Saxinger, W.C. (1987). Transmission of HIV by transplantation of a renal allograft, with development of the acquired immunodeficiency syndrome. *Annals of Internal Medicine*, 1987; 106:244-5.

Kresis, J. (1997). Breastfeeding and vertical transmission of HIV-1. *Acta Paediatrica*, 421 (Suppl.):113-117 (1985). HTLV-III infection in kidney transplant recipients. Lancet, 2:1361-2.

Lambert, J.S. (1996). Paediatric HIV infection. *Current Opinion in Paediatrics*, 8:606-614.

Lavreys L, Rakwar J P, Thompson M L, *et al.* (1999). Effect of circumcision on incidence of human immunodeficiency virus type 1 and other sexually transmitted diseases: a prospective cohort study of trucking company employees in Kenya. *The Journal of Infectious Diseases*, 180, 330-336.

Limpakarnianarat, K., Mastro, T. D., Yindeeyoungyeon, W., *et al.* (1993). STDS in female prostitutes in northern Thailand. *International Conference of AIDS*, 9, 687 (abstract no. PO-C10-2820).

Lindo, J.F., Dubon, J.M., Ager, A.L., De Gwurville, E.M., Gabriele, S.H., Karkalla, W.F., Baum, K.M. and Palmer, C.J. (1998). Intestinal parasitic infections in HIV-positive and HIV-negative individuals in San Pedrosula, Honduras. *American Journal of Tropical Medicine and Hygiene*, 58(4):431-435.

Lindgren, S., Anzen, B., Bohlin, A., Lidman, K. (1991). HIV and child-bearing: clinical outcome and aspects of mother-to-infant transmission. *AIDS*, 5:1111-6.

Ma, W. J., Wang, J.J., Reilly, K.H., Bi, A.M., Kumismith, W.G., and Wang, N. (2010). Estimation of Probability of Unprotected Heterosexual Vaginal Transmission of HIV-1 from Clients to Female Sex Workers in Kaiyuan, Yunnan Province, China. *Biomedical and Environmental Sciences*, 23: 287-292 (2010)

Mackelprang, R.D., Carrington, M., John-Stewart, G., Lohman-Payne, B., Richardson, B. A., Wamalwa, D., Gao, X., Majiwa, M., Mbori-Ngacha, D., Farquhar, C. (2010).

Maternal human leucocyte antigen A* 2301 is associated with increased mother-to-child HIV-1 transmission. *Journal of Infectious Diseases*, 202(8): 1273-7.

Mahiane, S. G., Legeai, C., Taljaard, D., Latouche, A., Puren, A., Peillon, A., Bretagnolle, J., Lissouba, P., Nguema, E.P., Gassiat, E., Auvert, B.(2009). Transmission probabilities of HIV and herpes simplex virus type 2, effect of male circumcision and interaction: a longitudinal study in a township of South Africa. *AIDS* 23 (3), 377-383.

Mamatha, M.L. and Merchant, H.R. (2010). Vertical Transmission of HIV–An Update. *Indian Journal of Pediatrics* (2010) 77:1270–1276 DOI 10.1007/s12098-010-0184-0

Marshal, M.P., Friedman, M.S., Stall, R., King, K.M., Jonathan Miles, J., Gold, M.A., Oscar G. Bukstein, G.O., Jennifer Q. Morse, J.Q. (2008). Sexual orientation and adolescent substance use: a meta-analysis and methodological review. *Addiction*. 2008; 103:546–556.

Mastro, T., Satten, G., Nopkesorn, T., Sangkharomya, S., Longini, I. (1994). Probability of female-to-male transmission of HIV-1 in Thailand. *Lancet*, 1994; 343: 204-207.

Masur, H., Michelis, M.A. and Greene, J.B. (1981). An outbreak of community-acquired *Pneumocystis carinii* pneumonia. *New England Journal of Medicine*, 305: 1431-1438.

Meyer, I.H. (2003). Prejudice, social stress, and mental health in lesbian, gay, and bisexual populations: conceptual issues and research evidence. *Psychological Bulletin*, 2003; 129:674–697.

Mimiaga, M.J., Case, P., Johnson, C.V., Safren, S.A., Mayer, K.H. (2009). Preexposure antiretroviral prophylaxis attitudes in high-risk Boston area men who report having sex with men: limited knowledge and experience but potential for increased utilization after education. *Journal of Acquired Immune Deficiency Syndrome*, 2009; 50(1):77–83.

Mimiaga, M.J., Noonan, E., Donnell, D., Safren, S.A., Koenen, K. C., Gortmaker, S., O'Cleirigh, C., Chesney, M. A., Coates, T. J., Koblin, B. A., Mayer, K. H.(2009). Childhood sexual abuse is highly associated with HIV risk taking behaviour and infection among MSM in the EXPLORE Study. *Journal Acquired Immune Deficiency Syndrome*. 2009; 51: 340–348.

Mimiaga, M.J., Reisner, S.L., Pantalone, DW, et al. An open phase pilot of behavioral activation therapy and risk reduction counseling for MSM with crystal methamphetamine abuse at risk for HIV infection. Paper Session 2. Presented at: Society of Behavioral Medicine 2010 Annual Meeting; April 7–10, 2010; Seattle, Washington. PowerPoint available at: http://www.sbm.org/meeting/2010/presentations/Thursday/Paper%20Sessions/Paper%20Session%2002/An%20open%20phase%20pilot%20of%20behavioral%20activation%20therapy.pdf. Accessed August 10, 2010.

Milam, J., Richardson, J. L., Espinoza, L., & Stoyanoff, S. (2006). Correlates of unprotected sex among adult heterosexual men living with HIV. *Journal of Urban Health*, 83(4), 669–681.

Mok, J.Y.Q. et al (1989). *Archives of Disease in Children*, 64:1140.

Mundy, D.C., Schinazi, R.F., Ressell-Gerber, A., Nahmias, A.J. and Randal, H.W. (1987). HIV virus isolated from amniotic fluid. *Lancet*, II: 459-460.

Mustanski, B., Garofalo, R., Herrick, A., Donenberg, G. (2007). Psychosocial health problems increase risk for HIV among urban young men who have sex with men: preliminary evidence of a syndemic in need of attention. *Annals Behavioural Medicine*, 2007; 34:37–45.

Newell, M.L., Dunn, D., Peckham, C.S., Ades, A.E., Pardi, G. and Semprini, A.E., (1992). Risk factors for mother-to-child transmission of HIV-1. *Lancet,* 339:1007-1012.

Newell, M.L., Peckham, C., Dunn, D. and Ades, A. (1994). Natural transmission of vertically acquired HIV type infection. *Paediatrics,* 94:815-819.

Neumayer, H.H., Fassbinder, W., Kresse, S., Wagner, K. (1985). HTLV-III antibody screening in kidney transplant recipients and patients receiving maintenance haemodialysis. *Transplantation Proceedings,* 19:2169-71.

Njoku, M.O (2004). Studies on the prevalence, seroepidemiology of Cryptosporidiosis and some cofactors in the immune responses and pathogenesis of HIV infection in North Central Nigeria. PhD thesis page 65.

Nkowane, B.M. (1991). Prevalence and incidence of HIV infection in Africa: a review of data published in 1990. *AIDS,* 5:S7-S16.

Ogundele, B. (2010). HIV/AIDS patients want court to stop promotion of condoms. Nigerian Tribune, Wednesday nov, 03, 2010. http://tribune.com.ng/index.php/news/13032-hivaids-patients-want-court-to-stop-pro.accessed 03/11/2010.

Oxtoby, M.J. (1990). Perinatally acquired HIV infection. *Pediatrics Infectious Disease Journal,* 9:609-19.

Padian, N. S., Shiboski, S. C. and Jewell, N. P. (1991). Female-to-male transmission of human immunodeficiency virus. *JAMA,* 266(12), 1664-1667.

Pasquier, C., Cayrou, C., Blancher, A., Tourne-Petheil, C., Berrebi, A., Tricoire, J., Puel, J. and Izopet, J. (1998). Molecular evidence for mother-to-child transmission of multiple variants by analysis of RNA and DNA sequences of human immunodeficiency virus type 1. *Journal of Virology,* 1998; 72: 8,493-8,501.

Peckham, C., and D. Gibb. (1995). Mother-to-child transmission of the human immunodeficiency virus. *New England Journal Medicine,* 333:298–302.

Peterson, C. (1992). Cryptosporidiosis in patients infected with the Human Immunodeficiency Virus. *Clinical Infectious Diseases,* 15: 903-909.

Plummer, F.A., Simonsen, J.N., Cameron, J.O., Ndinya-Achola, J.O., Kresis, J.K., Gakinya, M.N., Waiyaki, P., Cheang, M., Piot, P., Ronald, A.R. and Ngugi, E.N. (1991). Co-factors in male-female sexual transmission of HIV type 1. *Journal of Infectious Diseases,* 163: 233-239.

Pozio, E., Rezza, G., Boschini, A., Pezzotti, P., Tamburini, A., Rossi, P., Difine, M., Smacchia, A.C., Schiesari, A., Gattei, E, E., Zuccani, R. and Ballarini, P. (1997). Clinical Cryptosporidiosis and HIV-induced immunosuppression: findings from a longitudinal study of HIV-positive and HIV-negative former injection drug users. *Journal of Infectious Diseases,* 176: 969-975.

Price, R.W. (1996). Neurological complications of HIV infection. *Lancet,* 348:445-452.

Prompt, C.A., Reiss, M.M., Grillo, F.M., Kopstein, J., Kraemer, E., Manfro, R.C., Maia, M.H., Comiran, J.B. (1985). Transmission of AIDS virus at renal transplantation. *Lancet*, 2:672.

Provisional Public Health Service inter-agency recommendations for screening donated blood and plasma for antibody to the virus causing AIDS. *MMWR*, 1985; 34:1-5.

Pruss, A., Caspari, G., Kruger, D.H., Blumel, J., Nubling, C.M., Gurtler, L., Gerlich, W. H. (2010). Tissue donation and virus safety: more nucleic acid amplification testing is needed. *Transplant Infectious Disease*, 12 (5): 375-386.

Purcell, D.W., Johnson, C., Lansky, A., Prejean, J., Stein, R., Denning, P., Gaul, Z., Weinstock, H., Su, J., & Crepaz, N. (2010). Calculating HIV and syphilis rates for risk groups: estimating the national population size of men who have sex with men. Abstract #22896. Presented at: 2010 National STD Prevention Conference; March 10, 2010; Atlanta, GA. Available at:
http:// www.cdc.gov/hiv/topics/msm/resources/research/msm.htm. Accessed June 1, 2010.

Quarto, M.., Germinario, C., Fontana, A., Bartuni, S. (1989). HIV transmission through kidney transplantation from a living related donor. *New England Journey Medicine*, 320:1754.

Qian, M., Bui, T., Ho, R.J., Unadkat, J.D. (1994) Metabolism of 30-azido-30-deoxythymidine (AZT) in human placental trophoblasts and Hofbauer cells. *Biochemical Pharmacology*, 48(2): 383–389.

Quinn, C.T., Wawer, J.M., Sewankambo, N., Serwadda, D., Li, C., Wabwire-mangen, F., Meehan, M.O., Lutalo, T. and Gray, H.R. (2000). Viral load and heterosexual transmission of HIV-1. *New England Journal of Medicine*, 342:921-9.

Reinhardt, P. P., Reinhardt, B., Lathey, J.L. and Spector, S.A. (1995). Human cord blood mononuclear cells are preferentially infected by non-syncytiuminducing, macrophage-tropic human immunodeficiency virus type 1 isolates. *Journal of Clinical Microbiology*, 33:292–297.

Reynolds, S. J., Shepherd, M. E., Risbud, A. R., Gangakhedkar, R.R., Brookmeyer, R.S. (2004). Male circumcision and risk of HIV-1 and other sexually transmitted infections in India. *The Lancet*, 363(9414), 1039-1040.

Rogers, M.F., Ou, C-Y., Kilbourne, B., and Schochetman, G. (1991). Advances and problems in the diagnosis of human immunodeficiency virus infection in infants. *Pediatrics Infectious Disease Journal*, 10:523-531.

Royce, R.A., Sena, A., Cates Jr., W. and Cohen, M.S. (1997). Sexual transmission of HIV. *New England Journal of Medicine*, 336 (15): 1072-1078.

Ruan, Y. H., Qian, H. Z., Li, D. L., Shi, W., Li, Q.C., Liang, H.Y., Yang, Y., Luo, F.J., Vermund, S.H., Shao, Y.M. (2009). Willingness to Be Circumcised for Preventing HIV among Chinese Men Who Have Sex with Men. *AIDS Patient Care and STDs*, 23(5), 315-321.

Ryder, R.W., Nsa, W., Hassig, S.E., Behets, F., Rayfield, M., Ekungola, B., Nelson, M.A., Mulenda, U., Francis, H., Mwandagalirwa, K., Davachi, F., Rogers, M., Nzilambi, N., Greenberg, A., Mann, J., Quinn, T.C., Piot, P. and James W. Curran, J.W. (1989). Perinatal Transmission of the human immunodeficiency virus type 1 to infants of seropositive women in Zaire. *New England Journal of Medicine,* 320, 1637-1642.

Safren, S.A. and Heimberg, R.G. (1999). Depression, hopelessness, suicidality, and related factors in sexual minority and heterosexual adolescents. *Journal of Consulting and Clinical Psychology,* 1999; 67:859–866.

Safren, S.A., Sari, L., Reisner, A. H., Mimiaga, M.J. and Stall, R.D. (2010). Mental Health and HIV Risk in Men Who Have Sex With Men. *Journal of Acquired Immune Deficiency Syndrome,* 2010; 55:S74–S77.

Safren, S.A., Traeger, L., Skeer, M.R., O'Cleirigh, C., Meade, C.S., Covahey, C., Mayer, K.H. (2010). Testing a social-cognitive model of HIV transmission risk behaviours in HIV-infected MSM with and without depression. *Journal of Health Psychology,* 2010; 29:215–221.

Samuel, D., Castaing, D., Adam, R., Saliba, F., Chamaret, S., Misset, J.L., Montagnier, L., Bismuth, H. (1988). Fatal acute HIV infection with aplastic anaemia, transmitted by liver graft. *Lancet,* 1:1221-2.

Scarlatti, G., Lombardi, V., Plebanic, N., Vegni, C., Ferraris, G., Bucceri, A., Fenyo, E.M., Wigzell, H., Rossi, P. and Albert, J. (1991) Polymerase chain reaction, virus isolation and antigen assay in HIV-1-antibody-positive mothers and their children., *AIDS,* 5:1173-1178.

Semen banking, organ and tissue transplantation, and HIV antibody testing. *MMWR* 1988; 37:57-8, 63.

Schulz, T.F., Boshoff, C.H. and Weiss, R.A. (1996). HIV infection and neoplasia. *Lancet,* 587-591.

Scarlatti, G. (1996). Paediatric HIV infection. *Lancet,* 348: 863-868.

Schwarz, A., Hoffmann, F., L'age-Stehr, J., Tegzess, A.M., Offermann, G. (1987). HIV transmission by organ donation: outcome in cornea and kidney recipients. *Transplantation,* 44:21-4.

Sharp, P.M., Robertson, D.L., Gao, F. and Hahn, B.H. (1994). Origins and diversity of HIV. *AIDS,* 8 (Suppl. 1): S27-S42.

Siegal, F.P., Lopez, C. and Hammer, G.S. (1981). Severe AIDS in male homosexuals, manifested by chronic perianal ulcerative herpes simplex lesions. *New England Journal of Medicine,* 305: 1439-1444.

Simonds, R.J., Holmberg, S.D., Hurwitz, L.R., Coleman, T.R., Bottenfield, S., Conley, L.J., Kohlenberg, H.S., Castro, G.K., Dahan, A.B., Schable, A.C., Rayfield, A.M. and Rogers, M.F. (1992). Transmission of HIV-1 from a seronegative organ and tissue donor. The New England Journal of Medicine, March, 329:726-32.

Smith, D.K., Gwinn, M., Selik, R.M., Miller, K.S., Dean-Gaitor, H., Thompson, P.I., De Cock, K.M., Gayle, H.D. (2000). HIV/AIDS among African Americans: progress or progression? *AIDS;* 2000; 14(9):1237-1248.

Sperling, S.R., Shapiro, E.D., Coombs, W.R., Todd, A.J., Herman, A.S., McSherry, D.G., et al. (1996). Maternal viral load, zidovudine treatment, and the risk of transmission of human immunodeficiency virus type 1 from mother to infant. Paediatric AIDS Clinical Trials Group Protocol 076 Study Group. *New England Journal of Medicine,* 1996; 335:1621–9.

Stall, R., Paul, J.P., Greenwood, G., Pollack, L.M., Bein, E., Crosby, G.M., Mills, T.C., Binson, D., Coates, T.J., Catania, J.A. (2001). Alcohol use, drug use, and alcohol related problems among men who have sex with men: The Urban Men's Health Study. *Addiction*, 2001; 96:1589–1601.

Stall, R., Friedman, M., Catania, J.(2008) Interacting epidemics and gay men's health: a theory of syndemic production among urban gay men. In: Wolitski RJ, Stall R, Valdiserri RO, eds. Unequal Opportunity: Health Disparities Affecting Gay and Bisexual Men in the United States. New York, NY: Oxford University Press; 2008:251.

Stoneburner, R.C., Chiasson, M., Weisfuse, I.B. and Thomas, P.A. (1990). The epidemic of AIDS and HIV-1 infection among homosexuals in New York City. *AIDS*, 4: 99-106.

Strunnikova, N., Ray, S.C., Livingston, R.A., Rubalcaba, E. and Viscidi, R.P. (1995). Convergent evolution within the V3 loop domain of human immunodeficiency virus type 1 in association with disease progression. *Journal of Virology*, 69:7548–7558.

Suligoi, B., Raimondo, M., Regine, V., Salfa, M.C., Camoni, L.(2010). Epidemiology of HIV infection in blood donations in Europe and Italy. *Blood Transfusion*, 8(3): 178-85.

Sullivan, S. G., Ma, W., Duan, S. D., *et al.* (2009). Attitudes towards circumcision among Chinese men. *JAIDS Journal of Acquired Immune Deficiency Syndromes* 50(2), 238-240.

Sundaravaradan, V., Hahn, T. and Ahmad, N. (2005). Conservation of functional domains and limited heterogeneity of HIV-1 reverse transcriptase gene following vertical transmission. *Retrovirology*, 2005; 2: 36.

Tachet, A., Dulioust, E., Salmon, D, *et al.* (1999). Detection and quantification of HIV-1 in semen: identification of a
subpopulation of men at high potential risk of viral sexual transmission. *AIDS*, 13(7), 823-831.

Testing donors of organs, tissues, and semen for antibody to HLTV-III/lymphadenopathy-associated virus. *MMWR* 1985; 34:294.

The EXPLORE Study Team. Effects of a behavioural intervention to reduce acquisition of HIV infection among men who have sex with men: the EXPLORE randomised controlled study. *Lancet*, 2004; 364:41-50.

Tovo, P.A. and de Martino, M. (1988). Epidemiology, Clinical features, and prognostic factors of paediatric HIV infection. *Lancet*, ii: 1043-1045.

Transmission of HIV through bone transplantation: case report and public health recommendations. *MMWR*, 1988; 37:597-9.

Turner, B.J., Hauck, W.W., Fanning, T.R. and Markson, L.E. (1996). Cigarette smoking and maternal-child HIV transmission. *Journal of AIDS and Human Retrovirology*, 14: 327-337.

UNAIDS (2010). Global Report. UNAIDS Report on the global AIDS epidemic. Copyright © 2010 Joint United Nations Programme on HIV/AIDS (UNAIDS).

U.S. Centers for Disease Control and Prevention. (2002). Surveillance of health care personnel with HIV/AIDS. Retrieved May 15, 2008, from http://www.cdc.gov/ncidod/dhqp/bp_hiv_hp_with.html.

Van Griensven, F. and de Lin van Wijngaarden, J.W. (2010). A review of the epidemiology of HIV infection and prevention responses among MSM in Asia. *AIDS*, 24 Suppl. 3: S30-40.

Van de Perre, P., Simon, A., Msellati, P., Hitimana, D.G., Vaira, D., Bazubagira, A., Van Goethem, C., Stevens, A.M., Karita, E., Sondag-Thull, D., Dabis, F. and Lepage, P. (1991). Postnatal transmission of HIV type 1 from mother to infant. *New England Journal of Medicine*, 325: 593-598.

Varghese, B., Maher, J.E., Peterman, T. A., Branson, B. M. and Steketee, R. W. (2002). Reducing the risk of sexual HIV transmission: quantifying the per-act risk for HIV on the basis of choice of partner, sex act, and condom use. *Sexually Transmitted Diseases*, 29(1), 38-43.

Wang, L.D. (2009). *AIDS*. 1st ed. Beijing: Beijing Publishing House.

Wang L, Wang N, Wang L Y, *et al.* (2009). The 2007 estimates for people at risk for and living with HIV in China: progress and challenges. *Journal of Acquired Immune Deficiency Syndromes*, 50(4): 414-418.

Ward, J.W., Holberg, S.D., Allen, J.R., et al. (1988). Transmission of HIV by blood transfusions screened as negative for HIV antibody. New Eng J Med, 318:473-8.

Wawer, M. J., Gray, R. H., Sewankambo, N. K., *et al.* (2005). Rates of HIV-1 transmission per coital act, by stage of HIV-1infection, in Rakai, Uganda. *Journal of Infectious Diseases,* 191(9): 1403-1409.

Wawer, M.J, Makumbi F, Kigozi G, *et al.* (2009). Circumcision in HIV-infected men and its effect on HIV transmission to female partners in Rakai, Uganda: a randomised controlled trial. *The Lancet* 374(9685), 229-237.

Wells, M.A., Wittek, A.E., Epstein, J.S. et al., (1986). Inactivation and partition of human T-cell lymphotrophic virus, type III, during ethanol fractionation of plasma. *Transfusion*, 26:210-3.

Winkelstein, W. Jr., Lyman, D.M., Padian, N., Grant, R., Samuel, M., Wiley, J.A., Anderson, R.E., Lang, W., Riggs, J. and Levy, J.A. (1987). Sexual practices and risk of infection by the Human Immunodeficiency Virus: The San Francisco Men's Health Study. *Journal of American Medical Association*, 257: 321-325.

Wolinsky, S. M., Wike, C.M., Korber, B.T.M., Hutto, C., Parks, W.P., Rosenblum, L.L., Kunstman, K.J., Furtado, M.R. and J. L. Munoz. (1992). Selective transmission of human immunodeficiency virus type-1 variants from mothers to infants. *Science*, 255:1134–1137.

World Health Organisaztion (1989). HIV-2 working Group: Criteria for HIV-2 serodiagnosis, Marseille, France.

World Health Organization and Global programme on AIDS, WHO/GPA (1994). The HIV/AIDS pandemic: Overview. WHO/GPA/TCO/SEF/94.4.

Xu, J. (2009). Prospective cohort study to the incidence of HIV/STIs among FSWs in Kaiyuan City. PhD [dissertation].Beijing, China: China Center for Disease Control and Prevention.

Yu, M. and Vajdy, M. (2010). Mucosal HIV transmission and vaccination strategies through oral compared with vaginal and rectal routes. *Expert Opinion on Biological Therapy*, 10(8): 1181-1195.

9

Affectation Situation of HIV/AIDS in Colombian Children

Ana María Trejos Herrera, Jorge Palacio Sañudo
Mario Mosquera Vásquez and Rafael Tuesca Molina
Fundación Universidad del Norte, Barranquilla
Colombia

1. Introduction

Acquired immunodeficiency syndrome (AIDS) is a global emergency and one of the most formidable challenges to human life and human dignity. The Declaration of Commitment on HIV/AIDS, adopted unanimously by the member states of the United Nations at the Special Session of the General Assembly (UNGASS) in New York and the Millennium Declaration, adopted by 189 nations and signed by 147 heads of state and government called for global action to build a global response to HIV/AIDS. (United Nations General Assembly Special Session on HIV/AIDS [UNGASS], 2001).

Globally, the number of children under 15 living with HIV has increased from 1.6 million [1.4 million – 2,1 million] in 2001 to 2.0 million [1.9 million-2, 3 million] in 2007, while young people between 15 and 24 represent an estimated 45% of new HIV infections worldwide. (Joint United Nations Programme on HIV/AIDS [UNAIDS] & World Health Organization [WHO], 2007).

With an adjustment in early 2006, the National Institute of Health (NIH) reported 54,805 cases of Colombian HIV infection and AIDS. The general behavior of the notification has been toward increased, with the rate for the period 1983-2005 to 5.36 cases per 100,000 population and for the last decade 1995-2004 to 7.85 cases per 100,000 population. The reported annual incidence should be used with caution in response to underdiagnosis, the underreporting and delayed reporting that characterized the passive surveillance of HIV/AIDS in the country. (Programa Conjunto de las Naciones Unidas sobre el VIH/SIDA [ONUSIDA] Grupo Temático para Colombia & Ministerio de la Protección Social de Colombia Dirección General de Salud Pública, 2006).

This chapter aims to analyze the situation of involvement for HIV/AIDS in Colombian children based on a study conducted in five cities - Colombian regions: (1) Barranquilla, Santa Marta and Cartagena, (2) Cali and Buenaventura (Instituto Colombiano de Bienestar Familiar [ICBF], Save the Children, Unicef & Universidad del Norte, 2006). The study shows that the delivery of HIV/AIDS diagnosis in children affected is not an established practice in the Colombian context. The low rate of disclosure indicates that within the integrated health management is a priority to develop strategies or clinical models of revelation that support processes of professionals who provide health services to affected families.

This project arose from the need to understand the situation of involvement and quality of life of children and adolescents seropositive for HIV in five Colombian cities, to articulate and assess the scope of the public policies at the time. Our study included children under 18 years of age with three situations of HIV/AIDS affectation: (1) children seropositive or seronegative for HIV, orphans HIV/AIDS (father, mother or both who had died from the disease), (2) children seropositive for HIV and, (3) children seropositive or seronegative for HIV, having lived with HIV positive people.

In 2006, only (3.8%) for 11 children in five Colombian cities were aware of their diagnosis of HIV/AIDS seropositivity compared with [96.2% (n=275)] who were unaware of the situation of HIV/AIDS affectation. The reasons for delaying the delivery of diagnosis that were reported by health professionals and caregivers of affected children, are related to prevent psychological harm or emotional stress to the child; situations cause fear of stigmatization and discrimination against the inadvertent disclosure of the child to others, and lack training regarding the procedure and age to provide this information by professionals providing health services to these children.

Furthermore, due to the importance of quality of life related to health (HRQOL) of children and their caregivers affected in the diagnosis, care and treatment of HIV/AIDS, the chapter will also address the evaluation of the following dimensions of quality of life: (1) Mobility, (2) Personal Care, (3) Activities of Daily Living, (4) Pain/Discomfort and (5) Anxiety/Depression using EuroQol (EQ-5D) instrument, as necessary to make decisions regarding front the care of these children.

Although current antiretroviral treatments managed to increase survival and quality of life of people affected by HIV/AIDS, it is also true that as a chronic disease requiring ongoing treatment, not exempt of adverse effects, to which should be add an important psychosocial impact. Based on this, relevant psychosocial variables have been also analyzed, such as family function instrument employing the Family Apgar and the perception of social support both children and their caregivers using the instrument Social Support (MOS) and scan variables Clinic children were seropositive for HIV/AIDS, which are also explored throughout this chapter.

Similarly results are displayed on the levels of information about the disease who have children who are aware of their diagnosis of HIV/AIDS seropositivity, as well as the caregivers of children who are still unaware of their situation involvement, which will allow to assess the degree of knowledge or misinformation that has this affected population and how can this affect or not confronting the diagnosis. In the same way, will address findings related to usage patterns and access to health services and education which will show that the health and education services in the Colombian context must overcome some obstacles in ensuring not only access to care but also increase the availability, fairness, integrity and quality from the perspective of rights and in order to benefit the child population under 18 years affected with HIV/AIDS.

This will be discussed by combining data from both quantitative and qualitative methodology, provided by the research tools employed and by the focus groups conducted with: (1) children who are aware of their diagnosis of HIV/AIDS, (2) caregivers of children who know their status of involvement for HIV/AIDS and (3) Professionals who provide health services to children affected population, which contain relevant evidence that allow further appreciation of the difficulties felt by the affected children in our country.

2. Illness status disclosure to children with HIV/AIDS

One of the factors that most worries the caregivers of children with HIV and professionals who provide health services is the issue of who, when and how they will reveal to the child that he/she has a chronic and stigmatizing disease that requires demanding treatment and involves the issue of death. (Nagler et al., 1995) explain that the HIV/AIDS carries stigma, which has profound psychological, social and emotional implications for the sufferer. For this reason, too many families make the decision to hide the child's HIV diagnosis, including members of the same family.

FACTORS THAT INHIBIT ILLNESS STATUS DISCLOSURE

1. *Cause damage or psychological harm to the child.* (Abadía-Barrero & Larusso, 2006; Bikaako-Kajura et al., 2006; Boon-Yasidhi et al., 2005; Davis & Shah, 1997; Instituto Colombiano de Bienestar Familiar [ICBF], Save the Children, Unicef & Universidad del Norte, 2006; Instone, 2000; Lester et al., 2002; Lipson, 1993; Myer et al., 2006; Oberdorfer et al., 2006; Tasker, 1992; Wiener et al., 1996; Wiener & Figueroa, 1998; Wiener et al., 1998).

2. *Concern about child discloses his/her HIV illness status to others.* (Bikaako-Kajura et al., 2006; Boon-Yasidhi et al., 2005; Davis & Shah, 1997; Instituto Colombiano de Bienestar Familiar [ICBF], Save the Children, Unicef y Universidad del Norte, 2006; Instone, 2000; Kouyoumdjian et al., 2005; Meyers & Weitzman, 1991; Oberdorfer et al., 2006; Tasker, 1992; Ledlie, 1999; Lester et al., 2002; Lewis et al., 1994; Waugh, 2003; Weiner & Figueroa, 1998; Weiner et al., 1998).

3. *Caregiver's difficulty accepting that the child is old enough to understand HIV diagnosis.* (Abadía-Barrero & Larusso, 2006; Bikaako-Kajura et al., 2006; Boon-Yasidhi et al., 2005; Flanagan-Klygis et al., 2002; Kouyoumdjian et al., 2005; Oberdorfer et al., 2006) .

4. *Parental guilt.* (Lee & Johann-Liang, 1999; Lipson, 1993; Ledlie, 1999; Tasker, 1992; Waugh, 2003).
   Fear about having to answers painful and difficult questions. (Cohen, 1994; Davis & Shah, 1997; Lee & Johann-Liang, 1999; Lipson, 1993; Tasker, 1992; Waugh, 2003; Weiner & Figueroa, 1998; Wiener et al., 1998)

5. *Fears that disclosure will negatively affect their child's health or cause hastening disease progression.* (Lipson, 1993).

6. *Fear that the child associate to caregiver with socially disapproved behaviors such as homosexuality and promiscuity.* (Kouyoumdjian et al., 2005)

7. *Belief that child will feel the same emotional reaction that caregiver felt when knew the bad news.* (Lipson, 1993).

Fig. 1. Factors that inhibit illness status disclosure to children with HIV/AIDS.

Colombian caregivers were afraid that the child would get depressed, be isolated, anxious or worried about having this chronic disease. Caregivers also fear that once the illness status is disclosed, the child will tell others, which will lead him and his family to situations of stigma and discrimination with potentially serious consequences such as expulsion from residence, school, and refusal to play with the child, among others. Similarly, professionals who provide health services to these children showed a lack of consensus on the procedure and age for disclosing illness status.

Researchers found that children were aware of their illness and impending death, despite their parent's stance of protective communication. (Hardy et al., 1994). Given the number of visits they make to the hospital or clinic and the acquaintances they meet, complete unawareness by a certain age is doubtful. Although kept in secrecy, children often showed curiosity or knowledge about their treatments (Lee & Johann-Liang, 1999). They may listen in on a conversation about AZT treatment between the doctor and their parent or ask other patients about their condition (Lipson, 1993). The stigma of HIV/AIDS leads families to keep the diagnosis secret from the child, other family members and schools.

The American Academy of Pediatrics guidelines for the illness status disclosure to children and adolescents with HIV infection says it is imperative that all adolescents have knowledge of their illness status and that disclosure should be considered for children under school age according to their level of cognitive development, age, family dynamics, psychosocial maturity and other clinical variables (Committee on Pediatric AIDS [COPA], 1999).

Disclosure of HIV diagnosis to children is becoming increasingly important because antiretroviral therapy becomes more widely available, however internationally rates of disclosure seem to be low. Some factors can inhibit and facilitate the decision making of caregivers to disclose illness status to their children with HIV/AIDS (See Figure 1).

Disclosure of HIV diagnosis should be viewed as a process, rather than an event, it is related to the child's cognitive development and aims to provide him/her with age appropriate information.

3. Health-Related Quality of Life (HRQOL) in children affected with HIV/AIDS

Advances in HIV treatment have allowed that quality of life of people affected with HIV/AIDS increased. Quality of Life related to Health subscales provides an overall vision of health and allows make important decisions about patient care. To have a benchmark of the health status of the pediatric patient should be a priority for institutions that provide health services.

For this reason we use EuroQol (EQ-5D) to estimate how Colombian caregivers perceive the Health-Related Quality of Life of their children. EQ-5D is a standardized instrument for use as a measure of health outcome. Applicable to a wide range of health conditions and treatments, it provides information about mobility, self-care, usual activities, pain/discomfort and anxiety/depression.

Results shows in Mobility subscale that 94.4% (N=269) of children with HIV/AIDS do not have trouble walking, 5.6% (N=17) have some problems or confined to bed. In Self-Care subscale, 96.1% (N=275) do not have problems bathing or dressing; 3.9% (N=11) of children have some problems or are unable to bathing or dressing. In Usual Activities subscale results shows that 96.1% (N=275) do not have problems to perform their usual activities, 3.9% (N=11) of children have some problems or are unable to perform their usual activities. In Pain/Discomfort subscale caregivers perceive that 84.6% (N=242) of their children do not have pain or discomfort, however 15.4% (N= 44) of children have some problems or may be experiencing pain and discomfort. Finally, caregivers perceive that 90.2% (N=258) of their HIV-positive children do not have anxiety or depression while 9.8% (N=28) may be experiencing anxiety or depression according to caregiver's report (See Table 1.)

Health-Related Quality of Life N=(286)	No Problems		Some Problems		Confined to bed/Unable to Perform	
	F	%	F	%	F	%
Mobility	269	94.4%	16	5.2%	1	0.4%
Self-Care	275	96.1%	7	2.5%	4	1.4%
Usual Activities	275	96.1%	8	2.9%	3	1%
Pain/ Discomfort	242	84.6%	40	14%	4	1.4%
Anxiety/ Depression	258	90.2%	25	8.7%	3	1.1%

Table 1. Health-Related Quality of Life (HRQOL) in Colombian children affected with HIV/AIDS measured by their caregivers.

The above results indicate that Colombian children affected with HIV/AIDS have a good level of health. Worth noting that all these children are affiliated to the social security health and are receiving Highly Active Antiretroviral Treatment (HAART). However, the highest percentage of problems found in Pain/Discomfort subscale with 15.4% of children who have some problems or may be experiencing pain and discomfort according to caregiver's report.
(The World Health Organization [WHO], 2003) defines health as a state of complete physical, mental, and social well-being and not merely the absence of disease or infirmity. It follows that measurement of health must not only include estimates of the frequency and severity of diseases, but also well-being and quality of life. This is particularly true for patients with HIV/AIDS because of the chronic and debilitating nature of the illness, stigma, and a high rise of premature death (Nojomi et al., 2008).

4. Family Functioning and social support in families affected with HIV/AIDS

Family Functioning play a very important role in coping with HIV illness. Understanding aspects of this interaction between children's health and their family is important to keep and increase quality of life, coping and adherence to treatment, well-being and psychological adjustment for a HIV-positive child. A family with good parental relationships would mean the family members are willing to solve problems together, showing concern for each other, and there will be fewer quarrels. In this sense, it is necessary for a child with a chronic illness such as HIV could find in his/her family some solid foundations that allow him/her to deal with this diagnosis.
For estimated this variable, we used Family Apgar to assess a family member's perception of family functioning by examining his/her satisfaction with family relationships. 73.8% (N=211) of Colombian children are in a norm functionality family. This mean, responder's perception about his/her family has the basic features to be functional and harmonic in the domains: adaptation, partnership, growth, affection and resolve. 18.2% (N=52) of families

affected with HIV/AIDS report moderate dysfunction while 8% (N=23) families report severe dysfunction (See Table 2).

In every family has a complex dynamic patterns governing their living and functioning. Of this dynamic is appropriate and flexible, in other words, functional, contribute to family harmony and provide its members the ability to develop strong feelings of identity, safety and welfare (Sherboune & Stewart, 2003; Cohen et al., 1985).

Family Functioning N=(286)	F	%
Norm Functionality	211	73.8%
Moderate dysfunction	52	18.2%
Severe dysfunction	23	8%

Table 2. Family Functioning in families affected with HIV/AIDS.

Interest in the concept of social support has increased dramatically over the last few years, due to the belief that the availability of support may impact favorably on a person's health and emotional well-being (Sherbourne, 1988). Consider the psychological impact of HIV/AIDS social support may play a small but potentially important role in helping HIV-positive people to cope with illness.

(Leserman et al., 1992) found that subjects primarily coped with the threat of AIDS by adopting a fighting spirit, reframing stress to maximize personal growth, planning a course of action, and seeking social support; satisfaction with one's social support networks and participation in the AIDS community were related to more healthy coping strategies (e.g., fighting spirit, personal growth). These results suggest that health professionals should encourage more adaptive coping strategies, help the patients to use existing sources of positive social support, and assist patients in finding community support networks.

The availability of someone to provide help or emotional support may protect individuals from some of the negative consequences of major illness or stressful situations (Barrera, 1981).

Investigators (Brandt & Weinert, 1981; Brown & Brady, 1987; Broadhead et al, 1988; Cohen & Syme, 1985; Cohen & Wills, 1985; Duncan-Jones, 1981; House & Kahn, 1985; Norbeck et al., 1981; Reis, 1988; Sarason et al., 1983) have attempted to measure the functional components of social support under the belief that the most essential aspect of social support is the perceived availability of functional support. (Cohen & Hoberman, 1983; House & Work, 1981; Wills, 1985). Functional support refers to the degree to which interpersonal relationships serve particular functions.

The functions most often cited are (1) emotional support which involves caring, love and empathy, (2) instrumental support (referred to by many as tangible support), (3) information, guidance or feedback that can provide a solution to a problem, (4) appraisal support which involves information relevant to self-evaluation and, (5) social companionship, which involves spending time with others in leisure and recreational activities. (Ahumada et al., 2005; Fleming et al., 2004; Gill et al., 2002; Sherbourne, 1988).

A 20-item MOS questionnaire was administered to all participants. This questionnaire limits the evaluation scale of the entire network of the interview subjects; participants performed their social support excluding people that do not have a good relationship. Four degrees of functional social support (Call et al., 2000): An emotional/informational, tangible, affectionate, and positive social interaction were administered and shows a Global Index of families affected with HIV/AIDS. 74.1% of families have a maximum social support, 22.7% have a medium social support and 3.1% have a minimum social support (See Table 3).

Social Support N=(286)	F	%
Maximum	212	74.1%
Medium	65	22.7%
Minimum	9	3.1%

Table 3. Social Support in families affected with HIV/AIDS.

5. Clinical status of children with HIV/AIDS

Health-related quality of life (HRQOL) is increasingly recognized as an important measure for assessing the burden of chronic diseases (Hays et al., 2000). HIV-specific parameters, such as low CD4 cell count and high virus load, have previously been shown to adversely affect HRQOL in some studies of HIV-infected patients (Casado et al., 2011; Niuwerk et al., 2001).
Other studies show weak HRQOL associations with disease stage and CD4 cell count (Niuwerk et al., 2001). Similarly, the effect of HAART on HRQOL has been assessed with some studies (Call et al., 2000).
According to international definitions on the concept of childhood affected by HIV/AIDS, participating minors must comply with the following affectation categories as criteria of population inclusion, nonexcluding amongst themselves: 1. HIV/AIDS seropositive and/or seronegative children, and adolescents, orphaned by HIV/AIDS (father, mother, or both deceased because of the disease). 2. HIV seropositive children and adolescents. 3. HIV seropositive and/or seronegative children and adolescents, cohabitating with HIV seropositive individuals.
80 children were HIV-positive in five Colombia cities. 80% (N=64) were receiving antiretroviral therapy and most 34.9% (N=30) had HIV load undetectable or low 20% (N=15) (See Table 4). As we mentioned earlier, Colombian children affected with HIV/AIDS have a good level of health because all these children are affiliated to the social security health and are receiving Highly Active Antiretroviral Treatment (HAART); 80% (N=64) children are receiving HAART (See Table 4).

Viral Load N=(80)	F	%
High	10	13.8%
Medium	8	10%
Low	15	20%
Undetectable	30	34.9%
Unclassified	17	21.3%
Antirretroviral Therapy (N=80)	F	%
YES	64	80%
NO	14	17.5%
Unknown	2	2.5%

Table 4. Viral Load and Antiretroviral Therapy in HIV-positive children.

6. Health service utilization and barriers to health services in children with HIV/AIDS

The results of this investigation shows the dynamics of the demand of services by children affected with HIV/AIDS, and the information will be useful in planning and organizing care for families with HIV. We found in Colombian families affected with HIV/AIDS a pattern of frequent use (50.8% N=145) of the health service (See Table 5).

Health Services Utilization (N=286)	F	%
Frequent	145	50.8 %
Regular	74	25.9 %
Occasional	37	12.9 %
Sporadic	30	10.4 %

Table 5. Health Services Utilization in Colombian families affected with HIV/AIDS.

Families affected with HIV have to face some barriers in health service provision such as: Arrival Time to heath service (half hour to an hour or more than an hour) 60.4% (N=138); Waiting Time exceeding 30 minutes in 53.8% (N=154) and 85.7% (N=245) of the children affected are not receiving Home Care even though they needed it; Health professional argue against this latter finding that caregivers do not provide personal information for fear of discrimination (See Table 6).

No significant results were found for other barriers explored: Respectful and Friendly Service; Discretion and Confidentiality Service; Subsidizes Antiretroviral Therapy; Acquisition of Antiretroviral Therapy with own money and Transportation, however many of the families reported in the focus groups did not have resources for transportation to health service (See Table 6).

Barriers to Health Services	Category	N	%
Arrival Time (N=286)	Less than half an hour	148	51.7%
	Half hour to an Hour	102	35.7%
	More than an Hour	36	12.6%
Transportation (N=286)	One Bus	127	43.6%
	More than one Bus	25	9.1%
	Mototaxi	35	12.5%
	Particular Transport	29	10.5 %
	Other: (walking; bike)	70	24.3%
Waiting Time in Service (N=286)	Immediately (15′)	39	13.6%
	Family should wait (15′ A 30′)	93	32.6%
	More than 30′	154	53.8%
Respectful and Friendly Service (N=286)	Yes	259	70.6%
	No	26	29.1%
	Sometimes	1	0.3%

Barriers to Health Services	Category	N	%
Discretion and Confidentiality Service (N=286)	Yes	265	92.7%
	No	20	7%
	Sometimes	1	0.3%
Home Care (N=286)	Monthly	4	1.4%
	2 to 3 months	14	4.9%
	Every 6 months	7	2.4%
	1 time per year	16	5.6%
	Never	245	85.7%
Entity that subsidizes Antiretroviral Therapy (N=64)	Subsidized by the foundation	4	6.5%
	Subsidized by the health lender (EPS)	6	10.4%
	Subsidized insurance scheme (ARS)	33	50.6%
	Subsidized by distrital or departamental health secretary	21	32.5%
Acquisition of Antiretroviral Therapy with own money (N=64)	Yes	4	6.7%
	No	60	93.3%

Table 6. Barriers of Health Services in Colombian families affected with HIV/AIDS.

87.4% of Families affected with HIV reports that health attention has not been denied (See Table 7).

Denial of Health Services (N=286)	F	%
YES	36	12.6 %
NO	250	87.4 %

Table 7. Denial of Health Services in Colombian families affected with HIV/AIDS.

7. Conclusion

The low rate of disclosure of HIV status to children found in the study indicates that it is a priority to develop disclosure clinical model in the Colombian context. For this reason since 2008 our institution is conducting the investigation: "Evaluation of the effects of a disclosure clinical model in HIV-positive children 7 – 18 years old in adherence to treatment and psychological adjustment". Research Project awarded with the Fellowship for Research from the Department of Research and Projects. Awarded in the 2008 Call for Proposals for Doctorate Programs at Universidad del Norte

This research aims to provide a clinical model to help affected families overcome fears that lead them to delay the delivery of HIV diagnosis. Mainly, caregivers want to avoid psychological or emotional harm to child and they fear that child tell the diagnosis to others and be discriminated against.

According to the above, health professionals do not know for sure at what age a child should know their HIV diagnosis. Some believe that at 10 years a child is old enough to manage this information. Some believe that children should learn about biosecurity practices and adherence to treatment without knowing the diagnosis in a playful way, through stories, comics and other fun techniques. Health professionals recognize that children perceive that something happens with his/her bodies by going through periods of illness and drugs.

Caregivers and health professionals explain to children that drugs are for flu, pneumonia, heart problems, fever and other low-impact diseases, but do not tell the child that he/she has HIV/AIDS.

Colombian families interviewed showed a positive degree of satisfaction with Family Functioning and Social Support. Children have good quality of life, low virus load and have access to Antiretroviral Treatment. Some barriers were identified in health services utilization.

On the other hand, we consider important to offer some recommendations to access to Colombian children affected with HIV/AIDS. Not all health services in the Colombia cities have pediatrics patients with HIV. Once identified health services, health teams evaluate the research protocol, this assessment could take 2 or 3 months. Also, it is important to know that caregivers take children to health services once a month and informed consent must be obtained through a detailed explanation of the research and get his/her signature as the child's legal representative.

Health services should provide to researches a private place for interviews. Many health services were not including in this study for lack of such space.

This type of researches must have a budget to be allocated to pay transportation costs of caregivers and HIV-positive children. These families have economic limitations to move to health services.

Another recommendation is to consider extending the running time for such studies because of the difficulties identified in the location and recruitment of subjects.

8. Acknowledgment

The authors acknowledge the support of the financial organizations and especially the willingness of those who made this study possible: children and adolescents affected by HIV/AIDS and caregivers of the five cities: Cali, Buenaventura, Barranquilla, Santa Marta y Cartagena.

Moreover, we extent our heartfelt thanks to all institution that offer services to families affected with HIV/AIDS, especially those who were agreed to cooperate with aims of this research:

In Cali city: Emsanar, Lila Mujer, Fundamor and Casa Gami.

In Buenaventura city: Fundación Si Buenaventura.

In Barranquilla city: Fundación François Xavier Bagnoud, Fundación Esperanza por la Vida, Susalud EPS, Fundación Grupo Estudio Barranquilla and Unidad Especial de Salud y Ambiente (UESA).

In Santa Marta city: Heres Salud E.U., Fundación Luz de Esperanza and Sistemas Integrales de Salud de Colombia (SISCO).

In Cartagena city: Unidad Médico Quirúrgica, Fundación Amigos Positivos, Sistemas Integrales de Salud de Colombia (SISCO) and Vivir Bien.

9. References

Abadía-Barrero C & Larusso M. The Disclosure Model versus a Developmental Illness Experience Model for Children and Adolescents Living with HIV/AIDS in São Paulo, Brazil. *AIDS Patient Care and STDs* 2006. Volume 20, Number 1.

Ahumada R, Castillo L, Muñoz B y Moruno M. Validación del Cuestionario MOS de Apoyo Social en Atención Primaria. *Medicina de Familia (And)* Vol. 6, N.º 1, abril 2005

Barrera M. *Social support in the adjustment of pregnant adolescents: assessment issues.* In Social Nerworks and Social Support (Edited by Gottlieb B.). Sage, Beverly Hills, CA 198 1.

Bikaako-Kajura W, Luyirika E, Purcell DW, Downing J, Kaharuza F, Mermin J., et al. Disclosure of HIV status and adherence to daily drug regimens among HIV-infected children in Uganda. *AIDS Behaviour* 2006, 10(Suppl. 4), S85-S93.

Boon-Yasidhi V, Kottapat U, Durier Y, Plipat N, Phongsamart W, Chokephaibulkit K & Vanprapar N. Diagnosis Disclosure in HIV-Infected Thai Children. *J Med Assoc Thai* 2005.

Brandt P. A. & Weinert C. The PRQ-A social support measure. *Nurs. Res.* 30, 277-280, 1981.

Broadhead W. E., Gehlbach S. H., DeGruy F. V. and Kaplan B. H. The Duke-UNC Functional Social Support Questionnaire: Measurement of social support in family medicine patients. *Med. Care* 26, 709-721, 1988.

Brown S P., Brady T., Lent R. W., Wolfert J. and Hall S. Perceived social support among college students: Three studies of the psychometric characteristics and counseling uses of the social support inventory. *J. Counseling Psycho/*34, 337-354, 1987.

Casado A, Consiglio E, Podzamaczer D, Badia X. Highly active antirretroviral treatment (HAART) and health-related quality of life in naïve and pretreated HIV-infected patients. *HIV Clin Trials* 2001; 2:477–82.23.

Cohen S & Hoberman H. Positive events and social supports as buffers of life change stress. *J. appl. Sot. Psycho/*13, 99-125, 1983.

Cohen S., Mermelstein R., Kamarck T. & Hoberman H. *Measuring the functional components of social support.* In Social Support: Theory, Research and Applications (Edited by Sarason I.). Martines Nijhoff. Holland, 1985.

Cohen FL. Research on families and pediatric human immunodeficiency virus disease: A review and needed directions. *Developmental and Behavioral Pediatrics* 1994, 15(3), S34-S42.

Cohen S. & Syme S L. *Issues in the study and application of social support.* In Social Support and Health (Edited by Cohen S. and Syme S. L.). Academic, Orlando, 1985

Cohen S. & Wills T. A. *Stress, social support, and the buffering hypothesis.* Psychol. Bull. 98, 310-357. 1985.

Committee on Pediatric Aids. Disclosure of illness status to children and adolescents with HIV infection. *Pediatrics* 1999.103:164-166.

Call SA, Klapow JC, Stewart KE, et al. Health-related quality of life and virologic outcomes in an HIV clinic. *Qual Life Res* 2000; 9:977–85.

Davis J K & Shah K. Bioethical aspect of HIV infection in children. *Clinical Pediatrics* 1997, 36, 573-579.

Duncan-Jones P. The structure of social relationships: Analysis of a survey instrument-Part 1. Sot. *Psychiaf.* 16, 55-61, 1981.

Flanagan-Klygis E, Ross LF, Lantos J, Frader J & Yogev R. Disclosing the diagnosis of HIV in pediatrics. *AIDS and Public Policy Journal* 2002, 17(1), 3-12.

Fleming C, Christiansen D, Nunes D, Heeren T, Thornton D, Horsburgh R, James M , Graham C and Craven D. Health-Related Quality of Life of Patients with HIV Disease: Impact of Hepatitis C Coinfection. *Clinical Infectious Diseases* 2004; 38:572-8

Gill CJ, Griffith JL, Jacobsen D, Skinner S, Gorbach SL, Wilson IB. Relationship of HIV viral load, CD4 counts, and HAART use to healthrelated quality of life. *J Acquir Immune Defic Syndr* 2002; 30:485-92.

Hardy MS, Armstrong FD, Routh DK, Albrecht J & Davis J. Coping and communication among parents and children with human immunodeficiency virus and cancer. *Developmental and Behavioral Pediatrics* 1994, 15(3), S49-S53.

Hays RD, Cunningham WE, Sherbourne CD, et al. Health-related quality of life in patients with human immunodeficiency virus infection in the United States: results from the HIV Cost and Services Utilization Study. *Am J Med* 2000; 108:714-22.

House J. S. & Kahn R. *Measures and concepts of social support.* In Social Support and Health (Edited by Cohen S. and Syme S. L.). Academic Press, San Francisco, 1985.

House J. S. *Work, Stress and Social Support.* Addison- Wesley, Reading, MA, 1981.

Instituto Colombiano de Bienestar Familiar [ICBF], Save the Children, Unicef y Universidad del Norte. *Calidad de Vida, Apoyo Social y Utilización de Servicios de Salud y Educación en niños, niñas, adolescentes y acudientes afectados con VIH/SIDA en cinco ciudades-región colombianas: (1) Cali y Buenaventura y, (2) Barranquilla, Santa Marta y Cartagena.* Informe Final de Investigación 2006. Departamento de Investigaciones Universidad del Norte (DIP): Barranquilla.

Instone SL. Perceptions of children with HIV infection when not told for so long: implications for diagnosis disclosure. *J Pediatr Health Care* 2000. Sep-Oct; 14(5):235-43.

Joint United Nations Programme on HIV/AIDS [UNAIDS] & World Health Organization [WHO], 2007). Aids Epidemic Update. 27/08/2010. Available from: http://data.unaids.org/pub/epislides/2007/2007_epiupdate_en.pdf

Kouyoumdjian F, Meyers T & Mtshizana S. Barriers to disclosure to children with HIV. *Journal of Tropical Pediatrics* 2005. Vol. 51. No 5.

Lee CL & Johann-Liang R. Disclosure of the Diagnosis of HIV/AIDS to children born of HIV-infected mothers. *AIDS Patient Care and STDs* 1999, 13(1), 41-45.

Ledlie S. Diagnosis Disclosure by Family Caregivers to Children who have Perinatally Acquired HIV Disease: When the Time Comes. *Nursing Research* 1999. 48(3):141-149.

Lester P, Chesney M, Cooke M, Weiss R, Whalley P, Perez B, Glidden D, Petru A, Dorenbaum A & Wara D. When the Time Comes To Talk About HIV: Factors Associated With Diagnostic Disclosure and Emotional Distress in HIV-Infected Children. *JAIDS Journal of Acquired Immune Deficiency Syndromes* 2002. 31:309-317.

Leserman, J, Perkins, DO, Evans, DL. Coping with the threat of AIDS: the role of social support. *Am J Psychiatry* 1992 149: 1514-1520.

Lewis SY, Haiken HJ & Hoyt LG. Living beyond the odds: A psychosocial perspective on long-term survivors of pediatric human immunodeficiency virus infection. *Developmental and Behavioral Pediatrics* 1994, 15(3), S12-S17.

Lipson M. *What do you say a child with AIDS.* The Hastings Center Report 1993. 23; 2: research library core. Pag. 6.

Meyers A & Weitzman M. Pediatric HIV disease: The newest chronic illness of childhood. *Pediatric Clinics of North America* 1991, 38(1), 169-194.

Myer L, Moodley K, Hendricks F & Cotton M. Healthcare provider's perspectives on discussing HIV status with infected children. *Journal of Tropical Pedia*trics 2006, 52(4), 293-295.

Nagler S, Adnopoz J & Forsyth B. *Uncertainly, stigma and secrecy: psychological aspects of AIDS for children and adolescents.* In: Andiman W, Geballe S, Guende, eds. Forgotten Children of the AIDS Epidemic 1995. New Haven, CT: Yale University Press; 1-10.

Niuwerk PT, Gisolf EH, Reijers MH, Lange JM, Danner SA, Sprangers MA. Long-term quality of life outcomes in three antiretroviral treatment strategies for HIV-1 infection. *AIDS* 2001; 15:1985-91.

Nojomi M, Anbary K & Ranjbar; M. Health-Related Quality of Life in Patients with HIV/AIDS. *Arch Iranian Med 2008*; 11 (6): 608 – 612.

Norbeck J. S., Lindsey A. M. & Carrieri V. L. The development of an instrument to measure social support. *Nurs. Res.* 30, 264-269, 1981.

Oberdorfer P, Puthanakit T, Louthrenoo O, Charnsil C, Sirisanthana V & Sirisanthana T. Disclosure of HIV/AIDS diagnosis to HIV-infected children in Thailand. *Journal of Pediatrics and Child Health* 2006. 42:283-288.

Programa Conjunto de las Naciones Unidas sobre el VIH/SIDA (ONUSIDA)., Ministerio de la Protección Social de Colombia y Dirección General de Salud Pública (2006). Infección por VIH y Sida en Colombia. Estado del Arte 2000-2005. *Pro-Offset Editorial Ltda: Bogotá D.C.*

Reis J. A factorial analysis of a compound measure of social support. *J. clin. Psychol.* 44, 876890, 1988.

Sarason I G., Levine H. M., Basham R. B. and Sarason B. R. Assessing social support: The social support questionnaire. *J. Person. Sot. Psvchol.* 44, 127-139, 1983.

Sherboune C & Stewart A. The MOS social support survey. *Sot. Sci. Med.* Vol. 32, No. 6, pp. 705-714, 1991.

Sherbourne C D. The roll of social supports and life stress events in use of mental health services. *Med. Care* 27, 1393-1400, 1988.

Tasker M. How can I tell you. Secrecy *and disclosure with children when a family member has AIDS.* Bethesda, MD 1992: Association for the care of children Health.

The World Health Organization [WHO], 2003. WHO Definition of Health. 23/02/2011. Available from: http://www.who.int/about/definition/en/print.html

United Nations General Assembly Special Session on HIV/AIDS. Declaration of Commitment on HIV/AIDS. Resolution A/Res/S-26/2, 27 June 2001 (www.unaids.org/UNGASS/docs/AIDSDeclaration_en.pdf), hereinafter cited as Declaration of Commitment.

Waugh S. Parental Views on Disclosure of Diagnosis to their HIV-positive Children. *AIDS Care* 2003. Vol. 15 No 2, pp. 169-176.

Wiener L, Battles H, Heilman N, Sigelman C & Pizzo P. Factors associated with disclosure of diagnosis to children with HIV/AIDS. *Pediatr AIDS HIV Infect* 1996. 7(5):310-324.

Wiener LS & Figueroa V. Children speaking with children and families about HIV infection. In P. A. Pizzo & C. M. Wilfert (Eds.), *Pediatric AIDS* 1998: The challenge of HIV infection in infants, children and adolescents (pp. 729-758). Baltimore: Williams and Wilkins.

Wiener LS, Septimus A & Grady C. Psychosocial support and ethical issues for the child and family. In P. A. Pizzo & C. M. Wilfert (Eds.), *Pediatric AIDS* 1998: The challenge of HIV infection in infants, children and adolescents (pp. 703-727). Baltimore: Williams and Wilkins.

Wills T. A. *Supportive functions of relationships*. In Social Support and Health (Edited by Cohen S. and Syme S. L.). Academic, Florida, 1985.

Permissions

All chapters in this book were first published by InTech Open; hereby published with permission under the Creative Commons Attribution License or equivalent. Every chapter published in this book has been scrutinized by our experts. Their significance has been extensively debated. The topics covered herein carry significant findings which will fuel the growth of the discipline. They may even be implemented as practical applications or may be referred to as a beginning point for another development.

The contributors of this book come from diverse backgrounds, making this book a truly international effort. This book will bring forth new frontiers with its revolutionizing research information and detailed analysis of the nascent developments around the world.

We would like to thank all the contributing authors for lending their expertise to make the book truly unique. They have played a crucial role in the development of this book. Without their invaluable contributions this book wouldn't have been possible. They have made vital efforts to compile up to date information on the varied aspects of this subject to make this book a valuable addition to the collection of many professionals and students.

This book was conceptualized with the vision of imparting up-to-date information and advanced data in this field. To ensure the same, a matchless editorial board was set up. Every individual on the board went through rigorous rounds of assessment to prove their worth. After which they invested a large part of their time researching and compiling the most relevant data for our readers.

The editorial board has been involved in producing this book since its inception. They have spent rigorous hours researching and exploring the diverse topics which have resulted in the successful publishing of this book. They have passed on their knowledge of decades through this book. To expedite this challenging task, the publisher supported the team at every step. A small team of assistant editors was also appointed to further simplify the editing procedure and attain best results for the readers.

Apart from the editorial board, the designing team has also invested a significant amount of their time in understanding the subject and creating the most relevant covers. They scrutinized every image to scout for the most suitable representation of the subject and create an appropriate cover for the book.

The publishing team has been an ardent support to the editorial, designing and production team. Their endless efforts to recruit the best for this project, has resulted in the accomplishment of this book. They are a veteran in the field of academics and their pool of knowledge is as vast as their experience in printing. Their expertise and guidance has proved useful at every step. Their uncompromising quality standards have made this book an exceptional effort. Their encouragement from time to time has been an inspiration for everyone.

The publisher and the editorial board hope that this book will prove to be a valuable piece of knowledge for researchers, students, practitioners and scholars across the globe.

List of Contributors

Jose M. Varela, Francisco J. Medrano and Enrique J. Calderón
Instituto de Biomedicina de Sevilla and CIBER de Epidemiología y Salud Pública, Internal Medicine Service, Virgen del Rocío University Hospital Seville, Spain

Eduardo Dei-Cas
Parasitology-Mycology Service (EA4547), Centre of Biology Pathology, Lille-2 University Hospital Centre, Faculty of Medicine, Univ. Lille Nord de France, France
Biology & Diversity of Emerging Eukaryotic Pathogens, Institut Pasteur de Lille, Lille, France

Kennedy Daniel Mwambete and Mary Justin-Temu
Muhimbili University of Health and Allied Sciences, Tanzania

Natasha Potgieter and Tendayi B. Mpofu
Department of Microbiology, University of Venda, South Africa

Tobias G. Barnard
Water and Health Research Unit, University of Johannesburg, South Africa

Samie A. and Bessong P.O.
AIDS Virus Research Laboratory, Department of Microbiology, University of Venda, Thohoyandou, South Africa

Obi C.L.
Academic and Research Directorate, Walter Sisulu University, Nelson Mandela Drive Eastern Cape, South Africa

Dillingham R. and Guerrant R.L.
Centre for Global Health, University of Virginia, Charlottesville, USA

Roos E. Barth and Andy I.M. Hoepelman
University Medical Centre Utrecht, Department of Internal Medicine and Infectious Diseases, The Netherlands

Lilian María Mederos Cuervo
National Reference Laboratory TB/Mycobacteria Collaborate Center PAHO/WHO Tropical Medicine Institute Pedro Kourí (IPK), Cuba

Veeranoot Nissapatorn
University of Malaya, Malaysia

Goselle Obed Nanjul
School of Biological Sciences, Bangor University, UK
Applied Entomology and Parasitology Unit, Department of Zoology, University of Jos, Nigeria

Ana María Trejos Herrera, Jorge Palacio Sañudo Mario Mosquera Vásquez and Rafael Tuesca Molina
Fundación Universidad del Norte, Barranquilla, Colombia

Index

Printed in the USA
CPSIA information can be obtained
at www.ICGtesting.com
JSHW051351091023
49903JS00006B/109